Elements of
Research in
Physical Therapy

SECOND EDITION

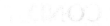

Elements of Research in Physical Therapy

SECOND EDITION

Dean P. Currier, Ph.D.

Professor of Physical Therapy
Department of Physical Therapy
University of Kentucky
Lexington, Kentucky

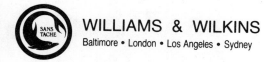

WILLIAMS & WILKINS
Baltimore • London • Los Angeles • Sydney

Editor: George Stamathis
Copy Editor: Florence Forbes
Design: Joanne Janowiak
Illustration Planning: Wayne Hubbel
Production: Carol L. Eckhart

Accurate indications, adverse reactions, and dosage schedules for drugs are provided in this book, but it is possible that they may change. The reader is urged to review the package information data of the manufacturers of the medications mentioned.

Made in the United States of America

First Edition, 1979

Library of Congress Cataloging in Publication Data

Currier, Dean P.
  Elements of research in physical therapy.

  Includes index.
  1. Physical therapy---Research. I. Title. [DNLM: 1. Physical therapy.
2. Research. WB 25 C976e]
RM708.C87 1984   615.8'2'072   83-21874
ISBN 0-683-02247-4

Composed and printed at the
Waverly Press, Inc.
Mt. Royal and Guilford Aves.
Baltimore, Md. 21202, U.S.A.   85 86 87 88 89   10 9 8 7 6 5 4 3

To Joan
Wendy
Tracey
Brad

Preface to the Second Edition

Since preparing the first edition of this book, several events have occurred that enhance physical therapy research. More than one physical therapy journal is being published that devotes considerable space to research, more and more physical therapists are publishing their studies in a variety of health related journals, the Foundation for Physical Therapy was established to fund research, increased numbers of research abstracts are submitted yearly for presentation at the annual conference, more new entry-level programs are opening which expose students to research methods, and more physical therapists are obtaining graduate degrees requiring theses and dissertations. Physical therapy research is gaining in vigor and vitality that should contribute to many important findings and to new and improved approaches to patient care over the next decade.

The second edition has been updated to reflect change in physical therapy research. Each chapter has received changes that improve its value to students who are learning about the research process. Some reorganization of material has taken place to combine experimental research and hardware instrumentation. Chapter 9 was created to strengthen the book by emphasizing the importance of design in scientific investigation. Years of student input have helped make the book readable and appealing to those wanting to learn about physical therapy research. Readers of the book should be able to set up research projects and critically judge reported studies.

The assistance of Libby VanHook and the suggestions offered by colleagues have been immeasurable during the preparation of the second edition.

Preface to the First Edition

Physical therapy in North America has grown out of a need of service for patients having disease or injury affecting mobility of their body, and has developed sound educational techniques for teaching that body of knowledge which has evolved through the years. Only in recent years has proper experimentation and the nucleus of a synthetic rationale emerged to relate clinical procedures with scientific bases. Instruction in research methods has been included in the curricula for the initial preparation of physical therapists but yet textbooks for research methods in physical therapy are scarce.

The purpose of this book is to inform readers about the elements of research. The book was designed for a one-term course and must necessarily omit many aspects of research. For the undergraduate student, the book can reduce barriers of fear caused by lack of understanding of research and can shape favorable attitudes toward research. The book can assist the graduate student in development of the thesis. For the practitioner uninstructed in research methods, the book will provide an understandable review of various research methods and procedures. The contents provide a basis for appreciating clinical research, for interpreting the research literature, and for exposing the reader to techniques that have immediate application to clinical investigations. The organization of the contents is the result of the author's experience in teaching research methods and of student critique of the instruction.

The first part of the book calls attention to the what, why, who, and where of research; developing a research problem; and searching the literature. The discussion on the proposal should serve as a guide to the neophyte investigator for planning the research project. Because of the emphasis in recent years placed on the rights of subjects in research, the consent of research subjects is discussed. The second part of the book establishes the roots of research; that is, the basics of data and measurement, and the methods and instrumentation used in the research process. The third part discusses several statistical procedures for analyzing data from which inferences and conclusions are based. The statistical procedures do not require prior knowledge of algebra. Theorems and derivation of statistical formulas have been omitted. The final part of the book completes the process by discussing methods of reporting research.

I would like to express my appreciation to the American Physical Therapy Association for permission to reprint some material. I am grateful to Professor Barrie Pickles for paving the way for physical therapy research at the University of Alberta and to Donna McTavish for her patience and efficiency in preparation of trial copies of the manuscript. A very special thanks to colleagues who contributed time freely to review parts of the manuscript: Donna C. Boone, Elizabeth Davies Carruth, Carmella Gonnella, James E. Griffin, Don Lehmkuhl, Gary Holdgrafer, Shrawan Kumar, Mary Moffroid, James Vargo, and Steven Wolf.

Many of the quotations introducing the chapters are from Bartlett J: Familiar Quotations, ed 14. Boston, Little, Brown and Co, 1968, and Straus MB (ed): Familiar Medical Quotations. Boston, Little, Brown and Co, 1968.

I am grateful to the Literary Executor of the late Sir Ronald A. Fisher, F.R.S., to Dr. Frank Yates, F.R.S., to Longman Group Ltd., London, for permission to reprint Table C, Appendix, from their book *Statistical Tables for Biological, Agricultural and Medical Research,* ed 6, 1974, and to the *Biometrika* Trustees for permission to use Tables D and E, Appendix.

A bad book is generally a very easy book, having been composed by its author with no labour of mind what-ever; whereas a good book, though it be not necessarily a hard one, yet, since it contains important facts, duly arranged, and reasoned upon with care, must require from the reader some portion of the same attention and study to comprehend and profit by it, as it required from the writer to compose it.

PETER MERE LATHAM
(1789–1875)

Contents

Part One

DEVELOPING RESEARCH

1

Research and Physical Therapy

I keep six honest serving-men
(They taught me all I knew);
Their names are What and Why, and
When
And How and Where and Who.
Kipling
Just So Stories (1902)

Physical therapy is an expanding profession that is comprised of both art and science components. The growth and development of physical therapy is dependent on its science to uncover, modify, and accommodate new information. Art is the skill that takes place in the practice of physical therapy.

The use of techniques, procedures, and methods to achieve movement, function, and improved health is an art, not a science. Art and science are sometimes purported to be one and the same. Although related, the student must keep in mind that a fundamental difference exists between the two. The difference between art and science is that art is concerned with methods or ways of effecting certain outcomes, while science is concerned with theoretical truth.[1] A science can be defined as a body of knowledge gained through diligent and systematic study with concern for facts and principles.[2] Research is a method of science that supplies pieces of knowledge by finding answers to questions, hypotheses, theories, principles; research is an attempt to find the theoretical truth or answer, why?

Peat[3] has identified the art component of physical therapy as that of human relationships, the occurrence of vested interest, tradition, and the placebo effect. The intensive caring relationship that practitioners establish with their patients results in the patient's gaining confidence in the physical therapist. Techniques are sometimes taught through therapist-therapist interaction by a process analogous to "ecclesiastical succession" where the leader of a particular therapeutic approach teaches a few practitioners who in turn become qualified in the approach to instruct others. The relationship tends to justify the therapeutic approach on the basis of personal observation, "anecdotal justification." Vested interest occurs when practitioners cling to a belief that a certain technique is of value although no objective evidence is available to support such faith. Tradition may occur in some clinical situations where technique is the primary factor, whereas teaching and learning are technical events without benefit of the underlying physiological bases. The placebo effect takes place when the physical therapist convinces the patient that his or her therapy is of value.

Science in physical therapy aids in eliminating bias and enables reproducibility of results. It allows for universal communication by means of using terms that have a specific meaning and are used for all. Science permits accurate quantitative measurements of existing phenomena. Therapeutic approaches can be scientifically tested to validate their effectiveness which adds creditability to physical therapy. Scientific achievement of physical therapists can be judged by disseminating results of research through publication.[3]

Some professions claim to be scientific and, therefore, must develop their bodies of knowledge through research.[4] Is a profession a science? an art? must it encourage research? Perhaps defining a profession may help to answer the questions. A profession is an occupation whose members must possess a body of knowledge that is both identifiable and different from that of others, and the members must assume responsibility for adding to that body of knowledge.

According to Greenwood[5] a profession possesses certain elements distinct from those of a non-profession. The major distinction is the body of knowledge that has been organized into an internally compatible system upon which the skills that characterize the profession are formed. The body of knowledge is a system of abstract propositions that focus on the uniqueness of the profession. The body of knowledge (theory) forms the basis upon which the professional rationalizes his (clinical) practice. Mastery of the theory is essential before acquiring the skill to practice, and preparation for the profession must be an intellectual as well as a practical experience. The value and emphasis placed on the theory precipitates an activity that is not usually a part of a non-professional occupation; namely, formation of theory by means of systematic research. Research is required to develop valid theory that provides a firm base for the techniques and procedures used by the professional. Furthermore, in a technological profession a researcher-theoretician is a class of labor that gradually develops between the theory-oriented and the practice-oriented individuals.[5] Physical therapy has a body of knowledge and a clinical science which has been suggested as pathokinesiology.[6] The knowledge and principles of physical therapy must be developed, however, through research; and students of physical therapy must be aware of the whats, whos, whys, wheres and hows of research. How research is performed is considered essential for its understanding, for interpretation of the literature, and as an element for being identified as a professional.

WHAT IS RESEARCH?

Research has been defined as a method of science, but it needs clarification. Research is a diligent and systematic study that uses scientific inquiry or methods to compile or uncover facts, test hypotheses, and show relations. Kerlinger[7] has defined scientific research as being systematic, controlled, empirical, and critical investigations about the presumed relations among natural phenomena. He further defined research by its use of hypothetical propositions.[6] Research provides "sight" or truth, uncovers facts and causes, improves reasoning, and adds knowledge. Research is the process permitting description of individual attributes or events. Research is the process of asking and answering questions as well as the process of abstracting answers from observations.[8] It is "an activity designed to test a hypothesis and to permit conclusions to be drawn."[9] Although no simple definition really tells what research is all about nor is agreed upon by all disciplines, the following definition describes research as it is presented in this book.

> Research is the studying of a problem in pursuit of a definite objective through employing precise methods, with due consideration to the adequate control of factors other than the variable under investigation and followed by analysis according to acceptable statistical procedures.[10]

The reader must realize that good research can be reported without statistical analyses ever having been used and that good research can be performed without conforming to the guidelines presented herein. The above definition provides a baseline on which to begin and to establish operational elements of research.

Students are often overheard saying that they must go to the library to do research. Although a review of the literature is a pertinent activity or phase of performing research, the process of reviewing literature is hardly synonymous with most definitions presented. Also, research is sometimes referred to by colleagues as being synonymous with problem solving. A differentiation must be made between research and problem solving because their purposes and processes are different. Research is a search for new knowledge or verification of beliefs and has a definite objective through the controlled process of scientific inquiry. Problem solving is a systematic approach to the solution of a problem or objective through the process of action or thought. Problem solving does not require exact and precise elements of scientific inquiry nor does it require quantitative data analyzed by statistical procedures. Problem solving deals with "everyday" decisions.

The differences between research and problem solving then are contrasted by the degree of precision, control, or demand placed on their processes. Research is a more rigorous process than is problem solving and although both methods are important in physical therapy, they should not be used synonymously. Wandell[11] has stated that the purpose of research is to uncover new information, while the purpose of problem solving is to solve an immediate problem in a distinct setting.

TYPES OF RESEARCH

Research is often divided into two types, basic and applied. Basic research is often referred to as pure research. The research undertaken is usually selected because it will reveal knowledge about a wide area,[12] or knowledge which is common to all professions.[13] Basic research is implicitly or explicitly intended to increase understanding of the causes or function of whatever is being studied.[8] Pure research may be associated with experimentation on animals.[14] It tends to be abstract and general and although basic research may lead to practical application it is not begun with specific use.[15] Applied research is often called clinical research or clinical trials, and sometimes is called action research, particularly in educational circles. Applied research is often concerned with applying or gaining knowledge in the practice of physical therapy. This latter type of research very often attempts to determine the efficacy of therapeutic procedures, and is implicitly or explicitly intended to increase understanding of methods of therapeutic and educational delivery.[7] Ritchie[16] has pointed out, however, that it is no longer possible nor wise to make a distinction between pure and applied research, since the two are often combined in modern approaches to improving human welfare.

I would like to introduce the idea of micro and macro research. Micro research is when researchers investigate at the cellular, tissue, or organ levels to uncover causes of an event or condition. Macro, on the other hand, occurs when researchers determine associations between events or conditions, using statistics to show strengths or bonds between the associations. Both micro and macro research are in a sense applied because they strive to show why or how the events or conditions are linked together, the difference is only at the level of investigation.

WHY RESEARCH?

According to the definition of a profession, members have the responsibility to develop and add to its body of knowledge through research. Research is imperative for the survival of a profession[6,17] and is perhaps the cornerstone of a profession while excluded from an art or technology.

Only through research can a profession open its theory, principles, and procedures to inspection by the scientific community.

Watkins[18] referred to the 1944 report of the Baruch Committee on Physical Medicine when stating that more basic and clinical research was needed for the proper development of rehabilitative medicine. Physical therapy in North America has grown out of a need of health service for patients and has developed sound educational techniques for teaching that body of knowledge which has evolved through the years. The history of the development of the health professions and sciences show that the organization of teaching and of professional service preceded that of formalized research.[19] Research evolves from curiosity or a need to test the existing knowledge and procedures; thus, in a developing profession old information is often converted into a new frame of reference.[20] The rate of growth of a profession will be proportional to the rate at which its body of knowledge grows and the amount of energy that is given to research.[4]

The members of a profession cannot wait for things to happen or wait for bits and pieces of fact and information to filter down from the research of other disciplines.[6] A profession must incorporate the idea and identify the need for research in its curricula for the initial preparation of its members. The research instruction must not be supported only from an educational point of view but the educational institution must further support research through its line item budget.[17] The quality of the end product of research instruction during the educational preparation of members of a profession will be demonstrated by professional growth and application to the professions' service.

Since physical therapy was established because of an identified need and has subsequently developed its educational system and treatment procedures, research is needed to support and add to the present body of knowledge. The time has come to augment the art with the science so that physical therapy can emerge as a science with clinical relevance.[21]

To be minimally effective in clinical practice, a physical therapist must be able to determine a patient's condition (within or outside normal limits), to determine what rehabilitative approach to take, and to modify the approach whenever the patient's condition warrants change. Research provides the information essential for answering the therapist's questions, the reliable techniques for assessment, and the best approaches to patient management. Research is essential for developing a scientific approach to clinical practice; that is, establishing objectives clearly, establishing efficacy of new approaches to patient management, and being systematic in making observations of the patient's condition and reaction to treatment.[8] It permits judicious selection of treatment once the therapist has assessed the patient.

Research is essential for developing inquiring attitudes among physical therapists. The therapist must constantly be able to recognize and challenge authoritative thinking and insist on evidence (observations, tests, valid and reliable inferences) for such thinking and beliefs. Physical therapists must challenge techniques that are passed on from therapist to therapist (ecclesiastical succession).[3] Instruction in research can assist the student in how to effectively question and apply the methods of scientific inquiry. Research is essential for establishing positive habits of thinking, controlling, confirming, and acting; not just action through the richness of clinical experiences with thought and control. Physical therapists must not accept what others say or all that is written but ask—is this really so? After asking, solutions (research) must be pursued to answer the question.[16]

WHO SHOULD RESEARCH?

Members of the profession are likely to be the best researchers for building the body of knowledge of that profession. The members are likely to have a better idea of the needs for research, and can best design strategies to meet those needs of their profession.

The researcher must possess certain qualities to perform successfully. Interest in a particular area or problem of the profession is of paramount importance because an uninterested researcher is unlikely to advance new ideas.[12] The researcher must be motivated to endure tedious work and be willing to input much effort and time into the research endeavor. The researcher must possess considerable knowledge of the area being investigated, must be curious and ever asking, why? Creative thinking, and perceptive and critical observational abilities are also essential characteristics of the researcher. Of course, training in the procedures of conducting research and methods of analyzing the results generated by the research process are essential. The development of positive attitudes toward research among members of a profession is generally the responsibility of the programs offering the initial preparation for the professionals, while the molding and production of researchers is the responsibility maintained by programs of graduate studies. Opportunities to perform research during pursuit of graduate studies is conducive to learning because the student is no longer preoccupied with mastery of accepted knowledge, but attention can be directed toward solving the unknown.[22] Many physical therapists also learn research methods at their place of employment.[23] Fitness for the enterprise of research is best expressed in Table 1.1 by words supplied by the world renowned scientist, Walter Cannon.[24]

Although advanced study (master's or doctoral levels) is certainly helpful in research preparation, research must not be limited to just these levels or individuals. Research is a rational and reality-oriented process and belongs to those who can meet and handle the process appropriately; that is, the elements (qualifications) of scientific inquiry. The clinical researcher is the physical therapist who functions both as a clinical practitioner and as an investigator. As a clinician the therapist can best identify the needs for

Table 1.1
Qualifications of a Researcher

Curiosity	Knowledge of mathematics
Imagination	Observational ability
Critical judgment	Good memory
Honest	Patience
Variety of experiences	Ability to write clearly
Technical skill	Critical (tactful) judgments of peers
Ingenuity	Humility

research, the kinds of questions that need to be asked. As a researcher, the therapist can influence directions of therapeutic approaches. These roles can and should be performed simultaneously. Likewise, the roles of teaching and research should function together.

The clinical therapist might justly ask, "What are the benefits derived from adding research to practice?" The question can be answered in several ways. Clinical research makes the practice of physical therapy more stimulating and less routine than it would be otherwise. Clinical research is a source of positive reinforcement to the therapist because it provides a feeling of accomplishment derived from formulating a research question; observing or collecting and analyzing data; and reporting results to colleagues at meetings or in professional journals.[8] Research provides a more effective clinical practice because it provides answers for determining the most effective approach to patient care. Research provides a body of knowledge for improved quality of patient care.

Research provides the satisfaction of discovery, forms extensive friendships among colleagues or former students, provides practical and reliable approaches to direct patient care, and uncovers truth. Rewards of research are also gained through the recognition accorded by peers, and seeing the spreading influence from research results.[24] Research may provide the freedom to develop one's own ideas or give one a degree of concentration and interest in a certain question.[16] The ultimate goal of most researchers is simply to advance knowledge.

WHERE RESEARCH?

The School

Responsibilities for research in physical therapy must not be granted solely to the student. Faculty of programs of physical therapy must also engage in research. Treatment, education, and research are recognized basic functions of a comprehensive center of health activity,[25] and the faculty are functional components of the center. The attitudes of students and the quality of research emerging from the center are dependent upon the knowledge, astuteness, interest, motivation, and direction of the faculty. Faculty serve as role models to students and if students do not observe or participate in ongoing research in their own discipline, then they might conclude that research is not a priority activity of the profession and can be an activity eliminated from busy work schedules.

The Clinical Setting

Of course, the practitioner must play a vital role in the profession by also performing research where the application of research is essential. The practitioner has the same purpose as that of the students and faculty of physical therapy programs, that of building a body of knowledge for improved quality of patient care.

The student of research methods today may eventually become the director of a clinical department. If positive attitudes toward research are developed by the student, then physical therapy research activity in the clinic may someday become a commonplace function of the practitioner. The director of a department engaging in research should be trained in research and management.[25] Leadership in clinical physical therapy calls for certain criteria. Management must not only accept and approve of research activity in physical therapy, but schedule work so as to allow for time to conduct and analyze research, and arrange for adequate facilities which involve space, equipment, and money. In other words, the leader must establish and support a climate of "vigorous intellectual ferment."[26] Proper management also calls for careful selection of staff. Staff present ideas which facilitate creativity and develop the new, the daring, and the different. Staff must consist of individuals trained in research and motivated to perform research, yet willing to function in the regular capacity of clinical therapists. A collection of selected staff can stimulate and inspire each other; research enhances their job satisfaction and self-respect.[26] Clinical research will improve quality physical therapy.

The Association

The professional organization can provide impetus for research activity in the profession through direction, monetary support, and recognition. The Research Committee, the Section on Research, the Foundation for Physical Therapy and the journal, PHYSICAL THERAPY, are arms of the American Physical Therapy Association. The Research Committee has developed long-range plans for fostering research within the profession, while the Foundation for Physical Therapy has been established to endow research activity. Other physical therapy associations have similar mechanisms. The Chartered Society of Physiotherapy has a Research Advisory Board;[27] but in 1975, the Specific Interest Group of the Association of

Chartered Physiotherapists in Research was formed. This latter group promotes research activity among physiotherapists in the British Isle and has made considerable progress.[28] The Canadian Physiotherapy Association's counterpart is the Clinical Studies Division.[29]

DIFFICULTIES ENCOUNTERED IN PHYSICAL THERAPY RESEARCH

The Clinic

Practitioners often hesitate to attend presentations of original research or read research reported in their professional journal because they do not understand what is being presented. The formal education of practitioners prior to 1965 did not regularly include instruction in research methods.[23] The lack of instruction in research has produced an understanding gap between authors of research reports and physical therapy practitioners who often do not understand research reports.[30] Some suggestions for correcting the problem of an understanding gap are (1) that practitioners return to academic institutions periodically to freshen up their academic knowledge and to learn about research, and (2) that researchers conduct workshops for orientation in research methods and interpretation.[31] An insufficient understanding of research is not necessarily unique to practitioners but may also be a shortcoming among students and faculty. The lack of understanding may have been a deficiency of the philosophy of the profession, but is being corrected.[23] Problems confronting schools, students, and physical therapy clinicians are presented separately only to call attention to specific difficulties or situations. The difficulties in research are not universal and are being alleviated in many areas.

Difficulties encountered by clinical therapists conducting research are different from those encountered by faculty members. Physical therapists are employed to treat patients and therefore, most of their time is expected to be directed in patient-oriented activities. Physical therapists have not educated the public, physicians, and administrators that they are researchers and that research is an integral part of their duties. Since the process of research is not measured easily for its immediate results or productivity (for example, number of patients treated per day), the employer may be reluctant to allocate the therapist's time for research activity. Probably of great significance is the failure of research to contribute immediately to the financial success of a facility. Research will, however, increase costs of operation.

The responsibility of overcoming obstacles for clinical research is not only that of the department's leadership, but that of every department member. Physical therapists must organize educational and public information programs to dispel any misunderstanding about the therapist's role in research. The best approach to alleviating any adverse concepts by critics is to demonstrate the ability and effectiveness to perform research in the clinic. All clinicians should not conduct research but large clinics having several or more therapists should have one or two researchers who are permitted sufficient time and support to investigate clinical questions. Large departments of physical therapy may consider establishing a "research arm" which has a few therapists who devote a percentage of their time conducting research.

The School

Most schools in the United States and Canada providing the initial level of physical therapy education offer some degree of research instruction[23,32,33] This commitment to research instruction at the initial level of education will eventually put to rest the image of not doing enough research.[17,34] Some schools do not place emphasis on laboratory experiences where an atmosphere of research-like activities prevails. Perhaps a more common and dangerous problem is the lack of research monies in line item budgets of physical therapy schools. Some directors of schools have not established research as a high priority and consequently, have not received financial support for research activity within the program. Support monies often encourage student and faculty research. Often faculty who have not been trained in or have not engaged in research are appointed, or they are not sufficiently interested in or committed to research. Faculty often have excessive teaching commitments that prevent time for research. Some faculty believe their major responsibility is teaching and ignore the fact that educational information is derived from scientific inquiry. Research provides new ideas or knowledge and improved technology while dispelling or confirming previously accepted knowledge. If no research is performed by faculty then the same information is being passed on from year to year. Alternatively, what new information is passed on is borrowed from other professions and applied to physical therapy without being validated for physical therapy. As a result, therapists apply the information to treatments before the information is tested under rigidly controlled conditions. Groups that continuously borrow information and adapt it without the scrutiny of controlled experimentation are not professionals and thus, do not command recognition of the scientific community.

Students will perform research when research is demonstrated to be an integral part of their education. Research cannot be demonstrated through the curricular contents alone, but must be demonstrated by means of a departmental atmosphere of intellectual curiosity and scientific inquiry through action. Students gain experience and insight from scientific inquiry through required projects at the initial level of education and through required thesis work at the graduate levels. Enthusiasm for and participation in research by faculty are contagious and soon the condition becomes an indigenous characteristic of the educational program. The intent of exposure to or training in research is not to make all physical therapists researchers. An acceptable blend of theory, research, and techniques needs to be developed in physical therapists. Presently, however, the needs for research are greater than the current supply of researchers. If the advancement of knowledge is dependent upon research and intelligence and if participation in research is a requirement of physical therapy, then intelligence must be a principal criterion for admission into physical therapy education.[4] The entry-level curriculum must continue to produce graduates who will critically evaluate and compare clinical procedures. The universities must be successful in producing such students if physical therapy is to continue its growth and take its place among respected health disciplines.[3] Since the majority of physical therapists do not go on to higher levels of education, they must learn the research process at the entry-level or through continuing education. The efforts of the universities may be paying dividends because the submission of research papers to the annual conference has reached a point where many good papers are rejected on the basis of volume and competition.[35]

Perhaps the response of an anonymous student when asked about the problems of performing research in physical therapy epitomizes the situation:

> The greatest area of concern in productive research for physical therapy is the lack of therapists involved or qualified to perform research. Our educational system does not always provide the necessary background for the student to have a precise understanding of research. As students, we are more concerned with learning treatment techniques which are already established. We concentrate in these areas because our grades are dependent upon learning concepts. Even though we might have a problem which needs research, we push it aside to get the grades to obtain a degree. Once we are out working, we again push it aside because our employer is more concerned with services and economics. Our educational system needs to provide the background emphasis for research and make known the opportunities available for students interested in performing research or becoming researchers.
>
> Anonymous Student

STIMULATION TO ENGAGE IN CLINICAL RESEARCH

During the initial education of physical therapy students, frequent laboratory sessions in most courses or units tend to stimulate students.

Students learn to measure, test, assess, and make conclusions as a result of laboratory exposure. Assignment for interning in facilities having therapists who engage in research is another approach to stimulating interested individuals.[34]

Administrators of the clinical facility and faculty of the physical therapy school must be convinced that therapists do have a role in clinical research. Only when encouragement and support by clinical administrators and faculty are given will the research atmosphere flourish.

NEEDED AREAS OF RESEARCH

Physical therapists traditionally function as clinicians for direct patient care, educators, administrators, and as consultants. All areas of function germane to physical therapy are areas requiring research. Since physical therapists are predominantly providers of health services, then substantial energies should be directed toward the science aspects of the profession and of the delivery of physical therapy services.

Some specific areas identified for research are:

1. The efficacy and value of therapeutic procedures and physical agents.[34,36-38] Facilitation and mobilization techniques, electrical stimulation, lasers, biofeedback, therapeutic exercises and aids to enhance muscular strength, and comparison of physical agents and of their combinations for treatment of specific conditions are examples.
2. Tests and measurements in the assessment of physical conditions and in the analysis of motion[34,36,38] Development of improved clinical techniques for measuring muscular strength, gait, edema, and treatment effectiveness are needed along with demonstrated validity and reliability of the techniques and instruments of measurement.
3. Rehabilitation engineering of devices for assisting the physically handicapped,[36] and for achieving optimum design of the therapist's equipment.
4. Growth and developmental defects and ways of improving physical function.[38]
5. Practices of accreditation, registration, licensure;[4] and standards for physical therapy services.[39]
6. Curriculum construction, legislative planning, cost studies,[40] competencies of practice, and effectiveness and impact of specialization.

The April 1979 issue of PROGRESS REPORT of the American Physical Therapy Association invited ideas on priorities in physical therapy clinical research. The report of the mail-in survey listed the priorities as: (1) treatment outcomes, (2) physiological effects of treatment, (3) methods of patient assessment, (4) pathological mechanisms, (5) delivery of services, and (6) psycho-social aspects. Later in June 1979 the Research Committee held a clinical research hearing in which individuals presented testimony on research priorities. These results indicated that treatment outcomes were suggested most as needing research.

ESTABLISHING RESEARCH

The establishment of research in a facility (clinic, school, program) requires thorough and deliberate planning,[25,41] administrative support,[8,25] and employment of therapists prepared to practice, research, and teach.

The development and implementation of any new activity within a facility must necessarily derive administrative support. Research requires trained personnel, ideas, money, space, and "a climate of vigorous intellectual ferment."[26] Each criterion is administratively related. Above all, the administrators must be convinced of the necessity and value of physical therapy research. The administrator can be identified as the director of a department or program, or as the director of a hospital or school.

Administrative Support

When establishing research in the clinic, some attention must be given to the administrative aspects. Without the support and encouragement of the clinical administration, the aspiring researcher has a harder than usual task to conduct research.

The therapist's working conditions can encourage or discourage research. The researcher needs security of job with guarantees that an approved research project can be completed.[24] Many researchers were hurt financially (unemployment) when federal funds were reduced or withdrawn in the late 1960s because their salaries and projects were funded solely by research grants ("soft monies"). Freedom to perform without undue interference from administrators is helpful to the researcher, as is the absence of administrative pressure and reduced numbers of written reports. Uncompromising deadlines or measurable end products can destroy pilot or burgeoning research. Access to pertinent literature is very important. Professional in-service programs are beneficial to the researcher because they provide a forum for ideas and communication. Also, sympathetic official attitudes are most encouraging because they condone the objectives and activity of the researcher, provide an "aire" of endorsement, and negate prejudices.[24]

"I do not have enough time to do research because I am expected to treat patients," is often voiced as a deterrent to clinical investigations. Since when has intellectual curiosity been confined to certain periods of the day? Do ideas or questions of clinical nature occur only when certain periods of the day are designated for thought peculiar to research? The answer to these questions should be obvious, but time is essential to perform literature reviews, write proposals for approval by administrative and research personnel, analyze data, and report results. Efficient therapists find time during the work day for activities other than direct patient care. Research can and should be integrated into your regular patient care program. Research is really a part of direct patient care because it answers questions and improves quality of care. Finding time to do research is the responsibility of the individual rather than that of the administrator. Silvermann[8] has provided suggestions for selling the research idea to administrators. Results obtained and published from research provide a means of accountability. Published reports can be counted and the findings can be used in the administrator's talks to community groups or the board of directors. Ongoing research is likely to convey local, state, and national recognition to the facility and therapists. This type of recognition is looked upon favorably by administrators because it brings notoriety and possibly attracts gifts of money.[8]

Research is an excellent way of evaluating clinical programs and revealing objective information. After all, practitioners do assess, observe, and measure so a systematic approach with controls built in could deliver important findings for supporting objectives. The systematic approach would probably not interfere with ongoing activity because it is really what physical therapy is about. Data gathering is part of any effective treatment program.[8]

Research Funding

Research studies require the use of instruments that invariably require financial support for construction, operation, or maintenance. Large amounts of money are needed for some studies in which purchases of equipment must be made and in which salaries of research assistants must be paid.

Monies are either obtained internally, from sources within the institution or facility, or externally, from sources outside of the institution. Internal funding is usually made in small amounts to assist pilot studies, while external funding is obtained from sources such as government, organizations, and foundations. The latter sources award large amounts of money, but are very competitive and require special applications and time. A researcher can usually expect one year to elapse between submission of a grant application and initiation of the project if successful in obtaining external funds. The researcher is advised to plan research projects well in advance of anticipated target dates for starting when planning to obtain external funding, but also be prepared for possible rejection of financial support. The interested researcher can find assistance in grant writing by means of personal assistance from: those having experience, books, and workshops.

Table 1.2
Cumulative Summary of the Research Processes Presented

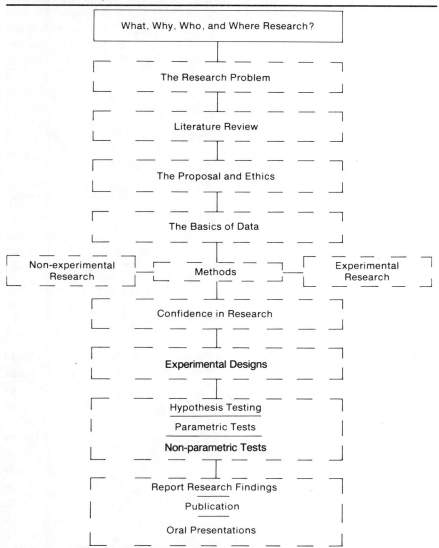

HOW RESEARCH?

Many different methods are described for use in research; some are identical in purpose and technique but are given different names by different disciplines. Different methods are devised for studying different content areas because one method may not be adequate or flexible enough to fulfill the needs of all areas of interest. All methods of research do, however, have commonalities. All methods require the collection of information relevant to the subject undergoing investigation; the collected data must be verified, analyzed, and interpreted, and the findings must be presented in some orderly fashion. Some hows or methods of the research process are presented in the following chapters.

SUMMARY

This chapter has provided an introduction to the scientific method of research by discussing the what, why, who, and where of research, and discussing the types of research. Attention was called to areas of needed research in physical therapy and problems that may be encountered in establishing or conducting research. Table 1.2 provides an overview of the research process which is discussed in this book.

REFERENCES

1. Fowler HW: A Dictionary of Modern English Usage, E. Gowers (ed), ed 2. New York, Oxford University Press, 1965
2. Random House Dictionary of the English Language, Unabridged ed. New York, Random House, 1983
3. Peat M: Physiotherapy: art or science? Physiother Canada 33: 170–176, 1980
4. Worthingham C: The development of physical therapy as a profession through research and publication. Phys Ther Rev 40: 573–577, 1960
5. Greenwood E: The elements of professionalization. In Vollmer HM, Mills DL (eds): Professionalization. Englewood Cliffs, NJ, Prentice-Hall, Inc, 1966
6. Hislop HJ: The not-so-impossible dream. Phys Ther 55: 1069–1080, 1975
7. Kerlinger FN: Foundations of Behavioral Research, ed 2. New York, Holt, Rinehart and Winston, Inc, 1973
8. Silverman FH: Research Design in Speech Pathology and Audiology: Asking and Answering Questions. Englewood Cliffs, NJ, Prentice-Hall, Inc, 1977
9. The national commission for the protection of human subjects of biomedical and behavioral research: the Belmont Report: ethical principles and guidelines for the protection of human subjects of research. Washington, DHEW Public Health Service, 78-0013, 1978
10. Report of the American Public Health Association Task Force. Am. J Public Health 47: 218–234, 1957
11. Wandelt M: Guide for the Beginning Researcher. New York, Appleton-Century-Crofts, 1970
12. Wilson EB Jr: An Introduction to Scientific Method. New York, McGraw-Hill Book Co, 1952
13. Steinhaus AH: Why This Research? In Hubbard AW (ed): Research Methods in Health, Physical Education, and Recreation. Washington, Am Assoc Health Phys Educ, 1973
14. Campbell EWR: Introduction: The purpose of research. Physiotherapy 56: 480–481, 1970
15. Cox RC, Best WL: Fundamentals of Research for Health Professionals. Laurel (MD), RAMSCO Pub. Co., 1982
16. Ritchie AE: Considering research. Physiotherapy 56: 110–112, 1966

17. Basmajian JV: Professional survival: the research role in physical therapy. Phys Ther 57: 283–285, 1977
18. Watkins AL: Some research problems in physical therapy. Phys Ther 29: 443–447, 1949
19. Hines HM: What research means to a profession—its growth and continuation. Phys Ther 31: 450–451, 1951
20. Houtz SJ: Challenge of the scientific method. Phys Ther 31: 465–467, 1951
21. Gowland C, Clarke B: Research: Why bother! Physiother Canada 32: 270–274, 1980
22. Hellebrandt FA: Graduate study—a key to research and writing. Phys Ther 40: 257–260, 1960
23. Currier DP: Research in Physical Therapy Schools. (Unpublished survey.)
24. Cannon WB: The Way of an Investigator: A Scientist's Experiences in Medical Research. New York, Hafner and Co, 1965
25. Moffroid MT, Hofkosh JM: Development of a research section. Phys Ther 49: 1208–1214, 1969
26. Greenblatt M: Conducting a research department. Hosp Community Psychiatry 13: 580–581, 1962
27. The Research Advisory Board. Physiotherapy 52: 126–127, 1966
28. Partridge CJ: Progress in research. Physiother 68: 353, 1982
29. Clinical Study Council. Physiotherapy Canada 23: 184, 1971
30. Lehmkuhl D: Let's reduce the communication gap: Part I, the question what and why? Phys Ther 50: 61–63, 1970
31. Ruffer WA: Who should make research applicable? J Health Phys Educ 40: 41–42, 1969
32. Currier DP: Research in programs of initial physical therapy education. Physiotherapy Canada 29: 211–213, 1977
33. Report of the Royal College of Physicians of Edinburgh on co-operation between medical and other health professions. Physiotherapy 63: 228, 1977
34. Griffin JE: What's the answer. Phys Ther 50: 259, 1970
35. Michels E: Paper submissions hit all-time high. Progress Rpt 10: 5, 1981
36. Basmajian JV: Research or retrench: The rehabilitation professions challenged. Phys Ther 55: 607–610, 1975
37. Fowler WM: Physical therapy and research. Phys Ther 49: 977–982, 1969
38. Hislop HJ: The doctorate in physical therapy. Phys Ther 48: 1325–1326, 1968
39. Chase HC: Some current research in the allied health professions. Phys Ther 51: 771–776, 1971
40. Magistro CM: The 1976 presidential address. Phys Ther 56: 1227–1239, 1976
41. Schrenk R: Research: Stepchild of medicine. Am J Clin Pathol 34: 268–269, 1960

2

The Research Problem

If research is a process used to find facts or add to a body of knowledge (theory), then the process must have a beginning. Accumulating facts without any preconceived idea of what facts to gather or which are relevant would be disastrous. An organized plan is essential for gathering the facts. The first step in the plan for beginning research is to formulate the research problem.

WHAT AND WHY A RESEARCH PROBLEM?

Definition (What?)

The simplest way to define a research problem is to state that it is a question. The question must be answerable; that is, a solution to the question must be possible. A problem can be an "irritation" which stimulates a person into doing research in order to answer the question or to eliminate the irritation.[1] The problem can be something that needs solving, an unresolved situation. The problem can be an idea which a person has for developing an approach to treatment or a new product.

We all have had questions to which we have sought answers. Often we asked another person, perhaps a teacher or a peer, and received a satisfactory answer. Sometimes we did not get a satisfactory answer to our question and had to seek a solution or answer by library or textbook search. Our questions in these illustrated situations were answered by simple methods; however, not all of our questions or problems may have simple answers or solutions.

Too often people do not seek answers to their questions or problems unless the answer or solution is quickly and easily available. These persons are not curious and are not potential researchers. The persons who search for an answer, establish a formal organized plan to acquire an answer, and use methods of scientific inquiry to get the answer are researchers. The researcher is motivated to eliminate the irritation by obtaining a satisfactory answer to his question. Thus, research begins when answers to the question cannot be found.

The Value of the Research Problem (Why?)

The unanswered question is important because it directs or stimulates the curious and motivated person into seeking an answer and can be responsible for starting research or scientific investigation. The stated problem can help direct the researcher and lead to an investigation through which a scientific approach is used for its solution. The specific information or findings resulting from the research enables the researcher to make generalized statements based on the specific empirical observations from the research process. The reasoning process is deduction. The results of the research can serve as a basis for prediction and control of the phenomena studied.[2] The basic value of the research problem is to stimulate research that will lead to new scientific knowledge through the finding of answers or solutions to the problem. Also, research findings often lead to other interesting and significant problems to be studied.

IDENTIFYING A PROBLEM

How does one go about identifying or locating a research problem? For some, identifying a research problem or asking a research question may be more difficult than solving it or answering the question. Since various circumstances may serve as starting points for identifying an answerable question, certain attributes or activities can assist the student in identifying or locating a research problem. Suggestions on how to locate or identify research problems may be valuable for the conduct of research necessary to complete a course in clinical investigations, a thesis, or a dissertation.

Necessary Attributes for a Researcher

In Chapter 1 the desirable qualities of a researcher were discussed and listed. Some of these qualities are repeated for the purpose of emphasizing their importance in research.

One of the first considerations is the student's or researcher's attitude toward the scientific method or the advancement of the profession. A positive attitude consists of interest, curiosity, and motivation. Perhaps interest is the key characteristic that will aid in identifying the problem and seeking a solution. The student must be enthusiastic or interested in a particular area or the research process will be a distasteful experience. Having an interest in a particular problem can help direct the student in the pursuit of a solution and help the student to enjoy the experience. A student who finds routine dissection distasteful might develop interest in dissection when it becomes a means of seeking the solution to a defined problem of considerable personal interest. Usually, students with enthusiasm and interest in what they are doing will find the research experience enjoyable. Some students may even want to continue research as a result of this initial experience or exposure to research. The disinterested researcher does not usually contribute new ideas to research or a body of knowledge.[3]

Technical knowledge in the area of planned research is of paramount importance.[4-9] That is, the student must know a body of knowledge well in order to identify situations or areas which require additional facts or information before improvement can be achieved. The experienced researcher has little difficulty in identifying problems in a particular body of knowledge; his trouble is that he usually cannot find enough time to conduct the experiments necessary for answering all of his questions or solving the identified problems in his field of interest. The experienced researcher identifies new problems every time a research project or study is in progress.

The individual who knows the deficiencies that exist in a particular area will have an easier time in the formulation of the problem to be solved through research. The student must be able to identify problems requiring research and he must know how to design an experiment which will answer the question being asked. He must know how to select and operate the instrumentation used to measure or collect data. He must know how to record data and interpret the findings in light of the evidence collected. He must be able to adequately describe the problems, the methods, and the design used to collect data, and to present the results through oral and written presentations.

By far the most important attribute is thinking. Ritchie[4] has stated: "Don't accept what people say or write; ask yourself, or others, or the literature—is this really so, what is the evidence, how good is it, could I verify or disprove that point, how would I go about it and what would I need?" The selection of a research problem requires study, thought, and planning guided by imagination and critical judgment.[2] Thinking requires time and its process often gives the impression of idleness. Administrators often frown on this aspect of research because some do not consider this process productive to service; thinking is difficult to measure in terms of productivity. Thinking is essential because it is the process that puts pieces of the puzzle together for organizing and starting the research.

In addition, the identification of a problem requires that the researcher have imagination, originality, and critical judgment.

Acquired Essentials of the Researcher

Training in methods of research is essential for the student undertaking a project of scientific inquiry. Academic programs of physical therapy are structured to help students in research.

The programs offering initial preparation in physical therapy are helping the student to develop positive attitudes toward research and are teaching the student how to interpret the research literature. Programs of graduate studies prepare physical therapists in how to conduct research and encourage research through course work, independent studies, and theses. If proper training is provided in research then clinical physical therapists will further their interest in research by establishing research in their clinical programs. Students of physical therapy at all levels could then be exposed to research during clinical affiliations. Physical therapy's body of knowledge would grow, methods of health delivery would improve, and development of new and improved approaches to quality care would flourish. Training in research methods is essential for the survival of a profession because trained individuals will continue the required efforts to build the profession's body of knowledge. This book will attempt to provide introductory training in research by covering elements of physical therapy research.

Although research is a tool of science, the skills of research must be learned just as the physical therapist learns anatomy and physiology. Research contains a body of knowledge that is composed of designs, methods of analysis (statistics), instrumentation, and writing. Each area of research requires degrees of competency which, in turn, commands time for acquisition. That is, competency in research is acquired over a long period of time and not by successfully completing a single course or thesis. Whatever extent the exposure is to research, each contributes toward gaining the necessary competency in research. On-the-job training and apprenticeships have proven to be excellent approaches to acquiring research skills.

Acquisition of knowledge in a particular field builds competency. Several approaches to gaining knowledge can be taken by the potential researcher. The formal approach is to pursue course work in the area of interest by means of matriculation, workshops, or continuing education. The informal approach to learning is organized and continuous reading on a subject. This approach is very effective for acquiring knowledge in a specific area and has the advantage of flexibility; for example, reading predominantly research literature at the convenience of the researcher. Reading numerous research reports provides a variety of styles and inputs which enhances understanding. Enormous amounts of reading on a special subject will produce one area of competency essential for performing research.

Activities Leading to Problem Identification

An idea or problem may be born from a casual observation in the clinic. Therapists or student therapists encounter situations with equipment, assessments, procedures and techniques, curriculum, and peers or administrators, which may present difficulties.[6] These difficulties may be identified as research problems if immediate solutions are not available or if the identified questions cannot be answered by problem-solving methods. If physical therapists would record ideas and problems encountered during their daily experiences, research would become their primary activity. Many everyday difficulties do not have immediate solutions or answers because solutions or answers are unknown.

A problem might be the result of a gap in a body of knowledge. An example of such a problem might be expressed by the question: Are proprioceptive neuromuscular facilitation techiques effective in restoring muscular function when there has been brain damage in a patient? Filling gaps which exist in current knowledge could link theories with techniques. Because of these gaps, techniques used in the clinic often are not based on theory and facts.

A theory is a guess, conjecture, or a group of postulations. Many theories exist in physical therapy, and practitioners often conjecture about the best therapeutic approach to a particular patient problem. Theories are not facts and therefore contain generalizations which can and must be tested by rigorous scientific study. Researchable problems can be derived from theories, generalizations, and conjectures because they enable the researcher to make predictions about a wide range of circumstances. The results of investigating a postulation contribute to the theory by confirming or contradicting all or parts of the theory.[10]

Reading and analyzing the literature in a particular area of interest is perhaps the most satisfactory approach to identifying research problems.[1,4,6,7] As the studnet or researcher continues to read on a subject, a sizeable fund of knowledge will be built. As the reading program continues, not only is a stronger base of knowledge built but he becomes an authority on the subject because chances are great that he possesses more information on the subject than the "average" colleague. Constant reading and analyzing of the literature enables the student to identify deficiencies and strengths in knowledge, inconsistencies, and trends; most important, it may stimulate ideas for research. Research reports often suggest or indicate further studies which need to be conducted. Accumulating a list of promising research problems, in the form of index cards, is very helpful. The list can serve as a repository of reference and recall, and can be reviewed periodically by the researcher for selection of the most promising problems for initiating new research projects.

The student necessarily should confine literature reviews to the particular area that holds his interest. The literature is voluminous, so limiting reading to one or two areas of professional interest is a practical approach.

Controversial issues should be examined. Different points of view on issues or contradictory research findings may provide new ideas for solution of or resolving the controversy. The literature contains research reports in which controversies are frequently discussed in the introductory phase of the report. Controversies of note have been associated with research on isometric exercise, the role of the vastus medialis, the effects of propriocep-tive neuromuscular facilitation procedures, and the effect of faradic current in eliciting contraction of a denervated muscle. Professional exposure to intellectual discourse in courses, workshops, meetings, and informal dis-cussions may assist the student in identifying areas of controversy within the profession.[7] Research can be designed to help solve a particular controversy that interests the researcher.

Observing in other settings can be helpful in providing ideas or a fresh approach to a research problem.[1,4] Seeing research in progress or consulting with others who are engaged in research can be stimulating as well as helpful to the inexperienced researcher. Researchers usually enjoy discuss-ing their work because of their enthusiasm to advance knowledge and their willingness to gain or exchange knowledge with others. Exposure to other investigators or settings may also prevent duplication of efforts and costly equipment or convince the student of the vastness and complexity of a particular problem. Visitation and observations of research in departments outside of his own may enable the student to modify plans, abandon an idea, or provide the creation of a challenging problem to solve.

A final activity or source leading to a researchable problem is replication of previous studies. Many of the studies reported in the literature are "one shot" investigations that have not been replicated to show consistency of findings. The entry-level or master's student can often make a valuable contribution by repeating a study conducted by someone else to confirm results. Replication of findings of previous work strengthens theory and principles or occasionally uncovers doubtful or questionable conclusions. Borg and Gall[11] suggest that replication of a good study can be a better experience for some students than conducting an original study of poor quality but warn that replication should only be done if it can make a significant contribution or clear up questionable areas in the original study, and when doubt is cast about the accuracy of a previous work.

CONSIDERATIONS IN SELECTING A PROBLEM

Once a problem has been identified, the researcher must examine it thoroughly for certain considerations before reaching a decision for pro-ceeding with its study.[7] Some departments (clinic, program) or facilities (hospitals, universities) may have established criteria to be followed before beginning research. In the event no formal direction is required when selecting a research problem, a few considerations are suggested to assist the beginning researcher. Most of the considerations are interrelated.

Interest, Training, and Knowledge

These criteria have already received elaboration, but once the problem has been identified, the student or researcher must ask whether the problem is of sufficient personal interest to pursue further and devote the time required to seek the solution.[7] The researcher must be curious, motivated, and interested in the specific problem identified. Although a basic aim of research is to advance knowledge, most research is initiated because of the personal interest of the investigator in the specific problem being studied. Interest may be more of a difficulty for students in the academic setting than for physical therapists in the professional setting. The student is strongly advised to possess considerable interest in the problem before undertaking the required project.

The technical knowledge and skill of the researcher must be considered when doing research. In the case of a student, the question of whether the student possesses sufficient competency and training to handle the process of solving the problem arises, and approval is granted to proceed with a project. Usually projects are pursued near the end of a course of study; for example, the 4th year of an undergraduate student or the last year or term of a graduate student. Researchers often begin their research experience by collaborating with others such as an experienced researcher or faculty member. Some neophytes serve apprentice-like relationships before conducting research independently. The researcher's knowledge of a particular area is usually evident during the review process of a planned study. Inadequacy in any one of these criteria would be disastrous to the researcher and to the research particularly in terms of energy and time lost.

Sophisticated approaches to a solution of the problem should not be considered if the approaches require special training and knowledge that is not readily available to the student or if long periods of training would be required. Of course, the qualifications may be the reason the student enrolled in the program to begin with; for example, the student may have had the problem in mind and then selected a graduate program because of the faculty and capabilities of the facilities of the graduate program. The situation would be ironic if the student wanted to do research which required electromyographic equipment, but the program did not have faculty with sufficient competencies to teach or to direct research in electromyography.

Solvability of Problem

The student may select a problem that is of great interest, but the problem may not be answerable or cannot be solved for various reasons. Perhaps the problem is concerned with a condition or trait that cannot be defined sufficiently to plan an approach to its solution. The problem may be too broad or too complex for a solution within the capability of the available personnel or facilities. Therefore, it is necessary to select a problem for which a solution is possible within the framework of the facility and the time and background available to the student.

Professional Contribution

The value or gains of the research must be considered by the researcher before commencing a study or even before seeking approval for the study.[3,4,8] At some point the researcher must defend and justify the selected problem. The results obtained from the research process, answering the question, must be worthy of the energy, time, and costs incurred. The expected contribution does not have to be dramatic or world shaking; however, it should make some contribution to the profession by adding to the body of knowledge; improving the conditions or operation of techniques; improving instrumentation or quality of care; or in some way providing answers to questions which will decide an issue, stimulate further research, or be relevant to physical therapy.

The researcher must ask whether the problem is too small (trivial) to be of any value or whether the problem is too large (complex) to be answered in a single study. Administrators of research funding or committees granting approval for research are demanding accountability of the researcher and research more than ever before. Pursuing knowledge for its own sake is given scrutiny by those in authority to approve research; potential application of the research findings to improve human welfare is often given priority in approving research projects. The feasibility of all planned research must be challenged before proceeding with the research.

Availability of Technology, Equipment, and Facility

If the technical background of the researcher is inadequate in a specific area, consultation with experts must be arranged. For example, a statistician, electrical technician, or photographic technician might need to be consulted on experimental design and analysis, hardware instrumentation, or illustrations, respectively.

The problem may be selected which can be solved, but its solution may depend on expensive sophisticated equipment which is not available to the student. Sometimes arrangements can be made for the research to be conducted away from the student's department or through collaboration and direction of another advisor. Some research requires the purchase of equipment and supplies or the rental of space or costs for travel. The researcher must arrange for these necessities prior to commencing the project. The approving authority may be in a position to financially support the project or advise the researcher where monies can be obtained. Requests for grants to support the research may have to be made by the researcher. Equipment may often be borrowed.

The availability of the sample or population of subjects, events, or attributes to be studied must be considered. A problem may be identified but if the sample processing characteristics to be studied are not available or if the numbers are insufficient to answer the question, the research cannot proceed.

The researcher must also arrange his schedule so that sufficient time is available to complete the research process, problem through publication (Table 1.2). The idea in this section is to give the utmost consideration to the available technology and facility when selecting a problem for research.[7,8,12]

DELIMITING PROBLEMS

Once the problem has been identified for its research possibility, the problem must be delimited. One of the difficulties that students have in selecting a problem for their investigation is that their problem is too global. The student often does not realize that the selected problem is too complex or broad and that it cannot be solved through a single investigation. The problem must be narrowed so that the question can be answered. A general problem should be subdivided into many questions which should be solved separately; then information gathered can be pieced together.

The student might be interested in knowing how the knee extensors should be exercised for greatest enhancement, a complex or global problem. Subproblems of muscular force must be considered, such as type of exercise (static; dynamic-concentric, eccentric, isokinetic) and influencing factors (rate, repetitions, loads, frequency and sets). Positioning (joint angles, hand grasping, support, inclination of seat), effects of facilitation and assessment of strength also may be considered. If body positioning is selected as the problem, then the placement of the hands, angle of the hip joint, support or non-support for the back, the position of the knee (angle, static or dynamic type of exercise), and inclination of the thigh by inclining the seat angle or by use of a knee wedge must be given serious consideration. Each of the sub-problems could be used for a single investigation, but only the composite of all sub-problems could answer the question: How should the quadriceps be exercised for greatest enhancement of force? Table 2.1 shows an example of global and delimited problems.

The delimitations guide the research by establishing limits or boundaries, by narrowing the selected problem, and by defining the scope of the investigation.[9] Sweet and Moir[13] have suggested that the problem be defined by listing independent variables in four categories: (1) treatment variables (type, duration, intensity, consistency), (2) subject variables (age, sex, physical status), (3) therapist variables (age, sex, experience, employer, professional attitudes), and (4) condition variables, (type, severity, location, concurrent problems, intervening time between events). These authors' reasons for the listing of independent variables were to isolate variables to keep their effects constant (control), to determine effects of variables, and to achieve quantitative evaluation.[13] Assistance is usually required in

Table 2.1
Global and Delimited Research Problems

Global problem
  How can the muscular force of the quadriceps be enhanced?
Delimited problem (sub-problems)
  Types of Exercise
    Which type of exercise is best for increasing strength of the quadriceps? (static, dynamic-
      concentric, eccentric, isokinetic?)
    Do different exercises have specificity?
  Influencing factors in exercise
    What is best rate for performing dynamic exercises?
    What number of repetitions is best for increasing strength? (4, 6, 8, 10, 12, or 14 repeti-
      tions?)
    What number of repetitions is best for increasing muscular endurance?
    What is best load for achieving optimal strength gains? (40, 50, 60, 70, 80, 90, or maximum
      percentage of strength?)
    What is the ideal frequency of performing exercises? (1, 2, 3, 4, or 5 times/week?)
    What are the retention periods of strength gains? (weeks, months, or year?)
    What joint angles are optimal for performing static exercises?
  Stabilization Effects
    Do arm positions affect force generated?
    What effect do various hip positions have on the force generated?
    Does the backrest increase the ability of the quadriceps to generate force?
    How do design factors of equipment influence the force a muscle can generate?
  Facilitating Aids
    Does activation of reflexes during exercises influence strength gains?
    Does a wedge affect strength gains or force generated by the muscle?
    Does electrical stimulation of muscle during exercise affect strength gains?
    Do facilitating patterns of movement increase strength more than conventional positions?

delimiting the problem before the plan can be designed. Lloyd[14] has made some suggestions for breaking down of the research problem which may be of some assistance. He suggested an orderly arrangement of information about the problem as:

1. Identifying the field of science in which the problem is located.[14] The question of how to enhance quadriceps force during exercise can again be used as the problem identified. The problem may be associated with the interests of physical therapists, physical educators, and sports medicine personnel.

2. Listing known major variables.[14] Variables (things that can be manipulated or measured) might include: types of exercise; rate, repetitions and frequency of exercise; stabilization measures of hand grasping, hip angle, back support, inclination of seat; and force-generated.

3. Listing the type data required. This list requires thought on the specific variable or variables that are measured.[14] The data in our example of a global research problem are measurements of force, tension, or torque.

4. Locating methods of gathering the data.[14] The kinds of instruments and procedures which have been used for obtaining data of force, tension,

or torque must be considered and identified. The process of delimiting the problem involves assembling facts about the problem, verifying that the problem is real and answerable, and knowing how to go about resolving it. Once a problem has been identified we are ready to proceed with the process of verifying and organizing its solution.

LIMITATION

Limitations to a research project are not the same as delimitations. Limitations are conditions or variables that are not under the control of the researcher. The limiting conditions can influence the outcome of the investigation. Individual variations of the subjects undergoing study may cause limitations. The type of measuring device, the type of subject who volunteers for the study, or the method of selecting the subjects also may be limitations to the study and may influence the outcome. The economics of undertaking a solution to the problem and moral issues facing risk of subjects involved in the undertaking must be considered and could lead to certain limitations. The researcher, however, is obligated to control as many variables as possible.[7,9]

The delimiting of a researchable problem is the beginning of a process to converge on a specific issue within a general or broader subject area. Although a researchable problem requires a solution, it cannot be tested in question form. A question demands a response or reply which may still contain several ideas or concepts that have not been subjected to the trial or scrutiny of controlled experimentation. A delimited problem must be narrowed further; in other words, reduced to its component parts. In practice, the problem is identified for readers of the research plan (Chapter 4) or the published report (Chapter 12) as the gap in a theory, controversy of issues, or even the ineffectiveness of a treatment procedure. The component parts of the problem, hypotheses, and objectives serve to filter out surplus or unrelated information contained in the problem.[15] The formulation of hypotheses shaves the problem to conditional relationships which can be tested by the research process.

A hypothesis is a proposition that can be tested; it is a subdivision of a problem used in experimental research that involves causes and comparisons. A working hypothesis is a well written statement of the problem indicating the variables (measurements subject to change) of interest to the investigator. It may point out the particular relationship between the variables to be studied. The problem, for example, to be investigated may be the effect of moderate frequency electrical stimulation on the arterial blood flow to muscle. The variables to be studied are "moderate frequency electrical stimulation" and "arterial blood flow to muscle." The delimited problem may also be converted into a statistical hypothesis that can be precisely tested. An example of the latter form may be that no relationship exists between the variables studied and could be stated as: "No significant difference exists between measures of blood flow when using moderate frequency electrical stimulation and when not using moderate frequency electrical stimulation." Hypotheses and hypothesis testing will be discussed in detail in Chapter 10. The objectives or purposes define the boundaries

Table 2.2
Cumulative Summary of the Research Processes Presented

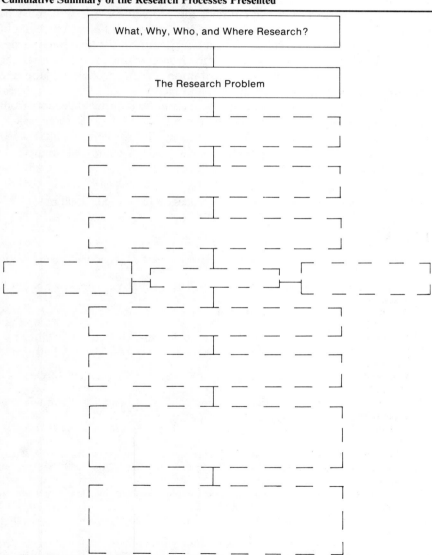

under which the investigation will be conducted and describe the end product which is expected to emerge from the research process.

SUMMARY

The research problem is a question that must be answered by some organized process. The problem may be identified by recognizing everyday difficulties and experiences: gaps in a body of knowledge and controversial issues in a profession. Once identified, the problem or question must be delimited to a form which can be solved or answered. Before engaging in further steps of the research process the investigator must take into consideration: his interest, training, and knowledge of the problem area; the solvability of the problem; its contribution to the profession; and the availability of technology, equipment, and facility.

Research is a process of thought and action, it requires direction from an identified problem. Remember the motto:

> "For everyone who does something, ten others had the same idea but they only thought about it."[14]

Table 2.2 summarizes the research processes presented thus far.

REFERENCES

1. Wandelt M: Guide for the Beginning Researcher. New York, Appleton-Century-Crofts, 1970
2. Trelease SF: How to Write Scientific and Technical Papers. Cambridge, MA, The M.I.T. Press, 1969
3. Wilson EG Jr: An Introduction to Scientific Research. New York, McGraw-Hill Book Co, 1952
4. Ritchie AE: Considering research. Physiotherapy 56: 110–112, 1966
5. Bernard C: An Introduction to the Study of Experimental Medicine. New York, Dover Publications, Inc, 1957
6. Van Dalen DB: Understanding Educational Research, ed 4. New York, McGraw-Hill Book Co, 1978
7. Clarke DH, Clarke HH: Research Processes in Physical Education, Recreation, and Health. Englewood Cliffs, NJ, Prentice-Hall, Inc, 1970
8. McLaren HM: So you want to conduct a clinical study. Physiother Canada 25: 219–224, 1973
9. Broer MR, Mohr DR: Selecting and Defining a Research Problem. In Hubbard AW (ed): Research Methods in Health, Physical Education, and Recreation, ed 3. Washington, Am Assoc Health Phys Educ Res, 1973
10. Gay LR: Educational Research: Competencies for Analysis and Application, ed 2. Columbus, OH, Charles E. Merrill Pub Co, 1981
11. Borg WR, Gall MD: Educational Research: An Introduction, ed 3. New York, Longman, 1979
12. Silverman FH: Research Design in Speen Pathology and Audiology: Asking and Answering Questions. Englewood Cliffs, NJ, Prentice-Hall, Inc, 1977

13. Sweet RL, Moir SB: Some elementary guides for performing research into the effects of physiotherapy treatments. Aust J Physiother 44: 85–90, 1973
14. Lloyd LE: Techniques for Efficient Research. New York, Clinical Publishing Co, Inc, 1966
15. Andrew CO, Hildebrand PE: Planning and Conducting Applied Research. New York, MSS Information Corp, 1976

3

Literature Review

There is a dead medical literature, and there
is a live one. The dead is not all ancient, the live
is not all modern. There is none, modern or ancient,
which, if it has no living value for the student, will
not teach him something by its autopsy.
Oliver Wendell Holmes
Medical Essays, "Medical Libraries"

The literature review is a fundamental ingredient of the scientific method and ranks high in its potential for contribution to the research effort. The importance of the review of literature has been mentioned as being valuable for locating a research problem. The literature review may even be the very first step in some research because the command of a body of knowledge may have been gained through reading or the inspiration of the research problem may have begun as a result of a literature review. The library is the vehicle of the literature review and exists for the purpose of information retrieval; it should be a part of the researcher's paradise.

Although students taking a first course of college English are usually introduced to the library, its contents, and its system of operation, the research tools may not be exposed as such. This chapter will offer suggestions which may assist the beginning researcher with the literature review. The literature review is a process of acquiring depth and understanding of the published information in a particular area of interest. The literature review may assist the student in locating and identifying a research problem; it will certainly be essential for a logical or chronological approach to the basis of the research which lies ahead.

WHY THE LITERATURE REVIEW?

Before proceeding with the writing of the formal research proposal (plan of research) a survey of literature relating to the problem must be undertaken. The reasons for this often laborious task are:

1. To ascertain originality of research. Although all research does not have to be original, the literature review can be used to determine whether comparable research has been published. The library is often used when

in pursuit of an answer to a question which has not been answered by associates or readily accessible reference sources. After reasonable or exhaustive but futile review of literature pertinent or allied to the question or problem, the researcher can reasonably be assured that the problem is original or at least the answer has not been reported in the literature. For example, in reviewing literature on how to increase the capacity for tension development in the quadriceps through resistive exercises, the researcher may have noticed that no research study had answered why a wedge was placed underneath the knee when a subject was performing strengthening exercises for the quadriceps. The scientific approach to answering the question could have been considered original by the investigator since a thorough review of the literature did not provide any evidence or reason why a knee wedge should be used in strengthening exercises. Justifying originality is not the most valid reason for the literature review. The researcher must know what has or what has not been published about the particular problem. If the solutions or answers to the problem had been reported to the extent the question had really been answered, then he might have been remiss in the selection and conduction of another study on the same problem. The review assists the researcher in the determination of feasibility of conducting a study on a particular problem.[1]

2. To provide ideas for solution of the problem. The investigator can formulate methods for answering the question by reading reports of studies which answered questions similar or allied to the question under review. Approaches in technique or instrumentation used in measuring or collecting data similar to that required by the investigator can be found in published research reports. Inadequacies of previous studies can be identified and can be avoided by the researcher with a thorough review of literature pertinent to his selected problem. Interpretations and discussions of other authors are important to the researcher in formulating a problem, or in seeking approaches to interpretation of the outcome in the research being planned. The theoretical information is valuable when the completed research is being written for publication. Information contained in the literature review helps to form background information for the examiner and assist in the interpretation of the results. Information gained from the review of literature will provide the researcher with insight into understanding the importance of the answers to his question and the importance of these answers to the area investigated. One of the contributions of any research report is the stimulus which a certain aspect of the study provides to another researcher. The findings of a study are like chain links because one researcher reviews literature to identify and formulate a research idea, and his completed report provides similar impetus to another researcher who, in turn, builds on to the body of knowledge.[1] Almost nothing is new in research, but reported findings of studies are extensions of what has already been done.

Literature reviews will often uncover controversies between reported findings of research or controversies in accepted concepts because of the lack of research replications. Reading continuously in a particular area of interest will increase the reader's knowledge of the subject.

3. To avoid repetitious findings. Occasionally a review of the literature uncovers several studies, similar in scope and design, that reveal insignificant findings. Replication of studies in order to confirm findings was mentioned earlier; however, when such repetitions occur several times in a specific area of the literature, they have outlived their purpose. Further replication of these studies serves no usefulness in research, and the student is discouraged to spend additional time with the particular problem. A strong possibility exists that additional studies using similar approaches in the particular area will yield insignificant findings.

PLANNING THE LITERATURE REVIEW

Primary Literature

Certain published materials are more appropriate than others for providing information about the particular problem or area of interest. These primary materials (periodicals, books) are written by members of your profession and, therefore, contain topics that are similar in nature and content to yours. For example, if the researcher is planning to study the effects of muscular length on force, the literature primarily concerned with the problem would be works containing studies central to the stated problem; studies of joint position on performance, studies of types of exercise, or perhaps studies of the velocity of motion. Primary sources are, therefore, those materials most central to the particular problem being investigated.

Secondary Literature

Materials allied or related to the problem or area of interest but more peripheral than central to the problem in question are secondary sources.[1] Materials containing studies which investigated muscles other than those under consideration, or studies which investigated other influencing factors on muscular force would be secondary to the example given above. One must realize that secondary sources for one problem may be primary for another study. The nature of the problem determines which sources are most central and of greatest value to the researcher and which sources are helpful but only for gathering background information. Secondary sources would be those in which abstracted information is sufficient as a reference, while primary sources might be those cited in detail in the written portion of the study or considered most pertinent to interpretation of or discussion of your results. Primary sources might also be the reprints or reproductions in your files. The secondary sources might be those materials skimmed over but containing some usable information.

REVIEWING PROCESS

Because of the voluminous amounts of literature, the task of reviewing it can become overwhelming unless the researcher has a plan to guide him in the review. Procedures used to conduct the review may vary with the individual, familiarity with the library, the demands of the subject or area being reviewed, and the detail desired.

Medical Subject Headings (MeSH), appearing as the second part in each January issue of the INDEX MEDICUS, is a most useful source for identifying key words used in a health science library. The MeSH enables the researcher to choose and categorize key words used in locating topics in INDEX MEDICUS and other indexes, automated reference services, card catalogues, and other primary sources that might contain pertinent information. These key words are useful later when preparing the research findings for publication. MeSH contains an alphabetized list of subject headings which is cross referenced for locating closely related words ("see," "see related," and "see under"), and a categorized list that provides general headings relating to the trends of the medical literature.

Listing any relevant main words associated with the statement of the selected problem is helpful. In seeking literature related to strength variations of the quadriceps with and without the use of a knee wedge during exercise, one could list such key words as: wedge, isometric exercise, strength, force, muscular tension, leg position, joint angles, joint motion, and knee. These key words are guides to indexes, card catalogues, books, and other primary sources that might contain pertinent information. Additional key words can be found following the titles appearing in the January issues of the INDEX MEDICUS, since this particular index is one of the most useful indexes of the library and to the researcher.

Bibliographies accompanying the pertinent research reports of others are valuable to the investigator. References are cited at the end of the pertinent articles and these can be used to locate more detailed information. Using the bibliographical information provided with each article of interest is an excellent means of obtaining additional information and references.

The examiner is often confronted with the decision of whether unpublished studies warrant review. The published report is usually given greater credit by editorial committes than is the unpublished report. Some editorial committes may be reluctant to accept an unpublished report or personal communication as a reference in published articles. Theses and dissertations are examples of studies which are often cited in the literature as unpublished reports. If a study is good enough to conduct and be cited as a reference, then it should be good enough to publish no matter whether the hypothesis was supported or was not supported by the outcome of the study. Unpublished reports that have been cited by an author are often difficult to obtain or may require excessive periods of time to acquire. Research is never completed until published, so unpublished studies may be viewed as uncompleted research. This point of view may be somewhat narrow because theses and dissertations can contain valuable literature reviews but because of their inaccessibility to many readers they are not readily accepted by many researchers.

The review should encompass major sources of literature published on the particular topic; major sources chiefly include periodicals but not exclusively. Pamphlets, published proceedings of seminars, and up-to-date books are also good sources for the literature review but must be valued for their excellence of pertinent information. The review will provide the researcher with the thoughts and actions of others on similar problems. Thus, the literature review is an essential resource for apprising the researcher of all pertinent writings of a particular time and on a particular subject. If you have any difficulties in the review process, like locating sources or a particular topic, consult a librarian.

A decision of when to terminate a literature review must be made by every researcher. The nature of the subject will often dictate the termination of the review; for example, only a few references may be available on a specific topic and this may lead to an early termination. The usual approach is to begin with current references and then work backward in time. Each published report that is reviewed will contain cited references of earlier work, and the researcher can judge their value and decide whether further review of the literature is necessary. Some journals may not accept references which go beyond 10 to 20 years from the current date. References reported many years earlier than the current year may indeed be valuable resources to the researcher and are acceptable in publications if given pertinence by the researcher. The researcher should terminate the literature review when enough support is available for providing sufficient background for pointing out the specific problem and its need for research. The literature review is flexible and may include few or many references which are current or go backward beyond 20 years. The point is that each and every reference used by the researcher must be of value to the planned study. In the published report the researcher cites the pertinent reference sources.

PERSONAL ABSTRACT FILE

Each potential reference reviewed should be indexed and filed in a personal reference file. Isolation of each reference on a single index card or attached cards is important because as review of the literature continues, considerable information is collected. The researcher should choose the size of the card (7.6 × 12.7, 12.7 × 20.3 cm) upon which to record bibliographical and abstract information and notes. Since different journals have distinct formats for listing literature cited, authors should follow the style for presentation of references of that journal for which the manuscript is being prepared. The bibliography usually includes the authors and co-authors' names as listed, title of article or book, periodical name or abbreviation (abbreviation according to INDEX MEDICUS or LIST OF JOURNALS INDEXED IN INDEX MEDICUS for the current year), volume number, pages, month, and year; or city of publisher, publisher of book, and year of publication.

Many research reports contain an abstract preceding the introduction of the report and this abstract is really a summary of the report conveying the essence of the report. The abstract provides sufficient information to determine whether the report is pertinent to the research problem. If additional information is required of any particular report, then the method, results, and discussion can be summarized and recorded on the card. Also, key words relating to the content of the report are good to list at the top of the card (right-hand corner). Because background information leading up to the purpose of the research and to the problem is often written in a chronological fashion, the cards might be arranged chronologically in the files. The cards can be used for instant retrieval of information. Extraction of all important information from each research report is essential during the initial review so that efficiency can be maintained.

INFORMATION RESOURCES

Abstracts

A number of journals provide their readers with an abstracting service which can save time in locating the original reports. Of course, abstracts are limited in the information provided, so one must exercise caution when using these resources. Abstracts should be considered as secondary sources of literature review. Abstracts of literature are generally located near the end of each journal issue. Chapter 12 discusses the content and format of published abstracts. Book reviews are also given space in many journals. The reviews usually call attention to the subject material contained in the book but do not provide as detailed information about a subject as do abstracts of literature. Such journals as PHYSICAL THERAPY, ARCHIVES OF PHYSICAL MEDICINE AND REHABILITATION, the AMERICAN JOURNAL OF PHYSICAL MEDICINE, PHYSIOTHERAPY CANADA, and PHYSIOTHERAPY provide abstracting services in most issues.

Biological Abstracts

This is a semi-monthly publication; each entry includes bibliographic citations and abstracts. Each issue contains an Author Index for retrieval of references based on authors or corporate names, a Biosystematic Index with references according to gross taxonomic categories, a Generic Index of the names of genus-species, a Concept Index of broad concepts, and a Subject Index for retrieval of references based on specific subject words. About 250,000 reports are covered yearly in BIOLOGICAL ABSTRACTS and BIORESEARCH INDEX. The latter is a monthly publication that indexes biology-related material not covered in BIOLOGICAL AB-STRACTS.

Excerpta Medica

This is a monthly international publication that monitors, abstracts, translates, classifies, and indexes biomedical literature. More than 5000 journals are routinely indexed; in addition, books, reported literature, and conference papers are also included. The index is divided into 42 sections covering the entire medical field and seven index sections which cover special areas. Sections may be subscribed to separately; for example, Rehabilitation and Physical Medicine. Usual arrangements are by subject but semi-annual and annual subject and author indexes are available.

Muscular Dystrophy Abstracts

This booklet is presented by the Muscular Dystrophy Association and EXCERPTA MEDICA, and is a service of abstracts from current world literature covering muscular dystrophy and related disorders and areas of basic science pertinent to their conditions. Twenty-two to 24 issues are published yearly along with an annual INDEX by Subject and Author.

JOURNALS

Listing all journals that might be of interest to physical therapists would be futile because of the diversity of interests and the numbers of available journals. Libraries have a master file of all journals contained in a particular library and this file is accessible to patrons. Since research is usually first reported in journal articles, journals are primary sources for seeking information for investigative work done on a particular topic. Selection of the journals most appropriate to the investigator's topic will depend on the subject being pursued. Individual issues of a journal preceding the current year are bound together into a cloth volume usually for each calendar year. The index for a particular year is located near the end of each bound volume. Issues for the current year are separate from the bound volumes of a particular journal and are usually placed on special racks or shelves.

Because current issues of journals for the present year are separate, the contents of each journal issue must be consulted individually. The current copies of a particular journal do not circulate or have restricted circulation. Special indexes for journals are available and are valuable sources for locating special articles.

INDEXES

Some journals have periodic indexes in addition to the volume index which is usually part of the December issue of the particular volume. The RESEARCH QUARTERLY, research journal of the American Alliance for Health, Physical Education, and Recreation had 10-year indexes beginning with 1930 and a 30-year-index from 1930 through 1959. These indexes are indexed by author and subject.

Fifty-year Cumulative Index: Archives of Physical Medicine and Rehabilitation

This index spans the years from 1929 to 1969. The index includes a 50-year history of the journal, cumulative indexes of authors and subjects, page index by volume and month, and a list of medical abbreviations.

Fifty-year Index of Physical Therapy

The FIFTY-YEAR INDEX OF PHYSICAL THERAPY, Journal of the American Physical Therapy Association contains a table of contents in addition to subject and author indexes. A pagination index lists the pages by volume and month and covers the years from 1921 to 1970.

Five-year Index of Physical Therapy

Five-year indexes have been published by PHYSICAL THERAPY since 1970. In each index a Table of Contents is used to list subject headings; an author index at the end of each publication cites the work of authors by a numbering system.

Current Contents

A weekly booklet that reproduces tables of contents of journals in various fields. Over 900 journals of the Life Sciences are covered with an equal or smaller number of journals covered in the physical sciences; chemistry; behavioral sciences; education; agricultural, food and veterinary sciences, and engineering and technology. Each issue also contains an Author Index providing addresses of authors of most articles for the convenience of writing for reprints.

Index Medicus

This is a comprehensive index to the world's medical literature and is published monthly. Several thousands of journals are indexed completely or selectively. Each issue contains a subject and author index. The Subject Index is alphabetized according to key subject headings with each subject heading containing the title of English language or translated articles; author; journal by special abbreviation; volume; pages; and date article was published. The Author Index contains the author's name and bibliographic information. The January volume lists the key words and all journals included in the indexing process.

CUMULATED INDEX MEDICUS is the annual INDEX MEDICUS which is a cumulation of monthly publications into author volumes and usually several subject volumes of citations. Subject headings, LIST OF JOURNALS INDEXED IN INDEX MEDICUS, and Bibliography of Medical Reviews are included in the annual editions. SCIENCE CITATION INDEX volumes are arranged as Citation Index and Source Index which list by first author those papers that are cited by other authors in the list of about 2600 journals that are covered. Each entry in the volume shows cited author, citing author, year cited article was published, name of publication, year article was cited, volume number, and pages. Separate sections of the Citation Index include a Corporate Index arranged by corporate name and a Cited Patent section arranged by the patent number.

Some suggestions for the use of indexes may help in locating research articles in journals:
1. Explore various subject headings by listing key words contained by the topic or related topics.
2. Begin with a specific subject heading before using general headings.
3. Start the literature search with the latest index volumes and then proceed to older volumes.
4. Explore each index volume systematically before proceeding to another volume.[2]

REPRINTS

If a published report is judged to be particularly useful, then a reproduction or reprint should be obtained. A reprint of an article is valuable to you in terms of convenience and efficiency in retrieving the information. A reprint can be placed in your personal file and is available to you immediately upon need. Reprints help to make maximum use of library time, contain complete references, and reduces errors caused by abstracting. Reprints of recent references (within the past 2 years) can be obtained by writing directly to the author and requesting a reprint of the article. Authors generally have reprints of their articles and are usually willing to send a copy upon request. The address of the author often accompanies the article at its beginning or ending. Figure 3.1 is an example of a postal card which can be printed or typed in advance, is economical, and is applicable to most requests for reprints. Pertinent information required for the postal card is illustrated. The label or printed address can be removed and used by the sender to address the envelope containing the requested reprint. This approach eases the mailing process for the sender.

BOOKS

Books on most any area of health are available in medical libraries or through a medical library. Books give basic material in breadth and varying degrees of depth according to the purpose of the particular book, but are not the most up-to-date sources of information. Books require more time to write and publish than do journals, thus losing some immediacy. Their bibliographies offer important sources on a topic.[3] Consult the card catalogue of your medical library for the book holdings of that library. The card catalogue uses either the Dewey decimal or the Library of Congress system for classifying and locating books. Card catalogues are arranged according to a cross-reference system which consists of subject, author, and title cards. Each card pertaining to a particular book contains identical information, but the order of information is peculiar to the function of the card. Remember the card catalogue contains only those documents which are owned by that particular library, and cards provide little information about the content of the books.

LIBRARY REFERENCE RESOURCE PUBLICATIONS

Books in Print

This is an annual index to general books currently available from about 1600 American publishers. Authors Index and Titles Index are arranged in separate volumes. The Author Index listing includes author, title, price, publisher, series, whether the book is illustrated, edition, year the book was published, and the type of binding. The Titles Index lists titles, author, price, and publisher. The Author Index is more inclusive than the Titles Index, but the Titles Index provides an alphabetical listing of American publishers. Both volumes cover paperback and clothbound books.

Subject Guide to Books in Print

Listings in this volume give author, title, publisher, current price, and year of publication. The listings represent books from more than 1900 American publishers under more than 37,000 subject headings and some 43,000 cross-references. Books in preparation are also listed.[4]

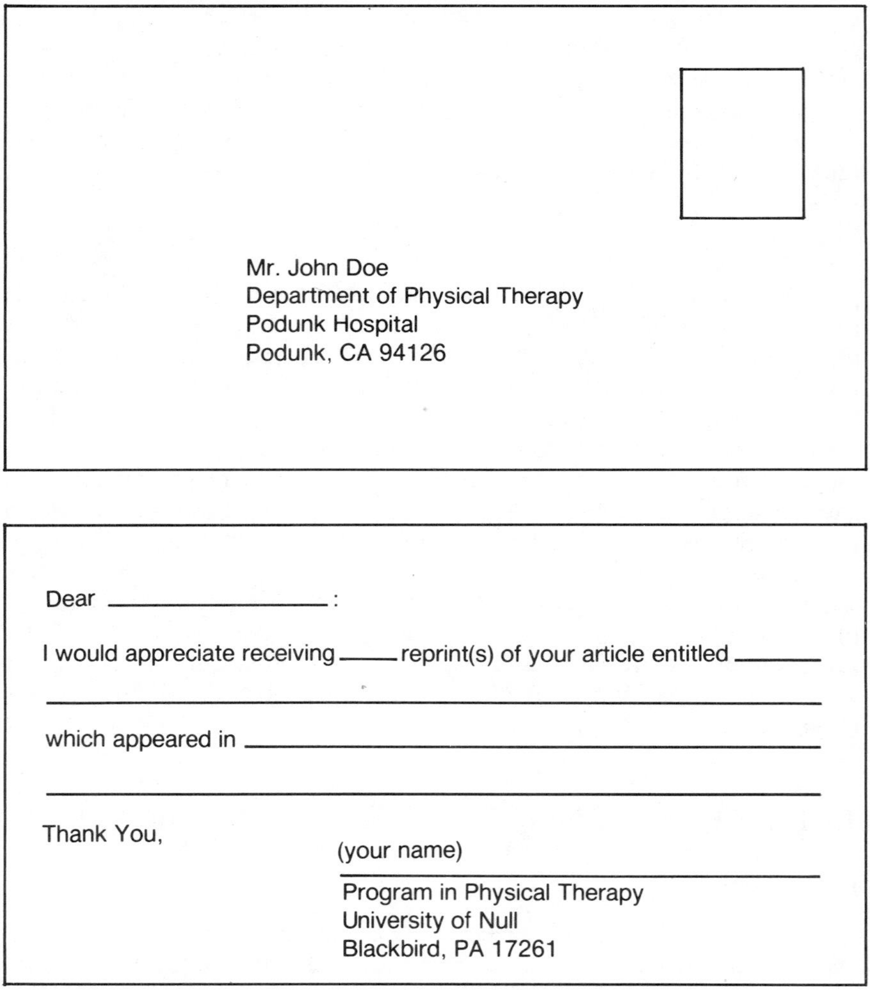

Mr. John Doe
Department of Physical Therapy
Podunk Hospital
Podunk, CA 94126

Dear _____ :

I would appreciate receiving _____ reprint(s) of your article entitled _____

_____

which appeared in _____

_____

Thank You,

(your name)
_____
Program in Physical Therapy
University of Null
Blackbird, PA 17261

Figure 3.1. Postal card for requesting reprints.

British Books in Print

This book is an annual index to general books offered currently by British publishers.

Bowker's Medical Books in Print

Medical books that are currently available from American publishers are indexed. This resource is published annually.

INTERLIBRARY LOAN

The purpose of this service is to make available for research, materials that are not owned by or are missing from the local library. The Interlibrary Loan service will usually provide photocopies of requested articles rather than make the journal available to you, but the service will not provide photocopies of entire publications (books). Books can be obtained by the local library from other libraries in the system with relatively short waiting periods (2 to 3 weeks). Usually there are no charges to users for loans or photocopies if the individual requests (numbers being requested) do not exceed a certain number, usually less than 10 articles per request. The library personnel will advise you if charges will be made. Theses, dissertations, and microfilmed copies of sources are also available through interlibrary services.

Special forms for requesting materials are available upon request at your library. Information usually requested on the special forms is your name and associated facility or department; status (student or faculty member); work phone number; complete bibliographical information of the requested book or article (Chapter 12 discusses bibliographical material); source of reference where book or article is indexed; and date when the library is to discontinue search if attempts to locate the requested material are unsuccessful.

The Interlibrary Loan system is a very valuable service to physical therapists working in small hospitals and towns where medical libraries are not available. The researcher should check the services of his local or secondary school library regarding interlibrary loans. Libraries make books and journals available to those researchers who cannot obtain materials at their own facilities. If interlibrary services are not available locally, contact the Regional Medical Library serving your state (Table 3.1).

OTHER MANUAL RESOURCES

Libraries contain many other resources for information which are not included in this book. Some defy the classifications given but are useful to the researcher. Two such resources are:

Electronic Industries Information Sources

This is a guide to research, developments, design, manufacture, and applications in electronics. References cover material from encyclopedias, dictionaries, directories, bibliographies, indexing, standards and specifications sources, governmental information sources, meetings, and conventions. References are listed by author, title, source index, and subject index.

Scientific Meetings

This is a listing of forthcoming national and international meetings of technical, scientific, medical, engineering, and management organizations. The listing is published three times a year.

AUTOMATED REFERENCE SERVICES

Literature review can be time consuming if exhaustive reviews are required. Even if reference materials are available to you in a large medical library, considerable time is spent in cross-referencing and checking the many sources to prevent exclusion of a particular report which may be of great value to you. One also finds that an overwhelming volume of literature exists on most topics. Automated systems have developed through the sponsorships of the Federal Governments of the United States and Canada to help the scientist to retrieve information from computerized storage systems. In cooperation with The National Library of Medicine in Bethesda, Maryland, and The National Science Library in Ottawa, Ontario, the libraries of government departments, agencies, and other research and special libraries in North America provide resources and services of great value to the researcher. These services are of value in terms of convenience and availability. The national libraries provide resources and services that are not always available locally. If the local library has access to the appropriate electronic equipment, publications or bibliographies can be transmitted immediately. Costs that are incurred for these services may be based on the number of years surveyed, whether the survey is "on-line" or "off-line" or simply on a flat fee basis. Arrangements for paying these costs will vary widely. In some cases the library budget has provision for these costs, while in others the department, to which the requester belongs, pays. Or the individual requester may have to pay in advance anywhere from five to twenty-five dollars. The requester is advised to determine the individual institution's policy regarding payment before making use of automated service.

Key words from INDEX MEDICUS (see Reviewing Process) are used in automated literature searches. Libraries offering these services will have a form to be completed. This form will require your listing key words that describe or categorize the topic that you wish searched for references. Library personnel are available to assist you in selecting your search words and planning your search strategy in the event that you are unfamiliar with the procedure.

Many universities have on-line computer terminals that link them to an information retrieval system such as Lockheed DIALOG, SDC/ORBIT, ERIC, and DATRIX II systems. Such systems increase the availability of multiple data bases which broaden the researcher's ability to retrieve citations, dissertations, and abstracts. Some data bases can be searched by the name of the author, key words in the article, date of publication, and titles. Charges vary from system to system based on computer time and printout entries. The user is advised to seek the librarian's advise on selecting pertinent data bases and costs.

Medlars

MEDLARS (Medical Literature Analysis and Retrieval System) is a computerized service of searching of journal articles listed in the INDEX MEDICUS. The service became operational in 1964 for the purposes of indexing the international biomedical literature and preparing bibliographies of scientific articles upon request. The bibliographies searched do not include articles published prior to 1964. Citations are given to the individual requesting the service and contain the title, author(s), journal, volume, pages, date, and whether the article is written in any language other than English.

Articles indexed are from INDEX MEDICUS, INDEX TO DENTAL LITERATURE, and the INTERNATIONAL NURSING INDEX, and contain citations to medical and health-related journals.

Regional Medical Library

The Regional Medical Library (RML) system has been established by the federal government and serves as the major medical library resource in each of the 7 regions in the United States. The RMLs provide library and ancillary services to libraries and health professionals in the form of interlibrary loans, reference service, and training. The RML system provides backup support to researchers and hospitals not having computers. Within the regions more than 300 medical libraries have terminals for MEDLARS. The location of the RML libraries by region are given in Table 3.1.

Medline

MEDLINE (MEDLARS on Line) is a newer and speedier version of Medlars. Because of its initiation in 1974, MEDLINE has a smaller data base than MEDLARS. The system is computerized and bibliographical information on a specific subject is available immediately from a computer readout. The citations span journals listed in the INDEX MEDICUS.

Microfilm

The microfilm provides the researcher with the original article. The reader can read any page of the article on a large viewing screen; the film

Table 3.1
Regional Medical Libraries

Regions	States			Libraries
1	CT	NH	RI	New York Academy of Medicine
	DE	NJ	VT	2 East 103 Street
	ME	NY	Puerto Rico	New York, NY 10029
	MA	PA		(212) 876-2531
2	AL	MS	VA	University of Maryland Health Sciences Library
	FL	NC	WV	111 S. Greene Street
	GA	SC	District of	Baltimore, MD 21201
	MD	TN	Columbia	(301) 528-7637
3	IA	MI	SD	University of Illinois at Chicago
	IL	MN	WI	Library of the Health Sciences
	IN	ND		P.O. Box 7509
	KY	OH		Chicago, IL 60680
				(312) 966-8974
4	CO	NE		University of Nebraska
	KS	UT		Leon S. McGoogan Library of Medicine
	MO	WY		42nd. and Dewey Avenue
				Omaha, NE 68105
				(402) 559-4326
5	AR	OK		University of Texas
	LA	TX		Health Science Center at Dallas
	NM			5323 Harry Hines Boulevard
				Dallas, TX 75235
				(214) 688-2006
6	AK	OR		University of Washington
	ID	WA		Health Sciences Library
	MT			Seattle, WA 98195
				(206) 543-8262
7	AZ	HI		UCLA Biomedical Library
	CA	NV		Los Angeles, CA 90024
				(213) 825-1200

can be advanced, dropped, or regressed at a rate controlled by the researcher. The film permits easy storage in lieu of the original copy which would require larger storage facilities. Consultation with the personnel at the information or circulation desk of your library will determine whether the service is available and to what extent.

Special Indexes

KWIC (Key-Word-In-Context) and KWOC (Key-Word-Out-of-Context) are computer-based systems for printing bibliographical titles according to a preselected series of key words. The key words of a title are sorted out and printed in alphabetical order and called a "permuted" index because every time a key word in a title is located the desired article will appear. The system was designed to be an efficient method of reducing

Table 3.2
Cumulative Summary of the Research Processes Presented

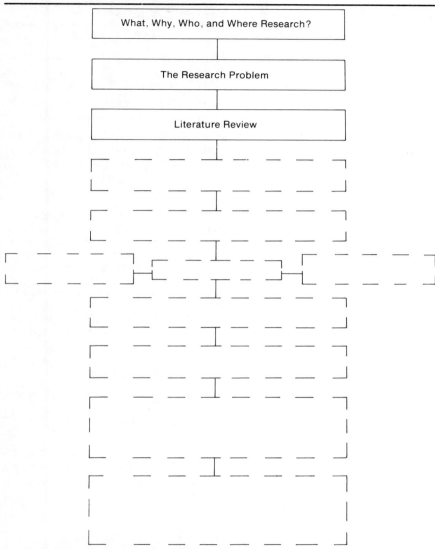

time required for scanning long titles or subjects; and, therefore, a long title will not be cited in its entirety. KWOC differs from KWIC by providing the complete citation in a single-entry listing (author, title, and source).[4,5] The student should consult with local library personnel for additional information about these systems and their availability.

SUMMARY

Without familiarity with the resources of a library or an organized approach to the library search, the process of literature review is difficult and time consuming. The researcher must be familiar with the valuable sources in the library such as the card and periodical files, indexes, reference resource publications, automated reference services, and interlibrary loan services. An organized plan that outlines the topics to be covered and various possible services providing information about the topics is necessary before beginning the library search. This section has provided a few guides for the literature review in preparation of an investigation. Used properly, the library can become a paradise for you in the research process. Table 3.2 provides a summary of the research processes presented thus far.

REFERENCES

1. Clarke DH, Clarke HH: Research Processes in Physical Education, Recreation and Health. Englewood Cliffs, NJ, Prentice-Hall, 1970
2. Treece EW, Treece JW, Jr: Elements of Research in Nursing, ed 3. St. Louis, C.V. Mosby Co, 1982
3. Prince B, Makrides L, Richman J: Research Methodology and Applied Statistics, Part 2: The Literature Search. Physiother Canada 32: 201–206, 1980
4. Herner S: A Brief Guide to Sources of Scientific and Technical Information, ed 2. Washington, Information Resources Press, 1980
5. Seefeldt V: Searching the Literature. In Hubbard AW (ed): Research Methods in Health, Physical Education, and Recreation. Washington, American Association of Health, Physical Education, Recreation, 1973

SUGGESTED READINGS

Leiper C, Richardson M: Aids to conducting a literature search. Physiother Canada 25: 225, 1973
Morton LT: Research and the library. Physiotherapy 56: 119–120, 1966

4

The Proposal and Ethics

What a man's work comes to! So he plans it ...
Robert Browning
Bells and Pomegranites

The proposal is an important component of the research process and serves as a foundation from which an investigator can begin to conduct a study. Although students should logically complete a course in research methods prior to beginning work on a proposal, the proposal is presented early so that for those courses requiring a written research proposal from students, sufficient time can be provided for its completion. Succeeding chapters will discuss necessary details that will enable the overall understanding of the research process and provide the essentials for completing the proposal. This section deals with a discussion of salient features of the formal research proposal, of the review process, and of its preparation. Some ethical considerations and guidelines for research on humans are discussed also.

WHAT IS A RESEARCH PROPOSAL?

A research proposal is a document that outlines a planned project or investigation. The proposal is sometimes called a protocol. The proposal is a design of a research study that outlines the problem, proposed procedures of data collection and analyses, and presentation of the resources for the investigation. It is an organized plan of the proposed research and serves the same function as a blueprint.[1]

WHY A PROPOSAL?

No research involving human subjects should be attempted unless some authoritative source representing the institution in which the research will be conducted reviews and approves the proposed study. Therefore, one of the main purposes of a research proposal is the production of a document for review prior to the initiation of the study; the document outlines the manner in which the investigation will be conducted. Because of legal aspects, a review of proposed research is necessary to determine that the rights and welfare of the subjects involved are adequately protected, and that the risks to a subject are outweighed by his potential benefits or by the value of the information to be gained.[2]

The general purposes of a written proposal are to: (1) place in writing the investigator's organized plan for conducting the project, (2) provide a guide for the investigator to follow during the conduct of the project, (3) provide a vehicle for review and a document which can be judged for its scholarly merits, (4) establish limits and criteria to be followed and adhered to throughout the conduct of the project, and (5) provide a measure of accountability of those involved in the project.

Placing the proposal in written form compels the researcher to organize ideas and think. Setting ideas down on paper reduces error and prevents important aspects of the study from being overlooked. The written proposal thus becomes a reference establishing controls and modes to be followed during the conduct of the study. The written proposal facilitates evaluation by others. The proposal should be reviewed by peers for their assistance prior to its being submitted for formal review by an appointed committee. Peer review can correct for flaws and assist in making improvements. Occasionally a great idea of the researcher's is not of value in the eyes of others, thus an informal critique by others of the proposal can save countless time, effort, and cost.

Research usually requires financial support which makes the proposal extremely important for acquiring funds. Funding sources require a proposal in which the procedures to be used are effectively described.[3]

The proposal may, in turn, be judged on: (1) its value or contribution to a body of knowledge; (2) the competency of the principal investigator; (3) the availability of facilities (time, space, equipment, funds, and personnel) to conduct the project; and (4) conformity to ethical or moral principles for human or animal investigations.

PROPOSAL REVIEW COMMITTEE

Most health-related facilities (hospitals, universities, organizations, and clinics) support the concept of, or a program of, scientific investigation, including applied and basic research. If such a program exists in a particular facility, a research committee or another body is usually established.

The review committee may be a permanent committee such as a utilization committee, ethical review committee, research committee, or a human assurance committee, or it may be established specifically for review of a research proposal. The committee might be composed of senior or recognized clinicians and investigators employed by or associated with the particular facility. The composition of the committee must command the respect of those submitting reviews as well as personnel of higher authority by means of its maturity, experience, and wisdom. A member of the committee cannot be involved in review of proposals in which he has a professional responsibility except to provide information upon request by the review committee.[2] The structure, tenure, and composition of the committee is established from need and is controlled locally.

The committee has the responsibility of reviewing research proposals and ensuring that all investigations conducted in the facility are conducted under the highest ethical, moral, and legal standards. The committee assures that the welfare and safety of all subjects undergoing study are adequately protected by the investigator and his co-workers. The committee assures that the risks to a particular subject are less than the potential benefits to the subject, or the importance of the research findings. In addition, the committee determines the acceptability of the proposed research in terms of feasibility, and standards and regulations of the facility and government. Where monies are available to support approved research proposals, the committee may have the added responsibility of establishing priorities of support.

The committee is usually responsible to a governing board or some group of higher authority. Minutes and actions of all committee meetings are recorded and maintained for review or audit whenever the need is presented.

The student will probably be faced with a different organizational structure for research activity at the university. Universities may have specific review mechanisms for research; a particular procedure for faculty to follow and a separate procedure for students. The university may decentralize the authority to its colleges for review. Universities, however, usually establish central committees that have the final authority for the approving of research studies. The decentralized reviews, in this structure, constitute peer reviews serving to improve proposals before reaching the central review committee for disposition. Student research projects, other than theses and dissertations, involving human subjects and animals can often receive an expedited review by delegated members of the central review committee. The review process may take 2 to 4 weeks before approval is given by the central review committee. Whatever the local situation may be, some form of review and approval is necessary to perform research studies where animal and human subjects are involved.

FORMAT OF THE PROPOSAL

Local facilities supporting research conceptionally and monetarily often have a specific or suggested format to be followed when submitting a research proposal. The format of the proposal presented here is a guide for those potential investigators who do not have a specific format to follow at their facility or who want to supplement an available format. The contents of any format should, however, provide pertinent information which would answer anticipated questions of the reviewers. A sample proposal can be found in Appendix, Table A.

In general, the entire proposal must be worded precisely so that the reviewer's time is not wasted by redundant or superfluous writings. Good writing is concise and a good proposal is worded to convince the reviewer that the proposed research merits approval. Avoid jargon or verbal gestures which merely add space or confuse the reviewer. Writing, like research, is basically a logical flow of reasoning and must flow smoothly and logically from step to step. Sufficient detail must be presented to answer anticipated questions by the reviewer and to avoid raising concerns about the problem or the investigator's scholarly ability.

The following subject headings are major divisions of the proposal, but are given only brief discussion here to clarify the headings. Detailed discussion of the contents or information essential to the writing of the proposal are provided throughout this book.

Title of Research Study

The words in the title should be concise but yet sufficient to give the reviewer a good idea of what the project is about or what is being proposed for study. The title may reflect the nature of the major problem or be a statement of a sub-problem of a major problem. Although the title must be free of excessive or redundant wording, brevity should not reduce clarity.

Name and Title of Investigators and Participating Facilities

The principal investigator's name and title are listed first and then names of other investigators follow in order of contribution to the study. An investigator's title may be the highest earned degree or position title that provides some indication of an investigator's scholarly ability or competence.

The participating facility is usually the place of employment of the investigator(s) or place where the research is to be conducted. This information is important to the reviewer who must judge the competency of the investigators and the adequacy and availability of the facility(ies).

Objective of the Study

A brief statement of the problem is helpful. If the statement is that of a major problem, then the sub-problem to which the proposal is addressed must also be stated. Not all studies have sub-problems, but many do, and a proposal is submitted for approval each time a sub-problem is to be studied. Sometimes sub-problems must be studied (pilot project) before the major problem can be solved or the major question can be answered. An example of a major problem is "How can the force of contracting muscles be increased?" A subproblem may be "What is the effect of various hip angles on the quadriceps force during dynamic resistive exercise?" The example of a sub-problem is related to the major problem and is one step in answering "How can the force of contracting muscles be increased." Perhaps the researcher is only interested in the effect of various hip angles on the force generated by the quadriceps; then the problem statement concerns the effect of hip angles and not other methods of increasing muscular force.

Perhaps the researcher does not wish to pursue further research in the area of enhancing muscular force during resistive exercise and is only interested in seeking an answer to "What is the effect of various hip angles on the quadriceps force during dynamic resistive exercise?" In this situation the only problem stated is "What is the effect of various hip angles on the quadriceps force during dynamic resistive exercises?"

Upon reading the problem statement, the reviewer has an idea of what is to be studied, but the reviewer does not know the aim or purpose for studying this particular problem. Purpose (goal, objective, aim) and problem statements are not the same.[4] A problem is defined as an answerable question and an objective is the purpose or aim for answering the questions. Objectives grow out of the problem statement or from previously researched questions and pave the way for gathering new information. Objectives can provide direction to the study.

If a single objective is to be achieved by the research, a succinct statement of the aim or purpose of the study should be stated. If more than one objective is to be achieved, the objectives should be listed in outline form to reduce wording and to catch the reviewer's attention. The objectives must be specific and listing them in order is helpful to the researcher and reviewer for establishing priorities of effort and emphasis.

The problem and objective must be delineated so that the plan of the study will enable data to be collected and analyzed in such fashion that answers to questions or tested hypotheses are possible.

A stated hypothesis or question in this section would take the place of a problem statement. The remainder of the proposal is built from the foundation provided by the stated problem and the objective of the study.

Significance of the Study

The investigator must explain why time and effort should be spent on the study. This section is a justification of why the research should be conducted or a defense of the stated objectives. An argument must be presented on what the study is expected to contribute to the problem or to a body of knowledge. The investigator's familiarity with the problem should be displayed during the discussion. The discussion must be in keeping with the objectives and the problem, and must not be too broad or overstated.

The investigator should provide supporting statements for the practical or theoretical importance of the research and state whether the proposed study is a replication of former research, a step in advancing knowledge (area of little or much research), or whether the answers to the problem will open up new areas of research.

Related Research

By this time the researcher has read many studies related to the study or is familiar with what research has been done in the area of interest. Only the most pertinent studies supporting the investigator's argument should be cited in this section, and then only the highlights of the cited studies are discussed. The investigator must present the information in a logical sequence, sometimes chronologically, to demonstrate his knowledge of previous research of his or others. The story must convince the reviewer that previous research has not answered the question or tested the hypothesis stated by the investigator.

If any current studies overlap the problem of the proposal, the investigator should show how his proposal differs from studies or how it will complement the other studies.

Technical flaws of previous research should be pointed out in the discussion. In the event that little or no previous work has been reported in the area of the proposed study, the investigator should cite studies most closely related to the proposed study.

Most of the discussion has implied importance only to original work. The student who is doing classroom projects or a master's thesis need not be so concerned about originality. Original studies require confirmation, especially if no other studies have been reported that refute or confirm the conclusion or inference. Replication of a study should be possible by reading the Methods section of a report. A replication of another study is treated similar to that of an original approach when writing the proposal. The reviewer must devote as much time to the review and render a judgment of the significance of the replication as he does for an original approach, so do not pass up a good opportunity to confirm or refute another's work. Read PHYSICAL THERAPY and many reported studies which need replication will emerge.

Procedure of the Study

This section is the principal part of the proposal and is, therefore, the part given the most detail; it should be organized and written well, but yet concise. Information included in this section will be given the closest scrutiny by the reviewer. The section should provide the operational aspects of the problem and objectives including method of selecting samples and gathering data, controls, measurements, statistical design, safeguards, and how the findings will be presented. Sometimes an outline form is preferred and reduces the length of the section for the convenience of the reader. Subheadings of various contents are desirable and assist in the ease of reading and identifying aspects of particular interest to the reviewer.

1. Sample. A brief description of the subjects (sex, age, physical or mental status) and welfare of subjects (safeguards, consent form) are to be included. If humans are not used, description of the sample characteristics and condition(s) is provided. The protection of the rights and welfare of subjects participating in an investigation is extremely important and a detailed discussion will follow at the end of this chapter.

Although the size of the sample is important, an accurate number of subjects required cannot be given at this point because needs for change or attrition of subjects often occur during the process of the study. The size of the sample affects the outcome of the experiment and should be sufficiently large; however, the size of the sample effects is dependent upon the type of experiment to be conducted. For example, few subjects may volunteer for projects involving noxious conditions, but many may volunteer for projects where conditions are pleasant and require minimal consumption of the subject's time. The investigator must be the judge about the size of the sample needed to meet the objectives of the study. Usually larger size samples are needed for relationship studies than are needed for comparative type studies. When using analysis of variance, a repeated measures design will conserve more on numbers required than will a randomized design. Chapter 5 contains more discussion on the sampling methods; Chapter 9, on design.

The rule is to provide sufficient information about the sample or the subjects' characteristics, how the subjects will be obtained, the approximate number of subjects needed, and how the subjects' welfare will be safeguarded (hazards to be encountered or ill effects). The nature of the consent form must be included with the proposal; a sample of a consent form is in Appendix, Table B.

2. Method. A description of how the study will be conducted should include controls to be used, units of measurement, tools or equipment, and techniques and conditions. These details are to be indicative of how data are to be gathered. If you merely state that a plethysmograph will be used to measure the arterial blood, you are not supplying enough information. Blood volume is measured by a venous occlusion plethysmograph. The instrument is air-filled, water-filled, or electronic, and is manufactured by several companies. The manufacturer's name and address may be footnoted in the published report so providing information now, although not essential, is helpful to the researcher for later use in writing the report for publication.

In case of a descriptive study, the measuring instrument might be the oral interview, mail questionnaire, or attitude scale. In thesis work the student is usually required to describe the type of instrument to be used, rationale for its selection, and its validity and reliability data. Submission of the paper instrument is a good idea so the reviewers can formulate judgments about the adequacy of the instrument for meeting the objective and problem of the study.

3. Design. The design of the study should be described. (see Chapter 9 for details) The character of the hypothesis, the variables involved, the method of selecting subjects, and the restrictions that might be placed on the study should be considered in the design. The design must permit the testing of hypotheses. For example, if the hypothesis involved comparing the effectiveness of training with isometric contractions versus contractions caused by electrical stimulation and combinations of these contractions with respect to increased muscular strength, the study might involve comparing the strength over time (final or posttest strength) of four groups. One group might serve as a control (no exercise), while the other three groups (isometric, electrical stimulation, and isometric plus electrical stimulation) serve as experimental groups. Thus, a design involving four groups would be required in the study. The availability of subjects and the residual effects of the training modes would determine whether the groups were to be randomly selected or whether the modes could be repeated over one group of subjects (see Chapter 5 for methods of selection). A brief description of the controls of the independent variables (Chapter 5) is recommended so provisions for minimizing variability of data during the data gathering are taken. Some variables are identified for the study by asking, "What effect does training by electrical stimulation of specific current characteristics have on the force developed by the quadriceps femoris muscle?"

Since the dependent variable (strength or force) might involve subject variation (motivation, size, sex, and age), administration of pretest strength should determine whether groups of subjects are similarly matched prior to beginning the various modes of training. The design should indicate the number of groups included in the investigation, how the groups will be selected, and whether there will be pretests and posttests.

In experimental research the investigator has a number of designs from which to choose. The complexity of designs depend on the number of independent (modes of exercise) and dependent variables (strength measures) involved in the study.

4. Analysis. The procedures for analyzing and synthesizing data are given. Although statistical designs are not mandatory in research, statistical methods are of paramount value to the researcher who deals with data containing variation. Often conclusions about data are based on a degree of uncertainty, and statistics enable the researcher to make a logical decision based on the most probable outcome which may not have been obvious to him without the assistance of statistical measures. The statistical design to be used in analyzing the data should be stated in name; for example, a two-tailed paired t-test at the 5% level of significance. Enough cannot be said for selecting the appropriate statistical design before the study begins. Many studies have been published in which the statistics were determined in retrospect to the collected data. Data should never be collected and then some statistical design found to fit the data; fit the data to the design. The full information contained in the data will not be obtained unless the researcher plans in advance the kinds of information he wishes to gather through selection of the types of tests, the test routines, and the appropriate methods of analyses. Once data are collected the researcher is limited to the choice of appropriate analyses because statistical designs are only appropriate to specific data-gathering designs. The planning and selecting of techniques for analyses of data are procedural and ethical issues which must follow rules of scientific inquiry.

Time, Space, and Availability of Equipment

1. Time. Researchers need a time frame to put them in perspective and keep the study on a schedule. The existence of deadlines and other commitments requires careful budgeting of time for research studies. A time frame or schedule consists of a listing of major phases of the study (e.g., proposal preparation, reviews, subject selection, gathering data, analyzing data, and report preparation) and the expected completion time associated with each phase. Allow time for the process of obtaining funds, purchasing, and delivery of equipment. Thus, allow for delays so that you can meet your completion date. The Gantt method is a chart listing major phases to be completed on the left-hand side and the time allowed for their completion across the top.[5,6]

Researchers frequently work on a 3-year schedule. That is, while they are collecting data for a study in the present year, they are also preparing the report of last year's study and writing the proposal for next year's study. The time schedule is of value when placed in the proposal because it permits the researcher to display his schedule for the conduction of the investigation, and it allows the reviewers to assess the appropriateness of the allotted times.

2. Space. Special rooms may be required for the study; appropriate negotiation for the use of the rooms may be necessary; if so, this should be indicated. Acquiring space may require special improvement funds for which approval must be made. If space is available, then so indicate in the proposal.

3. Availability of Equipment. The types of equipment to be used have been identified and described earlier, but what if the equipment must be purchased, borrowed, shared, or repaired? The reviewer must know whether the costs to be incurred are justified and/or whether equipment is immediately available or its use must be negotiated.

Cost Analysis

Every administrator is interested in costs of performing the research. Costs may be incurred indirectly in the salary of the physical therapist who requires time to conduct the research in lieu of time spent in treating patients. Costs may also be incurred in equipment and supplies, additional personnel, computer time for analyses of data or costs for a statistician to analyze the data, art work for illustrations and slides in presenting the findings, literature searches when computers are used for the search, renovation of rooms or special improvement, and construction of equipment not commercially available; and there may be hidden costs that have a habit of occurring after the study has been approved and funded.

Reviewers must make decisions about the proposal regarding the contributions that will be obtained and the costs of obtaining the information. The proposal is a form of advertisement to sell authorities on the merits of your efforts, time, and costs in doing the study. The manner in which the proposal is written is very important; you must convince others of your scholarly abilities in a single document. Sometimes you are invited to defend the proposal verbally or to answer questions of the committee. Many times these advantages are not available to the investigator. Granting agencies often require lengthy proposals written on special forms which they make available upon request. In the student's situation, the proposal must convince readers or a committee that you are ready and adequately prepared to perform the study in question. The situation would be ironic for a student majoring in sociology to request approval for a study in the biochemical effects of 10 minutes of ultrasound on ligamentous structures of rats. The researcher must also be aware of meeting review deadlines for submission of the proposal. Do not hesitate to seek assistance in writing the proposal or in performing the study.

THE PILOT STUDY

After identifying a researchable problem, the student or researcher may have some questions about its feasibility. Concerns may center on the data-gathering methods such as the adequacy of the measuring instruments and controls, scoring techniques, unanticipated flaws, and desire to try alternative procedures. The expenditure of time and costs in completing the study may also be of concern. The pilot study may be the solution for such concerns.

The pilot study is a preliminary trial of research. It requires most of the research process to be implemented but on a smaller scale than that of a major study. Pilot studies use fewer subjects than major research projects but each and every procedure is followed, including analysis of the gathered data. It serves as an evaluation of the researchable problem and is often used as a vehicle for assessing the quality of student theses and dissertations. Valuable experience can be gained by beginning researchers. The pilot study provides valuable information to the experienced researcher for improving the hypotheses and data-gathering procedures, for determining the time needed to complete a major study, for reducing flaws previously overlooked, and for obtaining feedback from subjects. The original research proposal will almost always be modified as a result of a pilot study. Information gained from the pilot study will improve the subsequent research. Many of the studies reported in the literature are results of pilot work but are not often reported as such. These "one shot" studies frequently need confirmation and larger numbers of subjects; therefore, further research.

STUDENT RESEARCH PROJECTS

Student research projects are a part of the curricula of many programs offering initial preparation in physical therapy. The purpose of student projects may be to acquaint students with the principles of the scientific method which involves identifying a research problem, developing a design for investigation of the problem, undertaking an investigation, and writing a report that describes the outcome of the project. Projects may include the methods and instruments discussed in later chapters. The learning that takes place during the project may provide the foundation for appreciating the elements of physical therapy research and may further serve to increase the understanding of research above that which is presented in a didactic course.

The procedures for developing and conducting the project follow the systems approach shown in Table 1.2 and elsewhere in the book. At this point you should be able to develop a research problem and be giving some thought to its organization and how to write a proposal. Although the proposal cannot be completed until after an understanding of the material presented in subsequent chapters, much of the proposal can be written now. In the event that some assistance is needed in identifying a research problem, the following section lists some titles of past student projects. No attempt has been made to select only quality project titles, the listing merely identifies areas that have interested previous students. The appropriate method for solving the identified problem follows each title.

Topics Selected by Students

Initial Preparatory Level.

From a Physical Therapy Affiliate Program[7]

Effect of massage in reducing edema of the hand. Sellers BJ, Haefner B (comparative)

Effects of stroking massage in reducing edema of the foot. Stearns L, Price S (comparative)

Effect of local massage on the skin temperature of the hand. Beattie DP, Christopher HR (comparative)

Thermal effects of massage to the hand using a power medium. Canfield J, Kluthe M (comparative)

From the Medical College of Georgia, Augusta, Georgia:

Determination of normal values for radial nerve conduction velocity. Humphries R, Currier DP[8] (comparative)

Physiological effects of passive exercise on cardiopulmonary function. Smith K[9] (comparative)

Physical therapy recipients in nursing homes: the criteria for selection. Adams P (survey)

Use of a backrest in strengthening knee extensor muscles. Richard G, Currier DP[10] (comparative)

Interrator reliability in manual muscle testing. Gunnels CA (correlational)

Validity of the orthokinetic cuff in reducing spasticity in the wrist. Freeman B (comparative)

Use of isometric maximum to predict one repetition maximum for progressive resistance exercise. Calzada A (correlational)

Connective tissue laxity in subject having Barlow's syndrome. Evans P (correlational)

Effect of adhesive strapping in the prophylactic care of the ankle joint. Rammel M (comparative)

Effect of the inverted position on the heart rate, blood pressure, and respiratory rate in the normal adult. Gilbert R (comparative)

Motor conduction of the anterior interosseous nerve. Craft S, Currier DP, Nelson R[11] (comparative)

Conditions of employment of the 1975 physical therapy graduating class in a four state area. Price S (survey)

From the University of Alberta, Edmonton, Canada:

Combined effectiveness of standardized physical therapy and biofeedback-induced foot warming exercise. Ogiwara S (comparative)

Short-wave diathermy combined with manual mobilization as a method of increasing range of motion in the treatment of "frozen shoulder." Strong M (comparative)

Comparison of two methods of post-operative management following geometric knee replacement. Woytiuk M (comparative)

Comparative effects of passive positioning and exercise on arterial insufficiency disorders. Anderson M (comparative)

Capsular lesions of the glenohumeral joint: a comparative study of active and passive treatment programmes. Millar B (comparative)

Comparison of the treatment of "tennis elbow" using ultasound with hydrocortisone and ultrasound without cortisone. Morgan F (comparative)

Assessment of the mobilization techniques of Maitland to increase the range of movement on the chronic "frozen shoulder." Crocker M (comparative)

From Lincoln Institute, Melbourne, Australia[12]:

Influence of motivation on the performance of an exercise (comparative)

Effects of three different exercise regiments on endurance (comparative)

Strength gain comparison between progressive resisted exercise and regressive resisted exercise (comparative)

Dosage time required for lengthening hamstring muscles (comparative)

From the University of Kentucky, Lexington, Kentucky:

Effect of increased abdominal muscle strength on forced vital capacity and forced expiratory volume. Simpson L[13] (comparative)

EMG activity in shoulder muscles during exercise in sagittal planes and diagonal patterns. Smiley C (comparative)

Do good physical therapy students make good physical therapists? Scott MJ (survey)

Normal values for two-point discrimination and reliability of a two-point discrimination instrument. Walder J, Bathke J (normative)

High voltage electrical stimulation and blood flow. Carlson D (comparative)

Energy cost during gait of a hemipelvectomy amputee. Kennedy PJ, Glasgow SC (case report)

Graduate Studies Level (Theses).[14]

Comparative study of selected aspects of today's basic professional education for physical therapy in India and the United States of America. Mapleton AJ

Electromyographic and cinematographic findings in a novel motor skill development by walking with a simulated below-knee pylon. Ho SBL

Comparison of the isometric strength of the extensors at the metacarpophalangeal joint. Barnes WJ

Circling behavior on the rate produced by direct drug stimulation of the globus pallidus and caudate/putamen. Springer AP

Effects of vibration on the Achilles tendon reflex. Coogler CE

Attitudes of physical therapists toward patients and health professionals. Sorensen AM

Evaluation of the back abdominal strength ratio with the cable tensiometer. Bendinsky A

Conservative management of low back pain in the chronic state: a comparative study of two different techniques of treatment. Fernando CK

SOME ETHICAL CONSIDERATIONS

Widespread concern about the ethics of medical research has evolved ever since the trials of Nuremberg. Ethical questions associated with the use of human and animal subjects are being raised more today than perhaps ever before. The welfare and rights of humans have been violated in medical research. Because of these violations the formulation of declarations have been developed to outline proper ethical principles involved in acceptable use of human and animal subjects in research.[15] In 1964, the World Medical Association established some guidelines for those engaged in research on humans (Table 4.1). This declaration has served as the basis of the regulations for testing new drugs under United States law and also as the basis of the guidelines of the Medical Research Councils of Great Britain,[16] the United States,[17] and Canada,[18] and of a great number of universities and hospitals. These approving bodies attach great importance to the ethical acceptability of experiments involving human subjects.

Laws have been written in response to political pressures caused by emotional reactions of the public to violations of ethical principles. The laws represent efforts to protect the rights and welfare of every human in society. Considerations for ethics arise because of uses to which research has been put, misdeeds of individuals conducting research, and appropriations of public funds to support research.[19]

Risk and Responsibility

Research often involves uncertainties which may in turn involve risks. Physical, psychological, and social injuries are considered as potential risks when a subject participates in activity involving uncertainties[19] Infringement of privacy and psychological damage such as emotional upset, public embarrassment and humiliation such as loss of self-respect or loss of dignity are considered potential risks as well as physical discomfort, exposure to pain, or other physical harm. Because people are protected from unjustifiable assault, research involving humans must be justified for its contribution to scientific knowledge.[20]

A proposed research study must be justified for its benefits to the subjects involved and to science. The term research applies to those procedures

Table 4.1
Declaration of Helsinki

I. Basic Principles

1. Clinical research must conform to the moral and scientific principles that justify medical research and should be based on laboratory and animal experiments or other scientifically established facts.

2. Clinical research should be conducted only by scientifically qualified persons and under the supervision of a qualified medical man.

3. Clinical research cannot legitimately be carried out unless the importance of the objective is in proportion to the inherent risk to the subject.

4. Every clinical research project should be preceded by careful assessment of inherent risks in comparison to foreseeable benefits to the subject or to others.

5. Special caution should be exercised by the doctor in performing clinical research in which the personality of the subject is liable to be altered by drugs or experimental procedure.

II. Clinical Research Combined with Professional Care

1. In the treatment of the sick person, the doctor must be free to use a new therapeutic measure, if in his judgment it offers hope of saving life, reestablishing health, or alleviating suffering.

If at all possible, consistent with patient psychology, the doctor should obtain the patient's freely given consent after the patient has been given a full explanation. In case of legal incapacity, consent should also be procured from the legal guardian; in case of physical incapacity the permission of the legal guardian replaces that of the patient.

2. The doctor can combine clinical research with professional care, the objective being the acquisition of new medical knowledge, only to the extent that clinical research is justified by its therapeutic value for the patient.

III. Non-Therapeutic Clinical Research

1. In the purely scientific application of clinical research carried out on a human being, it is the duty of the doctor to remain the protector of the life and health of that person on whom clinical research is being carried out.

2. The nature, the purpose and the risk of clinical research must be explained to the subject by the doctor.

3a. Clinical research on a human being cannot be undertaken without his free consent after he has been informed; if he is legally incompetent, the consent of the legal guardian should be procured.

3b. The subject of clinical research should be in such a mental, physical and legal state as to be able to exercise fully his power of choice.

3c. Consent should, as a rule, be obtained in writing. However, the responsibility for clinical research always remains with the research worker; it never falls on the subject even after consent is obtained.

4a. The investigator must respect the right of each individual to safeguard his personal integrity, especially if the subject is in a dependent relationship to the investigator.

4b. At any time during the course of clinical research the subject or his guardian should be free to withdraw permission for research to be continued.

The investigator or the investigating team should discontinue the research if in his or their judgment, it may, if continued, be harmful to the individual.

carried out on humans for the purpose of contributing to knowledge. Behavioral research and questionnaires are also included under many guidelines of research, since they involve human subjects. The researcher is, therefore, asked to show how subjects (normal or patients) will benefit from the experimental intervention, what controls will be exercised to ensure safety and the welfare and rights of the subjects, and how subjects will be informed about potential risks. Potential risks must be balanced against potential benefits. A new approach to treatment of a condition is not a guarantee that it will be effective or replace the old approach. Controlled trials are essential to determine the efficacy of the new approach. The researcher must have some justification for studying the new approach and a reasonable explanation of its potential benefits.

In general, the clinical therapist uses different and new therapeutic measures if in his judgment they are within the aims of the treatment requested by the referring physician. The therapeutic measures used must be consistent with "accepted" forms of therapy stated in licensure acts. The therapist obtains the patient's approval informally when rendering a full explanation of what the treatment is and what can be expected from the treatment. This situation does not require a formal written consent, only the written referral of the referring physician. The physical therapist can combine clinical research with professional care to the extent that the research is justified by its therapeutic value for the patients. In all incidences the therapist must obtain prior approval for controlled clinical trials (review committee, referring physicians, and patient via written consent). The objective of all new therapeutic approaches should be acquisition of fresh physical therapy knowledge in hopes of improving the quality of therapy.

Practitioners find the concept of withholding treatment from patients perplexing. If the treatment to be investigated is known to be effective, it is unethical to withhold it from the patient. If the effectiveness of the treatment is unknown or equivocal, it is unethical to continue its use or use it without appropriate controlled evaluation.[21]

When risks are unknown, a controlled trial using animals may be required. Ethics cover the use of animals, also. Principles of ethics safeguarding the comfort and humane treatment of experimental animals have been developed by the American Psychological Association, and a statement of how they will be treated in experiments is required in proposals that involve animals.[22]

The conduct of experimental studies is controlled directly by individuals and approving bodies at respective work facilities, and indirectly through meetings and journal articles. Opinions and discussion among professional groups generally precede the acceptance of resolutions, and principles or passage of rules.

Informed Consent

Explaining the nature and purpose of a treatment procedure to a patient is generally left to the judgment of the physical therapist, and the patient usually accepts this explanation without question. This approach does not fulfill the ethical codes or research protocols. When the treatment is novel or new, the physical therapist is wisely advised to make extra efforts for the patient's comprehension. Since the conduct of clinical research raises moral and ethical questions, informed consent is essential.[23] Today, facilities of employment require the therapist planning to engage in experimental research to obtain written consent of the subject prior to participating in the research study. In general, the researcher is obligated to give full details about risks and benefits involved in the research to those participating and those responsible for minors who will participate.

The information required in each informed consent form is given in Table 4.2.[2] Forms will vary from facility to facility but the information required will be similar. An example of a consent form is found in Appendix, Table B.

Guidelines for Research

Experimental and descriptive research involving human subjects is necessary to further scientific knowledge and to improve physical therapy. Some general rules of conduct are presented to assist the therapist who is interested in conducting research on humans; these rules serve only as

Table 4.2
Elements Required in the Informed Consent Form

1. Title of proposed study.
2. Principal investigator's name.
3. Description of study in narrative layman's language (200 words or less). Explain purpose, procedure, experimental effect.
4. Describe risks, benefits, and any discomfort that subjects can expect.
5. Indication of antidotes or alternative treatments available, that no form of compensation or medical treatment is available from researcher but is provided at expense of subject's health care insurer.
6. Offer to answer questions of subject about the study.
7. Inform subject of choice in withdrawal from participation in the study at any time without prejudice.
8. Indication that participation is voluntary and assurance of anonymity of data.
9. Signatures:
   Subject
   Witness
10. Date

guides. Specific rules are mandatory when applying for government research grants and for certain local institutions. The researcher must obtain the specific information concerning ethics and consent for particular applications.

Principles for Human Research:

1. Any research must be justifiable for its scientific value.
2. Even if the inquiry has scientific value, it must not be pursued if benefit is outweighed by risk to the subject.
3. The research must be conducted by scientifically competent people.
4. The research must be conducted under a sound design or proposal and be carried out according to the design, though the design may be modified on the approval of a review committee which had originally approved it.
5. Care must be taken throughout the study to see that the subject will not be harassed and the research must be terminated if risk of harm, physical or emotional, is apparent.
6. The subject should be entitled to withdraw at any time.
7. No subject should be used in research unless he has given his free consent after being fully informed. In the case of a child or mentally incompetent person the consent of his legal guardian should be obtained; and risks must be minimal in the case of these subjects. A child is usually defined as anyone under 18 years of age.[2,20,24]

Principles for Behavioral Research.

Sometimes a complete explanation in advance of the purpose of behavioral research may invalidate the results. These guidelines follow the ethical standards of the American Psychological Association.
1. When a person is involved as a subject in a research project. his permission must be obtained.
2. Whenever possible the nature, purpose, and results of the research should be described to those either directly or indirectly involved.
3. Individuals should not be coerced into participating in a research program, and they should be free to withdraw from such a program whenever they desire.
4. Only when a problem is significant and can be investigated in no other way is the investigator justified in giving misinformation to research subjects or exposing research subjects to physical or emotional stress.
5. When the possibility of serious aftereffects exists, research is conducted only when the subjects or their responsible agents are fully informed of this possibility and volunteer nevertheless.

6. The investigator seriously considers the possible harmful aftereffects and removes them as soon as permitted by the design of the experiment.[25]

Principles for the Use of Data Gathering Instruments.

The gathering of data such as answers to questionnaires, inventories, interviews, and other data-gathering instruments is descriptive research and is concerned with the matter of privacy.

1. Any research which includes the use of questionnaires should have scientific or other meaningful purpose and value.
2. Questionnaires should be designed and administered by competent people.
3. Care should be taken that insofar as is consistent with the purpose of the study, information to be acquired must be absolutely essential to the purpose of the study and should be as free as is possible from questions that might be embarrassing to the subjects.
4. Participation in such studies should be entirely voluntary, and care should be exercised in order to ensure that subtle pressures are not brought to bear in order to obtain participation.
5. Answers to questionnaires should be kept confidential, and when possible, anonymity should be afforded. Codes and ciphers must be kept in secure places; transfer of data between places (shipment and delivery) should have careful controls; and provision for the destruction of all edited and obsolete data on punched cards, printouts, tapes, and other records must be made. Computer transmission of data may be restricted in certain studies.
6. Subjects should be free to withdraw at any time prior to or during the administration of a questionnaire, and should be informed in advance of this right.
7. Subjects must be given a clear and understandable explanation of the purpose of a questionnaire prior to its being administered.[2,24]

The objective of laws, principles, and guidelines on research ethics is assurance of protection of the rights and welfare of the subject. Comparative and descriptive research represents a delicate balance between the health professions and public opinion and legal limitation. The researcher must accept responsibility for his actions by carefully weighing the manner in which the conduct of his research is discharged. The law, principle, or guideline can encompass every potential situation encountered in research.[22]

POLAR QUESTIONS ON ETHICS

Students pursuing instruction in research have been asked to state their position on two questions dealing with ethics in research. The questions deal with problems which are at opposite extremes (polar), and represent situations that students may face some day. The responses are those of students.

1. A professor performs and publishes research based on your proposal submitted in partial fulfillment of a course in research. What is your reaction?

> A professor's performance of research based on a student's proposal is perfectly ethical so long as the student is informed of the professor's intention and use of the proposal and has the expressed consent from the student for its use. If feasible and out of courtesy the professor should invite the student to participate in the experimental solution of his problem. The student will be somewhat limited in ability to complete the experiment so the collaboration would serve as a valuable learning experience to the student. When the report is published the person having greatest responsibility for the completion of the study should be the author listed first. Mutual agreement or a contract to this effect should be made before the study is begun.
>
> Anonymous Student

2. Student performs research in partial fulfillment of a course or thesis requirement and uses a professor's expressed research problem, laboratory, and equipment. What is your reaction?

> A professor should not be reluctant to allow a student to conduct research using the professor's idea, laboratory, and equipment. This arrangement permits a faculty member with research and teaching responsibilities to generate and oversee many more research studies than he would otherwise have time to complete on his own. This arrangement provides guidance to the student, while the student gains valuable experience. The professor usually has facilities and equipment at his disposal which may not be available to the student. Each contributor to the research should receive due credit. A mutual understanding of each other's role is necessary before the onset of the study. The interaction of student and professor in research allows for initiative, enthusiasm, and expertise which is necessary in the performance of research.

Table 4.3
Cumulative Summary of the Research Processes Presented

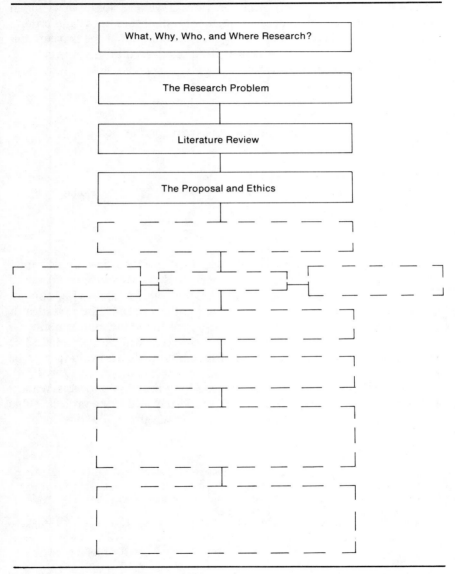

Anonymous Student

SUMMARY

The research proposal is a document that outlines a planned project or investigation. The proposal serves as a guide for the investigator to follow during the conduct of a project, provides a vehicle for review and a document which can be judged for its merit, establishes limits and criteria to be followed and adhered to throughout the conduct of the project, and provides a measure of accountability of those engaged in the project.

The proposal must be written concisely and convincingly. It should include the following information:

1. Title of the research study
2. Name and title of the researchers and participating facilities
3. Objectives of the study
4. Significance of the study
5. Related research
6. Plan of the study
7. Time, space, and availability of equipment
8. Cost analysis

Because the researcher asks questions, pries into the mind, and samples the physiological characteristics of an individual, the issue of ethics is raised by the public, legislators, and those responsible for approving studies. When writing the proposal and conducting the research, the investigator must consider the moral and ethical issues of the study, and state in the proposal how the rights and welfare of subjects will be protected. The researcher must obtain the consent of the individuals who volunteer to be studied.

Some titles of previous research projects have been listed to assist readers in formulating a research problem and proposing a title for a project. Table 4.3 provides a summary of the research processes presented thus far.

REFERENCES

1. Treece EW, Treece JW Jr: Elements of Research in Nursing, ed 3. St. Louis, CV Mosby Co, 1982
2. Code of Federal Regulations 45CFR46: Protection of Human Subjects (HHS). Washington, U.S. Government Printing Office, 1983
3. Makrides L, Richman J: Research methodology and applied statistics, Part 7: writing the research proposal. Physiother Canada 33: 163–168, 1981
4. Wandelt M: Guide for the Beginning Researcher. New York, Appleton-Century-Crofts, 1970
5. Archibald RD, Villoria RL: Network-Based Management Systems (PERT/CPM). New York, John Wiley, 1967
6. Gay LR: Educational Research: Competencies for Analysis and Application, ed 2. Columbus, OH, Charles E. Merrill Pub. Co, 1981

7. Schneiderwind W, Burke J: Physical Therapy Affiliate Program: An Introduction to Research. Carville, LA, US Department Health, Education, Welfare, 1970

8. Humphries R, Currier DP: Variables in recording motor conduction of the radial nerve. Phys Ther 56: 809–814, 1976

9. Smith K: Physiological effects of passive exercise on cardiorespiratory function. Phys Ther 56: 295–297, 1976

10. Richard G, Currier DP: Back stabilization during knee strengthening exercise. Phys Ther 57: 1013–1015, 1977

11. Craft S, Currier DP, Nelson R: Motor conduction of the anterior interosseous nerve. Phys Ther 57: 1143–1147, 1977

12. Wheeler JR: Student research projects: An innovative approach to learning. Physiother Canada 28: 99–101, 1976

13. Simpson L: Effect of increased abdominal muscle strength on forced vital capacity and forced expiratory volume. Phys Ther 63: 334–337, 1983

14. Theses and dissertations. Phys Ther 55: 58–60, 1975

15. Visscher MB: Ethical Constraints and Imperatives in Medical Research. Springfield, IL, Charles C Thomas Pub, 1975

16. Report of the Medical Research Council for 1962–1963 (Cmmd 2382). London, Medical Research Council, pp 21–25

17. American Medical Association Ethical Guidelines for Clinical Investigations. Chicago, Am Med Assoc, November 30, 1966

18. Medical Research Council; Extramural Programmes; 1966. Ottawa, Can, Medical Research Council, 1966

19. Michels E: Research and human rights, 2. Phys Ther 56: 546–552, 1976

20. Cox KR: Planning Clinical Experiments. Springfield, IL, Charles C Thomas Pub, 1968

21. Makrides L, Richman J: Research methodology and applied statistics, Part 6: ethics in human research. Physiother Canada 33: 89–94, 1981

22. Research Precautions of Ethical Standards. Washington, Am Psychol Assoc, 1963

23. Burdette WJ, Gehan EA: Planning and Analyses of Clinical Trials. Springfield, IL, Charles C Thomas Pub, 1970

24. Guidelines for Human Reseach: General Faculties Council. Edmonton, Canada, University of Alberta, 1972

25. Ethical standards of psychologists. Am Psychol 18: 56–60, 1963

SUGGESTED READINGS

Cox DR: Planning of Experiments. New York, John Wiley & Sons, 1958

Krathwohl DR: How to Prepare a Research Proposal. Syracuse, Syracuse University Bookstore, 1965

Slater SB: The design of clinical research. Phys Ther 46: 265–273, 1966

Wilson EB Jr: An Introduction to Scientific Research. New York, McGraw-Hill Book Co, 1952

Michels E: Research and human rights. I. Phys Ther 56: 407–412, 1976

Part Two

ROOTS OF RESEARCH

5

Quantification in Research

I often say that when you can measure
what you are speaking about and express it in
numbers, you know something about it; but, when
you cannot measure it in numbers your knowledge
is of a meagre and unsatisfactory kind; it may
be the beginning of knowledge but have scarcely
in your thought advanced to the stage of science
whatever the matter may be.

Lord Kelvin

A vital part of the research process is the gathering of measurements or counts in a form appropriate for deducing reasonable conclusions. A scientific premise is that if a phenomenon exists, it can be measured, and if it can be measured it can be understood. Research deals with existing phenomena and measured values of phenomena; therefore, it must deal with quantities, numbers, and facts.

The word "agree" means to correspond, conform, resemble, and concur[1] while the concepts of "objective" and "subjective" can be considered as degrees of agreement. Objective means to exist independent of thought or outside of the mind, and subjective is the opposite of objective and means to exist in the mind or dependent on thought.[1] The concepts of objective and subjective are often considered in terms of the amount or degrees of agreement. To be objective an event, trait, or quantity must be agreed upon unanimously; while to be subjective, the degree of agreement can vary with the event, trait, or quantity.[2] A group of physical therapists may "eyeball" the motion of a patient's glenohumeral joint and judge the range as being 155, 160, or 165 degrees, but upon measurement of the joint motion by an appropriate instrument the motion is found to be 160 degrees. In the first approach the 160 degrees of motion could have been the value most of the therapists agreed upon, but not all, while every therapist observed the measuring instrument and agreed with the value indicated on the instrument. We say the first approach was subjective because the measurement was a guess or a product of thought or experience, and the second approach is considered objective because the measurement resulted in agreement, but a difference in the process of agreement could be distinguished; degrees of agreement.

Instruments are used in education to measure the absorption of knowledge of a particular subject. Students are familiar with objective and subjective examinations. The former is objective because one response is correct and all others are incorrect to the question; in the latter instrument the results are somewhat dependent upon the judgment or mental belief of the professor (quality) and the process is considered to be subjective. The two examples are different degrees of agreement. Science is concerned with truth and reality; it is objective. Quantitativeness is objectivity.

Statistics is a branch of applied mathematics that deals with the organization, description, and interpretation of data obtained by observations and experiments. Examination and treatment of data with statistics enable the researcher to predict outcomes of related events or make generalities from the data with increased assurance of being correct.

Some dialogue must be made about the use of statistics in a book or course on research methods. Most students who have conveniently avoided taking more than a single course of college mathematics are usually terrified by the word mathematics. This book exposes the student to elementary statistics and scientific concepts because every physical therapist must know how to read and interpret the research literature in order to maintain professional competence. The therapist must think, act, converse, and write in scientific style. The manner of presenting the subject of statistics in this book should ease the apprehension of any student lacking mathematical background. Effort has been made to simplify the mathematical component. Eventually, the student seeking a career in scientific research must reckon with more sophisticated mathematical concepts than presented herein. Statistics is a valuable tool to the researcher who deals constantly with animate objects which have variations too complex and frequent to reason out with logic alone. Statistics is more often a friend to the researcher than not; the researcher works hard to build the body of knowledge of science so the student must understand some of the operations of the knowledge building process.

The use of statistics in research does not prove that the findings are true or real. Statistics never did, do not now, nor will they ever, prove anything. Statistics is a very valuable tool for helping the researcher to make correct decisions, conclusions, and inferences, but statistics do not prove anything. Data are variable; people are variable; characteristics, traits, events, and measurements are variable in the type of research physical therapists perform. Because of the variability of some methods of assuring accuracy, there is a need for increasing chances for making the correct decision or prediction, or instilling confidence in the research; statistics is the tool which helps determine the probability of making the right decision. You must learn what probability means in research and how statistics will assist with decision making.

Clinical therapists deal with patients who are different, but yet have similarities. Twenty patients may be diagnosed as having rheumatoid arthritis, which is a similarity between the patients, but upon examination of these patients you note dissimilarities. Your treatment plans may be based on the dissimilarities. The function of statistics in physical therapy is to make optimal use of numerical data concerning the disease, patients, and the efficacy of the treatments while considering the similarities and dissimilarities.[3]

This chapter will begin to establish the roots of scientific inquiry.

BASICS OF DATA

Variables

Research in physical therapy is concerned with animate and inanimate objects, and numerical facts derived from data. A datum is a single observable or potentially observable phenomenon; a datum is a fact and can be a number (*data* are more than one datum).[4] A single datum can be a single observation, a single value, or a single measurement. A single isolated observation or value does not usually command attention in science because it does not provide sufficient descriptive evidence of traits, events, or phenomena. Science deals with quantities of information because of the variation present in the universe; and, therefore, we deal with data and not usually a datum. Data are collections of individual observations of units, groups, or occurrences.

Data are a function of the problem or question and measuring instrument. Data vary from study to study but supply the researcher with the kinds of information needed to test the hypothesis or answer the question.[2] Data are quality or quantity which represent elements or observations in an experiment.

A measurable characteristic, trait, or property is called a variable and an individual measurement of a variable is a variate.[5] In a series of scores, effects, or characteristics, each unit may differ from another. A variable can change from one observation to another.[6] The differences between units of a variable are the quantities or qualities that are measured or assessed in research. Muscular force, heart rate, treatment time, latency, and methods of facilitation are a few variables that appear in physical therapy research reports. Most textbooks on statistics or research use the capital letters X and Y to denote variables.

Variables can be discrete or continuous. A discrete variable is a measurable characteristic that can assume only specific or limited values; exact numbers obtained by counting indivisible units. An integer (exact or whole number) is a discrete variable because it is a limited value. Real gaps exist between successive measures of discrete variables; the measures are not capable of infinite subdivisions. The number of patients sitting in the waiting room is an example of a discrete variable. Patients cannot be 5.5 or 10.3, they must number 5 or 10. If three transcutaneous electrical nerve stimulators are in use, and if an additional unit is put into service, the count goes from three to four without passing through any intermediate fractional values; at no time are stimulators slightly less than four or a little more than three. The measure of the variable is exact, and measurement proceeds by a series of gaps from unit to unit.

The number of hospital admissions, the number of physical therapy clinics in London, heart rate, glands, or number of days in a month are other examples. Attribute is the term given and used for labeling variables that cannot be measured directly as numerical values. Physical therapists conducting descriptive research might be working with qualitative data which deals with male or female, fracture or no fracture, levels of membership, or colors of clinical uniforms. When numbers or units are assigned to attributes, like a frequency count, statistical analyses can be made. If attributes are countable characteristics, they are also discrete variables. The numbers of diathermy units currently used in different parts of the country are attributes which may interest physical therapists in studies of sociology or human ecology.

Continuous variables might be muscular strength, distal latency of the median nerve, volume of water displaced by hands, and body weight. Measurable characteristics which can assume unlimited values are continuous variables:[7] approximate numbers obtained by measurement, capable of infinite subdivisions, without gaps existing between successive measures. If a therapist stimulates a nerve of a patient with 150 volts, the voltage is approximately 150 volts. The measured voltage may be more or it may be less than 150 volts; however, to increase the stimuli to 160 volts, the force must pass through infinite gradations between 150 and 160 volts.

A continuous variable may be limited to certain values in practice by the measuring device (defined range), but theoretically could take on any value (unlimited). For example, latency of nerve is measured to the nearest tenth of a millisecond (3.6 msec) but if electromyography were refined to a more precise procedure then the latency might read 3.589 msec. A group of young men may be measured for their O_2 intake during a specified activity; the recorded quantities of O_2 per unit of time could conceivably fall into a series of numbers (0.75, 1.15, 0.92, 0.87, 1.26 liters/min) with each having a different value. The series of different values constitutes a continuous variable, O_2 consumed per unit of time.

Variables can also be identified in research according to their function. Variables that will be manipulated in the study are independent variables and those measured as a result of the experiment are dependent variables. Examples of independent and dependent variables are shown in Table 5.1.

Derived Variables

Most variables in scientific inquiry consist of data recorded as output of various types of instruments which are direct measurements or counts.[8] Sometimes the values among two or more independently measured variables are best expressed as relationships. Derived or computed variables are expressions of the relationships between two or more quantitative variables: ratios, rates, and percentages.

A ratio can be a proportion or a relation between two similar variables. The ratio can be a single value like a quotient (0.5) or a fraction ($^{50}/_{100}$). The quotient is preferred for computational purposes because of its ease in mathematical manipulation. In the classical study by Inman and co-workers,[9] the glenohumeral joint was found to move two degrees for every one degree at the scapulothoracic joint. The relation was expressed as a ratio of 2:1.[9]

A state research question may be: Does the angle of the hip have any effect on the force generated by the quadriceps in strengthening exercises? The specific variables are identified from the question and shown in Table 5.2.

A percentage is a form of a ratio that is expressed as a proportion. The percent ratio is a variable expressed as a proportion of a whole, 100. The percent does not relate two variables.

Rates are also derived variables and are expressed as variables per unit of time. Rates are important in physical therapy. The distance a patient walks in a given unit of time or the time an impulse takes to travel over a segment of nerve are but two examples of rates.

Population and Sample

A population is commonly considered as the number of people living in a particular place or defined area. In research the meaning of population

Table 5.1
Examples of Variables

Independent	Dependent
Cause	Effect
Treatment	Physiological response
Abscissa, X	Ordinate, Y
Controlled factors	Outcome
Manipulated variable	Measured variable
Material taught	Test score
Whirlpool bath	Increased joint range
Angle of hip	Quadriceps force

Table 5.2
Identification of Variables from a Research Question—Does the Angle of the Hip have any
Effect on the Force Generated by the Knee Extensors?

		Independent	Dependent
Variable	A.	Angle of hip (degrees)	Muscular force (kg)
	B.	Type of exercise	
Variable factors	A.	Position of hands	Body size
		Support, no support to back	Cooperation
		Inclination of back support	Measuring instrument
			Researcher
	B.	Static	
		Dynamic	
		Concentric	
		Eccentric	
		Isokinetic	

may or may not refer to the number of persons residing in a circumscribed area such as a city, county, state, or country. A population is all groups, collections, or aggregates of people, animals, objects, materials, traits, measurements, events, or "things" in the world or universe. Population is the totality of observations of a defined variable, all individuals of a particular species. This type of population in which every member is considered is an infinite population. In practice, a researcher cannot measure or observe every member in the world having the defined trait, so often the population is defined to identify a specific group or size. If a physical therapist was interested in measuring the degrees of spasticity of the right biceps in every patient having a stroke, he could not complete the task in a lifetime even if people did not have strokes after the measurements began. Population is used in theory to include infinite variables, but in practice, the population is often redefined to meet the needs of the researcher for study and for making inferences. The therapist could, however, define the population about which inferences will be made from the data collected in the study. Population in this example could be all patients having strokes in Chicago where the totality of individual observations is confined to a circumscribed area which has been defined. The therapist could just as well have defined the population as all patients having strokes affecting their right-sided extremities and admitted to the therapist's hospital during the next two years. These types of redefined populations are called finite populations.

Also, in practice, not all individuals in a population can be measured because of economic, time, and physical constraints so the therapist decides only to measure a proportion of the subjects representing the population. The specific part or proportion of the population selected for measuring the variable is called a sample. The physical therapist who defined his population as all patients having strokes of the right side and being admitted over a period of 2 years may measure only a proportion of the total number appearing during the 2 years. The proportion of patients measured by the therapist constitutes a sample which will contain the numbers of patients established by the therapist arbitrarily. A sample is a subset of the population.[6]

Parameters and Statistics

If we were measuring a variable or variables among every individual or trait in the world, we would be dealing with a value or measure called a parameter. A parameter is a value that is characteristic of a population, and is the real or the true value. If heart rates of all physical therapy students could be measured during their first physiology examination the average heart rate for all physical therapy students in the world could be a parameter. Symbolically, in statistics, parameters are usually assigned capital or Greek letters. On the other hand, if the heart rates of all physical therapy students attending the University of Kentucky were measured under the same circumstances as above, the average value recorded would be a statistic. A statistic is a value that is characteristic of a sample. Since only the students attending a particular university were measured from all physical therapy students throughout the world taking their first physiology examination and since the students measured constituted a sample, the average heart rate characterized is a statistic. A statistic usually appears in small case or Roman letters.[6]

A caution should be given about the use of parameter in everyday verbal or written communication. Parameter is a mathematical term and defined as such[1] and should not be abused by misuse. Learn to communicate scientific terms appropriately, and do not use parameter unless discussing a value of a population in statistics.

Measurement

A substantial portion of research and clinical practice is spent assessing the subject and patient, respectively. Assessment requires measurement. Measurement is the assigning of numbers or quantities to behaviors, observations, functions, or objects according to rules.[10] Visual assessment and gross motor tests are common measurement systems used by physical therapists to assess motor functions.[11] The visual system does not include quantification of characteristics of the function, but practitioners may often support the soundness of the method by anecdotal justification for objective measurement in clinical or research situations. Measurements in either situation must be measured, recorded, and studied appropriately to eliminate subjectivity.

Levels of Measurement

Measurement and quantification exist at several levels, depending on the mathematical and logical assumptions that are fulfilled. Measurements and analyses of numbers based on the higher level of scales are considered more sophisticated than those of lower quality. The scale of measurement will determine the type of information that will be obtained from data.

Nominal Measurement. A nominal measurement is one in which numbers or labels have been assigned to differentiate, or represent, classes of objects, persons, or characteristics. The nominal scale is the weakest level of measurement because statements can only be made about presence or absence of equalities but not quantitative differences between members of the category. The numbers identify, classify, differentiate, or label members of the category. They have no other function and cannot yield additional information about the events, effects, or traits. Classifying types of arthritis which patients have into categories such as osteoarthritis, rheumatoid arthritis, traumatic arthritis, and gouty arthritis are nominal types of variables or attributes. Attributes are countable characteristics when numerical values are assigned. Labeling academic courses by numbers, people by phone or social security numbers, test subjects as numbers, addresses by postal-code numbers, and athletes by their uniform numbers constitute nominal types of values or discrete variables. Some scales of "activities of daily living" are assessed on the nominal level. A nominal measurement meets the minimal requirements of the definition of measurement, the assignment of numerals to objects or events according to defined rules.[12]

Ordinal Measurement. In ordinal measurement members of a category can be differentiated as having more of, the same, or less than, a particular quality or trait than another member. A conditioned muscle contains less lactic acid than a non-conditioned muscle after a given amount of work. The exact amount of difference between muscles does not fall within the capability of the ordinal measurement. Because the ordinal measurement is higher on the hierarchical scale than the nominal measurement, it must also possess those qualities of the nominal measurement in addition to its uniqueness of ordering or ranking its members along some scale or dimension. The quantity cannot be measured in magnitude but can only reflect the relative position between members on the scale. Therefore, statements about the quality of differences between members or the number of times one member is greater than or less than another are not possible.[7] If the researcher chooses the ordinal level of measurement, he can only state that subjects having an above-knee amputation have shorter stride lengths than normal individuals of similar height. Later, you will read about some statistics (median, percentiles, and rank-order correlation) that possess ordinal characteristics.

Interval Measurement. This level of measurement is more complex than the ordinal or nominal levels. Unlike the two levels of measurement discussed, interval measurements use a scale that has equal distances between points. The scale is given units of measurement, but the units of measurement are arbitrarily assigned. The interval scale is limited because the zero point is arbitrary. Temperature is the classical example cited. The distance between 10 degrees C and 20 degrees C is 10 degrees C; similarly the distance between 20 and 30 degrees C is 10 degrees C. One cannot, however, state that 20 degrees C is twice as warm as 10 degrees C. The difference in magnitudes and zero points can be conceptualized if Celsius, Fahrenheit, and Kelvin scales of temperature are compared. Another example of interval measurement is calender time because its zero point was assigned arbitrarily.[7]

Ratio Measurement. Ratio level measurement holds the highest position on the hierarchy and, therefore, possesses all the characteristics of the interval scale. The uniqueness of this measurement is its true or absolute zero point. This uniqueness enables the user to talk about the absence of something, for example, zero distance or time. Ratio judgments can be made about ratio data. One can state that something is two or three times as much as something else if it measures two or three times the number of units. The unit of measurement remains arbitrary, but the ratio scale allows you to multiply or divide each of the values by a specified number without changing the properties of the scale.[13] Many ratio level measurements are made in physical therapy research: nerve conduction velocity, length of a brace, treatment time, and volume of water displaced by an edematous hand. Few ratio level measurements are used by social or behavioral scientists since they cannot talk about zero intelligence or zero attitude.[14]

When a researcher discusses data, or results of a study, his statements must fit the scale or level of the data collected in the study. The researcher must be aware of the measurement level and avoid making statements or judgments at, for example, ratio levels when data are ordinal. An awareness of these levels will assist you in drawing appropriate conclusions about your data.

Rounding of Numbers

Before leaving basics of data, rounding of numbers in data should be mentioned. In published research reports, statistics are often reported to two figures to the right of the decimal point.

The rule in rounding decimal fractions to the nearest whole number is to drop the last place in the decimal fraction if it is less than 5. If the last place in the decimal fraction is greater than 5, the value to its left is raised by one. For example, the last figure to the right of the decimal is rounded up if the third figure is more than 5 (5.457 rounded up to 5.46) but is dropped if the third figure is less than 5 (25.342 dropped to 25.34).[15]

This rule holds true for whatever degree of accuracy is desirable. Rounding may occur for any value whenever a decimal is used. If an integer (whole number) is used, then rounding is not necessary; 36 is not rounded to 40 but stands by its own value. The accuracy or precision of the unit is usually dependent upon the measuring instrument. Stating a latency value of 2.9528 msec when using a clinical type electromyographic unit would be pretentious, since the instrument is not capable of yielding values of that precision. A value of 2.9 or 3.0 msec would be appropriate. The type of data, accuracy of the measuring instrument, or precision desired will help determine the rounding off procedure used in a research project.

ORGANIZATION OF DATA

Data obtained by way of surveys or experiments are very often an unorganized collection of numbers which, upon inspection, do not provide immediate information. For the collection of numbers to be meaningful to the researcher, the numbers must be arranged, summarized, or organized (arrays) so that pertinent information can be extracted.

Univariate Distributions

Univariate distributions are arrays that express a single variable. For example, suppose 10 people have the following strength values recorded from their left knee extensors; 50, 34, 26, 41, 37, 29, 45, 52, 30, and 46 kilograms (kg). These numbers, as a group, are not very meaningful to the reader, but if they are arranged in descending order of size they become more meaningful:

52
50
46
45
41
37
34
30
29
26

An arrangement of this kind is called an order or rank distribution, but has only the advantage of providing the order of scores. The order of scores represent an array of a variable or an univariate distribution.

Additional meaning or information may be obtained if the array (data) is classified or arranged into two groups. Those having knee extensor strength over 35 kg and those having strength under 35 kg (Table 5.3). If we knew that strength of the knee extensors over 35 kg was high for 15-year old girls, we then could gain additional information from the grouping (Table 5.3). By examining the table further we can make other interpreta-

Table 5.3
Strength Data of Ten People

Strength (kg)	People
Over 35	6
Under 35	4

Table 5.4
Frequency Distribution of Twenty Scores with a Class Limit of 0.3

Limits	Mid-points	Frequency	Cumulative Frequency
4.2–4.4	4.3	1	20
3.9–4.1	4.0	3	19
3.6–3.8	3.7	3	16
3.3–3.5	3.4	9	13
3.0–3.2	3.1	3	4
2.7–2.9	2.8	1	1

tions. We could say that 40% (4 of 10) of the people examined are under the cut-off point, or that 60% (6 of 10) were high for 15-year olds.

Frequency Distributions

Suppose we have recorded the latencies of the median nerve for 20 people as: 4.0, 3.5, 3.2, 4.0, 3.8, 4.2, 3.4, 3.5, 3.5, 4.0, 3.2, 2.8, 3.3, 3.8, 3.5, 3.4, 3.8, 3.4, 3.2, and 3.3 msec. Now the values are arranged by order and frequency:

X	f
4.2	1
4.0	3
3.8	3
3.5	4
3.4	3
3.3	2
3.2	3
2.8	1
	$20 = n$

By ordering the latencies you should have observed that several values appeared more often than once in the array. Grouping a series of numbers by their frequencies is a convenient method of arranging data. A collection of scores arranged by order of magnitude and accompanied by their frequencies is called a frequency distribution.[2] The latencies can be re-grouped in still another fashion:

X	f
4.2–4.4	1
3.9–4.1	3
3.6–3.8	3
3.3–3.5	9
3.0–3.2	3
2.7–2.9	1
	20 = n

This arrangement is a grouped frequency distribution which is composed of data arranged within class limits (sub-groups) to assist in the presentation of numbers.[16]

Research data can be presented by a group frequency distribution in still another fashion. (See Table 5.4.) The end points of the sub-groups (classes) are class limits, class boundaries, or class intervals (e.g., 3.3 − 3.5). The midpoint between the upper and lower class limits of a class is called the class midpoint (e.g., 3.4).

Class limits are equal sized divisions of the grouped frequency distribution; the lower (e.g., 3.3) and upper (e.g., 3.5) limits indicate the lowest and highest values that will be recorded in a particular boundary or interval. The class limits are determined by subtracting the lowest value of a set from the highest value (e.g., $4.4 − 2.7 = 1.7$) and dividing the quotient by the number of classes desired. In Table 5.4 the quotient 1.7 was divided by 6 ($1.7 \div 6 = 0.28$ rounded to 0.3) and 0.3 was established as the class size (the rule for rounding can be applied). The midpoint of a class is a value or measure halfway between the lower and upper limits of a class (e.g., $4.4 − 4.2 = 0.2 \div 2 = 0.1 + 4.2 = 4.3$).

The group frequency distribution is a convenient arrangement when dealing with large sets of data as sometimes used in sociology, education, and psychology. Although no rule has been established, the usual practice is to group data into 10 to 15 classes.[17] The data ($n = 20$) of Table 5.4 were used for illustrative purposes only and do not correspond to recommended practices of using grouped frequency distributions with large sets of data (e.g., $n > 100$). This distribution, however, requires different statistical methods than that of the simple frequency distribution or of raw scores and will not be discussed further in this book. The group frequency distribution is cumbersome when dealing with numbers that have many digits (2537.485 and 3516.983). Another disadvantage is that the identity of the individual raw scores is lost in the grouping process. For example, the values of 116.8 , 118.5, and 115.9 are lost in a class having limits of 115 to 119 and a midpoint of 117.

Bivariate Distributions

Bivariate distributions are arrangements of paired values or observations of two variables. The bivariate distribution is used when interest centers on the relationship of two variables and will be used in discussing correlation in Chapters 7 and 10.

Frequency distributions are used to reduce a mass of data for increased understanding and ease of presentation. Frequency distributions are used routinely to describe observations grasped quickly and for presentation in tables. You should remember that a series of numbers does not provide much information, but grouping the data into a meaningful distribution helped to extract additional information.

MEASURES OF CENTRAL TENDENCY

There are many other ways of describing data. Chapter 12 will discuss tables and graphs for presenting data for group performance. A branch of statistics called descriptive statistics is used to describe data of a group also. As mentioned earlier, a datum is of little value in applied research because one observed score or value is likely to be unstable, to be unrepresentative of the true situation or condition, or to be unauthoritative information. For example, if the physical work capacity of 100 children is measured and the range of scores varies from 500 to 1000 kg M/min, the child whose value is 1000 kg M/min may not be "typical" or representative of the group if the majority of scores were recorded between 525 and 750 kg M/min. For these reasons, large groups of numbers or scores are best for representing a characteristic or trait. Large groups of numbers or scores, however, become cumbersome or bulky; methods of descriptive statistics provide representation of a group of numbers with a single value, a statistic. Measures of central tendency are single values which supply information that typifies the central performance of an entire group.[6] Any measure indicating the center of an array or series of numbers is a measure of central tendency.

Mean

The arithmetic mean is the sum of a set of measurements divided by the number of measurements in the set.[7] The mean is a measure that describes a typical, representative, or "average" value for a set of observations. The mean is the balancing point in a series of numbers. If you could think of the force arm of a lever as a frequency distribution then the lever would be balanced if the fulcrum were at the arithmetic mean.[18] In other words, if the weight of the scores in the distribution are considered to be the forces and the distance of the scores away from the fulcrum to be the force arm of the level, then the force times the distance on one side of the arithmetic mean would exactly equal the force times the distance on the other side. The mean might be considered as a first class lever or teeter-totter.

You are familiar with batting average, average rainfall, grade point averages, and average patient load. Since the term "average" is used for other measures of central tendency, the term "mean" is used in statistics and in scientific literature so readers do not confuse the measures of central tendency.

The formula for the mean is:

$$\overline{X} = \frac{\Sigma X}{n}$$

Computation of the mean can be illustrated in the following example consisting of the strength values recorded from the left knee extensor muscles of 10 people. The sample contains 10 variates of the variable "strength".

X(kg)	
52	
50	$\overline{X} = \dfrac{\Sigma X}{n}$
46	
45	$= \dfrac{390}{10} = 39.0$ kg
41	
37	
34	
30	
29	
26	
$\Sigma X = 390$	

The Greek letter Sigma, Σ, is used to indicate the sum of these n observations. The symbol, ΣX, then directs you to sum all scores ($\Sigma X = 390$ kg). The formula for the mean directs you to divide the sum of scores by the total number of scores ($390 \div 10 = 39.0$ kg = mean). The symbol $\overline{X}$ (read X-bar) stands for the mean of the set of scores.

The mean has several important mathematical properties, but only two are discussed here. Any mean computed from a sample of size n is an estimate of a population mean, μ (pronounced mew). The sample mean is the most accurate and the most efficient estimate of the population's central tendency. The mean is affected by extreme scores in the distribution. The very small or the very large scores, which may not be typical of the majority of scores in the distribution, influence the outcome. For example, if a distribution consisted of five scores: 1, 10, 12, 15, and 100, the mean would be 27.6, which is not typical of the scores 10, 12, and 15. Since the mean of a sample is the best estimate of the population mean, it is used most frequently in scientific studies.

Median

The median of n numbers of scores, arranged in order of values, is the middle number of the distribution if n is odd, and the mean of the two middle numbers if n is even. The median is also that point on a scale of measurements above which and below which 50% of the scores fall. Examples of the median are:

Median of *odd* numbers of scores in a distribution (ranked): 4, 7, 9, 15, 20

The median is the middle number of the distribution. If n is *odd*; as shown here with 5 scores, the number 9 is the median.
Median of *even* number of scores in a distribution: 2, 3, 8, 12, 14, 60
The median is the mean of the two middle numbers if n is even; therefore, the median is found by first locating the two middle scores of the distribution which are the numbers 8 and 12. Next find the mean of these scores by summing the values (8 + 12 = 20) and dividing by 2 or 20 ÷ 2 = 10. Ten is the median of the distribution.

The median is not distorted by extreme scores as is the arithmetic mean. For example; 1, 10, 12, 15, and 900 are scores of an odd numbered distribution and 12 is the median which is rather representative of the majority of scores of the distribution. The median is very easy to calculate and define, and uses minimum mathematical computation. The median does not take into consideration the value of each score in the distribution. The median is an ordinal statistic because it ranks the score occurring in the center of a set of data as the "middle" score. This is, if scores are arranged in order, the score designated as the median has the same number of scores on either side of it.

Mode

The mode is the most frequently occurring value or score in a distribution. A distribution may have more than one mode. Examples of modes are: 2, 4, 4, 4, 5, 6, 6, 6, and 6 where the number 6 is the most frequently occurring number and the mode; or 2, 10, 10, 13, 20, and 20 where the numbers 10 and 20 occur with equal frequency and more than any other score so the numbers 10 and 20 are modes. The mode is a nominal statistic and does not depend on the values of measures or their order. The mode is a count or tally representing a particular trait; therefore, it is a nominal value as defined earlier in this chapter.

CHARACTERISTICS OF MEASURES OF CENTRAL TENDENCY

Mean

The mean is used appropriately for interval and ratio measures which can be added and divided because of equal units of division on their scales. The calculation of the mean also involves adding and dividing; it is a statistic which incorporates all scores of a variable in its calculation.[7] The mean can be used for subsequent arithmetical analysis of data.[6] The mean is the most stable or reliable measure of central tendency because it fluctuates less widely than the median and mode.[19] The mean is precisely defined and easy to calculate. It is the best estimate of its corresponding parameter of a population and is the only arithmetical measure that indicates size and postion in a frequency distribution. The mean is good for describing data because it is the balancing point of a set of data. Although the mean is the preferred measure of central tendency in scientific research, it is one of the most abused statistics. When extreme measures are present, the mean is not the best representative of the measures and should not be used. Suppose a set of data contained scores of 1, 55, 60, 48, 62, 51, 52, 58, and 200. The mean of these scores is 65.2, a value larger than most scores, and is not representative of the data as the "average" or balancing point.

Median

The median is used when a measure of central tendency is needed that represents the middle value of a distribution. The median is not distorted by extreme scores; therefore, it is preferred to the mean when the scores of a frequency distribution are grossly asymmetrical.[7] This statistic varies less than the mode on repeated measurements of a variable. Although mathematical procedures are available for its calculation, they are limited and less satisfactory than procedures using interval and ratio data.[6] The median is a measure of position only and not a measure of relative status. It does not incorporate the magnitude of particular scores of the variable in its calculations.

Mode

The mode is used to indicate which score in a distribution has the greatest frequency. When plotting scores along a continuum, the mode is the highest point. It is a crude average that is not unique because one or more modes may occur in a frequency distribution. The mode is a questionable measure of central tendency, since its value may be a low or high score.[20] Upon repeated measurements of a variable, the mode varies more than the mean or median; therefore, it is less stable. The mode could be nonexistent in continuous variables if the measuring instrument is precise enough to prevent two identical scores from being recorded.[17] The mode, when existent, is sensitive only to numerical counts.[6]

MEASURES OF VARIATION

Although the mean is the best measure for providing information about the central value of the distribution (centroid) and represents the entire distribution, the mean is only one point or measure of a distribution. Frequently the mean is not even a score contained among the scores of the sample. Other descriptive information about the distribution is, therefore, desirable. Perhaps you would like some information about how the scores in the distribution are spread or dispersed about the mean. The lowest and highest scores in the distribution or the scatter of scores in one sample as compared to those scores of another sample may be of interest. The researcher is usually concerned with the reasons for causing or contributing to the variation in the data collected in the study.

The various ways scores scatter or spread within a distribution can be expressed by measures of variation or variability. Below are three distributions, each having the same size ($n = 5$), and each having identical means and medians. A cursory observation soon reveals that the distributions are different. How are the distributions different if their size, means, and medians are the same? The distributions differ in their degree of variability.

A	B	C	
1	6	2	
2	7	5	$\Sigma X = 40$
8	8	8	$\overline{X} = 8$
10	9	10	Mdn = 8
19	10	15	

Range

The range is the least complicated measure of variability but is only a rough measure of scatter. The range is the difference between the largest and smallest scores in a distribution. The range for sample A is 18 (19 − 1 = 18), for B the range is 4 (10 − 6 = 4), and for C the range is 13 (15 − 2 = 13). By determining the ranges of the three samples you can easily determine which sample is more variable, sample A. The highest and lowest scores in the range are customarily reported in research studies.

The range has several disadvantages:

1. The range uses only a part of the available information contained in a distribution because it involves only two of the scores.
2. The range does not provide any information about the numbers that

are in a distribution or how the scores are distributed between the highest and lowest scores.
3. The range often becomes larger as the number of scores in the distribution are increased which makes distributions of unequal sizes difficult to compare with each other.

Variance

A student of the life and behavioral sciences soon realizes that measurable characteristics vary. The weight, age, heart rates, nerve conduction velocities, joint range of motions, strength, and lung volumes of patients vary. Life would be boring if variability of measurable characteristics did not occur. Thus, the researcher needs some statistic that will indicate the amount of variability in a set of data. The variance is a statistic that tells you how much the scores of a distribution deviate or scatter from the mean. A small variance indicates that most of the scores are relatively close to the mean, while a large variance indicates that most of the scores are some distance away from the mean.

Since the mean is the balancing point of a distribution of scores, basing the variations of the distribution on the mean as the starting point would seem logical. The variance is formed from the squares of deviation scores from the mean. If you subtracted all scores from the mean, you would notice that some score differences from the mean (deviations) would be positive because the scores were larger than the mean, and some scores would be smaller than the mean or negatively labeled. If all absolute differences (deviations) were added together, observing signs, the sum would be zero, but an old algebraic trick eliminates positive and negative signs by squaring the deviations. To illustrate:

X	Deviation $(X - \bar{X})$	$(X - \bar{X})^2$
2	-2	4
3	-1	1
$4 = \bar{X}$	0	0
5	$+1$	1
6	$+2$	4
$\Sigma = 20 \div 5 = \bar{X} = 4$	$\Sigma = 0$	$\Sigma = 10$

The formula which directs the above calculation is $\Sigma(X - \bar{X})^2$ and is known as sum of deviations squared or sum of squares. If the above formula is used in the calculation of the variance of a large set of data, the work becomes very tedious. Several formulas for calculating the sum of squares exist; these formulas use individual deviations from the mean when determining the variance, and they are equally good.[19] The formula for variance suggested here can be used easily with electronic calculators.

$$\text{Formula for Variance: } s^2 = \frac{\Sigma X^2 - \frac{(\Sigma X)^2}{n}}{n - 1}$$

Where, s^2 is the symbol for the variance of the sample which is the best estimate of the variance of the population, σ^2 (small sigma squared); ΣX^2 is the sum of all the squares (square each score and add up all the squares); $(\Sigma X)^2$ is the square of the sum (add up all the scores and square the sum; (e.g., $2 + 2 + 4 + 5 + 6)^2$); n is the size of the sample or number of scores (e.g., $n = 5$ in $2 + 3 + 4 + 5 + 6$); and $n - 1$ is a method, for certain algebraic reasons, of determining an unbiased estimate of σ^2. An unbiased statistic is one that will not show any systematic tendency or trend to be greater or less than the parameter of the population.

Table 5.5 is an example of calculating the variance from a sample. The result of the example shows that the variance is a descriptive index of how each score differed from every other score; the variance is an average of the squared deviations from the mean.[21] The variance is a measure of deviation (dispersion, scatter, or spread) of scores about the mean. The variance is sometimes referred to as the second moment;[16] is a measure of variability that is not related to the size of the sample, and is independent of the mean. That is, the variance reflects similarity or dissimilarity of the scores contained in the sample, and by examining the variance you cannot determine the balancing point of the distribution of scores. Unfortunately,

Table 5.5
Wound Size Before Physical Therapy (diameter in cm)

X (cm)	X^2		
5	25		
2	4	$\overline{X}$	= 6 cm
10	100	n	= 10
7	49		
6	36	s^2	$= \dfrac{\Sigma X^2 - \dfrac{(\Sigma X)^2}{n}}{n - 1}$
5	25		
4	16		
8	64		
7	49		$= \dfrac{404 - \dfrac{(60)^2}{10}}{10 - 1}$
6	36		
$\Sigma X = 60$	$\Sigma X^2 = 404$		
			$= \dfrac{404 - 360}{9} = \dfrac{44}{9}$
			$= 4.88888*$ cm^2

* Note: 4.88888 rounded up to two decimal points = 4.89 cm^2 = Variance.

the variance is not easily interpretable because its unit of measure is in squared terms of the variable. In the example, the variance of 4.89 is in centimeters squared (cm^2) but does not indicate area, since the original unit was measured as the diameter of the wound in units of centimeters. The researcher needs some statistic that will tell him about the size or magnitude of the variability throughout the distribution in the same unit as the values of the variable.

Standard Deviation

Since the variation is in squared units, a measure of variability that is not in squared units, but tells you something about the magnitude of the variation of the scores in the sample is desirable. The standard deviation is expressed in units of the raw data, and is the square root of the variance. The standard deviation is also defined as the square root of the mean of the squared deviations from the mean.[6]

The formula for the standard deviation is:

$$s = \sqrt{\frac{\Sigma X^2 - \frac{(\Sigma X)^2}{n}}{n - 1}}$$

where s is the symbol for standard deviation. The standard deviation is the measure of variability most frequently reported in the literature, although the variance is probably the most important measure of variability for statistical calculations. In the research literature the standard deviation is reported:

1. by spelling out the two words, standard deviation,
2. by abbreviating the two words, SD,
3. by reporting the value following the mean, 6.0 ± 2.21 cm,
4. or by using the symbol, s.

The standard deviation reflects the variability of scores within a sample and is based on how far the scores deviate from the mean. A large value for standard deviation indicates a large amount of variation within the sample, while a small value is indicative of little variation.

Coefficient of Variation

In practice, the researcher might wish to compare the magnitudes of standard deviations of similar populations; that is, you might wish to know whether scores of a certain motor development test are more variable than scores by the same group of children on another motor development test. Making these comparisons by using the standard deviations would be very risky, since the scores of the different samples might also have different means or units of measurement. The standard deviation is based on the squared deviations about the mean of a specific group of scores and when different standard deviations are compared with data having different means, the interpretations could be erroneous.

In order to compare the variability of different populations, a method of relative variation has been developed. The coefficient of variation is a ratio expression of the standard deviation and the mean in terms of a percentage; it has no units of measurement.

The formula for the coefficient of variation is:

$$CV = \frac{s}{\overline{X}} \times 100$$

A high percentage would indicate considerable variability in a set of data whereas a low percentage would indicate a small amount of variability in the data.

Using the results of a group of children on two different motor development tests, the coefficient of variation might be:

Test A:

$$CV = \frac{0.25}{5.00} \times 100 = 0.05 \times 100 = 5\%$$

Test B:

$$CV = \frac{5.00}{50.00} \times 100 = 0.10 \times 100 = 10\%$$

Comparison of the coefficients indicates that the children's scores were more variable on Test B (10%) than on Test A (5%).

The coefficients of variation were used in the study on recording electrode placement in median and peroneal nerve conduction studies in which latency and amplitude measurements were compared to ascertain the relative variability within the different measurements. Results of computing the coefficients showed that measurements of muscle action potentials were more variable than latency measurements, and therefore, the physical therapist using these measurements could place more reliance on values of latency than amplitudes of muscle action potentials when assessing the functional integrity of motor nerves.[22]

Percentiles, Percentile Ranks, and Quartiles

Often the description of the relative position of a score in a distribution is needed, particularly in descriptive research (Chapter 6). The standard deviation is not always the best way to describe the spread of scores in a distribution. Percentiles, percentile ranks, and quartiles describe the spread of observations in a sample[21] and their relative positions. These measures are ordinal level statistics.

A percentile is a score in the distribution which divides the frequency into hundredths (100 equal parts).[21,23] Suppose a certain percentage of individuals of a distribution have scores less than a specific value, the value below which the certain percentage of individuals lie is the percentile. If 76% of individuals on a 50-item test score below 38, the value of 38 is the 76th percentile (P_{76}). The calculation of percentiles in Table 5.6 can be made from data presented earlier under Frequency Distributions.

Each score has limits (−0.05 and +0.05) taken as one-half a unit below and above the reported value. For example, a value of 3.3 msec will have limits of 3.25 and 3.35 msec. In calculating the 30th percentile, the value below which 30% of the observations lie is six ($0.30 \times 20 = 6$). Looking at Table 5.6, the sixth observation or individual has a value of 3.3 msec and the upper limit is 3.35 msec. Thus, 3.35 msec is the value below which 30% of the observations lie, $P_{30} = 3.35$ msec. Any percentile desired can be determined similarly.

Percentiles are calculated according to particular ranks. Percentile ranks are calculated according to specific values or the reverse process of calculating percentiles.[7] Look at Table 5.6 and select the 13th individual whose score is 3.5 msec. The number of individuals having a latency below number 13 is 12 or 60% ($^{12}/_{20} \times 100 = 60\%$). Number 13 occupies one-half of the value or distance between 3.5 and the next higher value of 3.8 msec (number 14) or 2.5% ($^{1}/_{20} \times 100 = 5 \div 2 = 2.5\%$). The values between two observations must be considered for establishing percentile ranks corrsponding to exact values. If the 2.5% is added to the 60% already obtained, the percentile rank of the value 3.5 msec is 62.5. Percentile ranks are used to express scores obtained in survey instruments (Chapter 6).

Quartile is a generic term for a score dividing the distribution into four parts or quarters. The first quartile corresponds to the 25th percentile, the second to the median, and the third to the 75th percentile. The quartile deviation is a measure of variability which is defined as half of the difference between the 75th and the 25th percentiles. The formula for quartile

Table 5.6
Latencies of Median Nerve ($N = 20$) in Rank Order

Individual	Latency (msec)	Individual	Latency (msec)
1	2.8	11	3.5
2	3.2	12	3.5
3	3.2	13	3.5
4	3.2	14	3.8
5	3.3	15	3.8
6	3.3	16	3.8
7	3.4	17	4.0
8	3.4	18	4.0
9	3.4	19	4.0
10	3.5	20	4.2

deviation is:

$$Q = \frac{Q_3 - Q_1}{2}$$

where Q is the quartile deviation, Q_3 is the 75th percentile expressed as a quartile, Q_1 is the 25th quartile, and 2 divides the difference between the two quartiles in half. The 25th quartile of the data presented in Table 5.6 is 3.35 msec. This value was obtained by multiplying N by 25% and adding the one-half unit above the value for the upper limit ($20 \times 0.25 = 5$th individual or 3.3 msec; $3.3 + 0.05 = 3.35$ msec). The 75th percentile is 3.85 msec. The quartile deviation is then found by placing the quartile values in the formula and solving for Q.

$$Q = \frac{3.85 - 3.35}{2} = \frac{0.50}{2} = 0.25 \text{ msec}$$

The quartile deviation is used for computing the Thurstone attitude scale (Chapter 6) and provides a quick and easy descriptive measure of the variability.

PROBABILITY

Students who have not yet taken a course in research methods or statistics are often overheard saying that something is true because "it" was proven by a research study which was reported in some journal. This faith in reported studies is encouraging to those who report research studies, but yet may be harmful. Researchers deal with probability rather than certainty when reporting their findings of a particular research study.

What is probability? Kerlinger has said "Probability is an obvious and simple subject. It is a baffling and complex subject. It is a subject we know a great deal about, and a subject we know nothing about. Kindergartners can study probability, and philosophers do. It is dull; it is interesting. Such contradictions are the stuff of probability."[24] Probability is chance occurrence, likelihood, and randomness.

Probability is a concept and method of estimating what might or should happen in light of what has happened. That is, the researcher concludes or infers from what the collected data indicate; a risk is taken when making conclusions or inferences. Probability is not absolute, but an estimate or a chance of something or event occurring. The findings of one research study, unfortunately or fortunately, do not make the situation absolute. Conclusions are based on a chance occurrence and, therefore, the decisions or inferences are not absolute. Sustained study or replication of research projects is really needed. The possibility exists that a single report is wrong or that a replicated study refutes the original study; on the other hand, the original reported study may be true. Which study is then correct? Additional replication is essential to resolve the question. Often researchers ignore replication, thinking that only originality is meritorious. If the original report is never challenged then we continue to have faith in a concept that may really be false. For years the vastus medialis was believed to be solely responsible for the last 15 degrees of full knee extension. This belief was challenged with the use of electromyography and it is now believed that the vastus medialis functions in concert (phasically) with other components of the quadriceps to perform knee extension and that all components of the quadriceps contribute to full extension of the knee. This is an example of one study for which no replication was performed for many years following the acceptance of a tenuous concept; acceptance on blind faith.

No intent is made here to discredit reports in any way. To the contrary, this book supports research and its processes. The point being made is that the researcher bases conclusions on the probability that the conclusions are true. The reader must understand probability theory and realize that there is always some possibility that the conclusions based on data of a "one-shot" study may be erroneous. Fortunately, most of the time, reports are accurate and true and the authors of the report are truthful; conclusions are based in light of the collected data and the probability that the data are representative of the population or universe.

Historically, mathematicians developed the probability theory in efforts to win at gambling. Everyone has talked about his or her chances of winning something. Horse racing, card playing, batting in baseball, or staying alive while driving on a freeway are problems in probability.[7]

THE NORMAL CURVE

The theory of errors states that chance events or occurrences in large numbers tend to arrange themselves in the form of a bell-shaped curve. This curve is called the normal curve, the bell curve, the normal probability curve, and the normal distribution (Fig. 5.1). The normal curve is a mathematical paradigm or standard which permits the researcher to compare collected data to the "ideal" and then to make reliable conclusions, decisions, and predictions from the collected data. Few observable variables in research conform exactly to the normal curve when plotted, but frequently collected data approximate the normal curve. The normal curve offers convenience and practical application of mathematical theory through statistics.[24]

Figure 5.1 displays the normal curve which is smooth, and the ends never touch the baseline (asymptotic). Asymptotic implies that the distribution contains an infinite number of data which have no limits. The normal curve is representative of the population.

If you draw a broken line perpendicular from the midpoint of the peak

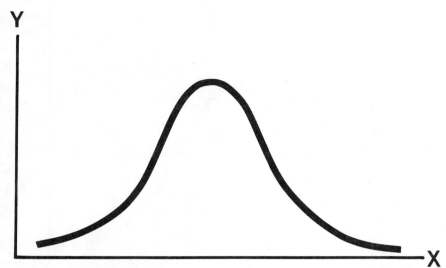

Figure 5.1.   Normal curve.

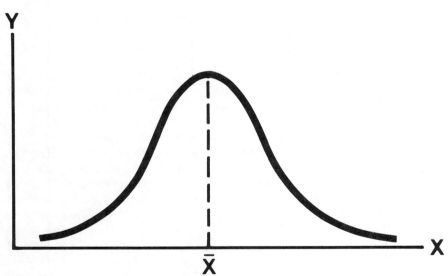

Figure 5.2.   Normal curve showing where the mean bisects the distribution.

to the abscissa (X), the point where the line bisects the abscissa can represent the mean of the distribution (Fig. 5.2). Each proportion on either side of the mean (broken line) will be ½ or 50% of the curve. If additional perpendicular lines (ordinates, Y line) are drawn from the inflexion points of the curve to the abscissa, the proportions can represent specific percentages or proportions of total area of the curve or probability (Fig. 5.3). An inflexion point is a point along the curve where the curve changes in

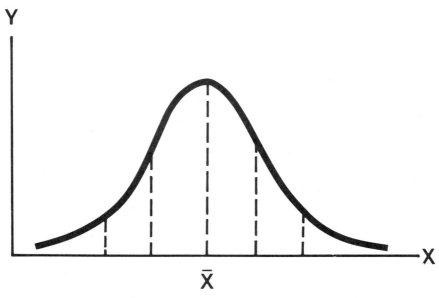

Figure 5.3. Broken lines are drawn from inflexion points to show proportional areas from the normal curve.

respect to the abscissa (*X* axis) from convexity (upward) to concavity (downward).[2] The proportions marked off along the abscissa correspond to standard deviation (SD) units because of the mathematical paradigm of the normal probability curve. In the normal curve the mean is designated as zero and units to the right or above the mean are labeled positively as +1, +2, and +3 standard deviation units. Units to the left or below the mean are labeled negatively as: −1, −2, and −3, respectively. The area between +1 and −1 standard deviation units represents about 68% (34.13 + 34.13%). The area between ±2 standard deviation units represents about 95% (47.72 + 47.72%) of the area, while ±3 standard deviation units are about 99% (49.87 ± 49.87%) of the total area of the normal curve (Fig. 5.4). Additional units can be calculated since in theory, the end lines of the curve are asymptotic (infinite) and never end, but in practice, ±3 standard deviation units are usually considered representative of the total area. The curve is symmetrical and extends from plus infinity to minus infinity. The curve can now be used to compare collected (obtained) research data to the ideal, or normal, or standard paradigm.

If we measured 50 young women for maximum isometric force of the quadriceps with the knee positioned at 60 degrees from full extension, and obtained a mean force of 60 kg and a standard deviation of 15 kg, we could interpret the data using the normal curve. We could say that about 68% of the scores should fall between 45 and 75 kg (±1 SD from mean;

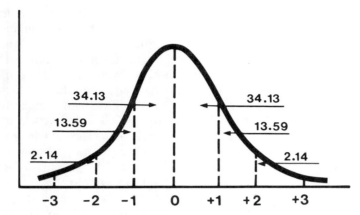

Figure 5.4. Normal curve showing areas (%) between ordinals at different standard deviations.

60 ± 15). If we continued to measure the quadriceps strength of thousands of equal sized samples of women under similarly controled conditions, we could plot the mean values of the samples and find that over the long haul (thousands) the mean values would follow a curve similar to the normal curve. Individual means will fluctuate by chance, but ultimately, the total group of means collected will cluster into the various proportions of the normal curve. Since testing infinite (population) numbers of subjects is not practical from a time and money point of view, small samples can be tested, the results can be compared with the normal curve, and reliable inferences can be made by the researcher about the population or quadriceps of all women in the world given rigid controlled limitations of the selection criteria (age, mass, health, and physical activities).

GATHERING DATA

The purpose of research is to learn something about people, about events, or about specific "traits". To learn about these traits we gather information by taking several of them and studying the characteristic or variable of interest. After our study, we come to some conclusion—physical therapists are good people, hot packs are useless, or eccentric exercise is effective. In order to come to the conclusion, we must sample characteristics or data. We must take a portion of the defined population for study and on the basis of the information contained in the portion selected, make a conclusion.

Making the correct choice of subjects or characteristics for the study will increase the likelihood of obtaining a representative population and, therefore, improving the generalizability of the results of the study. If a physical therapist wants to study the effects of ultrasound on "frozen shoulder" the logical choice of subjects would be patients with frozen shoulder. Any patient having frozen shoulder may not suffice for answering the question. Frozen shoulder resulting from disuse (fractures or muscular paralyses) may not be the same as that resulting from some acute inflammatory process. The point being made is that the study must be conducted on samples which are truly representative of a well defined population. No perfect method exists for choosing a sample which would assure an exact representativeness of the population. Successive samples taken from any population will differ among samples and from the population. The variation is called sampling variation and should be given consideration whenever conclusions are based on the data of a sample.[25]

An understanding of the concept of sampling is important to the researcher in order to avoid making incorrect conclusions from data gathered. The method used to gather the data can influence the outcome of the research and limit the statements made about the data of a sample (generalizability). The method selected for gathering data will also help in determining statistical design of the study.

Advantages of sampling have been cited by Daniel and Coogler.[26]

1. Reduced cost. Measuring a particular trait on every member of a population is economically impossible if the population consists of everyone in the universe. If the population is defined as all staff members of a particular hospital, then there is no need for sampling because all staff members can be measured economically. Sampling, however, reduces costs of research by involving fewer items than those contained in a large population.
2. Increased speed. Again, when dealing with a large population, you could not measure every member in a lifetime. Sampling enables the time commitment of the study to be within practical limits of the investigator's schedule.
3. Increased accuracy. By reducing the number of data in the study, all energy and time can be focused on the details of managing and interpreting the data.[26]

In research involving human subjects a biased sample threatens the accuracy of the findings. Sample bias can be prevented by observing proper probability sampling formats.[27]

Models of Samples

The Random and Independent Sample. The random and independent sample is a method of selecting a portion of a population. Random implies that each member of the population has the same chance (probability) of being selected into the sample, while independent means that the selection of any one member in no way affects the selection of any other member.[2] Random sampling is used to generalize results to the population, to comply with the assumed premises of certain statistics, and to reduce biases likely to result from selection of other procedures.[28] This type of sampling is impossible in practice if the population is defined as the universe. Each member does not have an equal chance of being selected into the sample because of the infinite number of members. When defined populations are small, the random sampling method is used commonly. For example, if you wished to sample the physical therapists graduating in a particular year, the names and addresses could be obtained, labeled, and a sample of desired size drawn from the complete listing. This procedure would be random and independent if every new graduate had an equal chance of being selected into the sample, and if a selected graduate in no way affected the next selection into the sample. Tables of random numbers are available for the purpose of random sampling. The researcher places a finger over a spot on the table of random numbers without looking; the number underneath the finger is selected and the graduate's name having the corresponding number is selected into the sample. The procedure is continued until the sample quota is reached. Another procedure involves placing all numbers into a hat and selecting concealed numbers from the hat (lottery).

The Stratified Random Sample. This method is used commonly in public polls. The population is divided into sub-groups or strata; each stratum contains a particular characteristic of interest, but only one characteristic is contained in any one strata. Each stratum is sampled randomly and the various subsamples collected from the strata are combined as the desired sample.

An example will help clarify the procedure. Let us say arbitrarily that the Canadian Physiotherapy Association has 6000 members consisting of 1% (60), members having doctoral degrees; 10% (600), having master's degrees; 35% (2,100), having baccalaureate degrees; and the remaining 54% (3,240), members having diplomas. Strata are represented by the numbers enclosed in parentheses. If the size of the sample was to be 10% (600) of the population (6000) then each stratum would contribute the percentage proportional to the population percentages. One percent (6) of 600 selected randomly from the doctorate stratum would constitute the partial sample representative of that portion of the population. Additional random samples would then consist of 60, 210, and 324 to compose the stratified random sample of members having various backgrounds of academic preparation. Stratified sampling is best when the variables of interest are closely related to the variables on which strata are based.[24]

Proportioning the strata is important if the researcher wishes to preserve the natural concentration of sections within the population. If 100 members of the Orthopaedics Section of the American Physical Therapy Association and 100 non-members of the Orthopaedics Section were surveyed to determine whether the Section should be given special status by the Association, the outcome would be obvious. The survey should maintain the proportion of the two groups if stratified random sampling is the preferred method of sampling. If there are 35,000 members of the Association and 7,000 are members of the Section, then the sample must include 20% from the Section and 80% non-members of the Section to maintain the proportion.

The Systematic Sample. This procedure is effective when a complete list of the members of the population is available for selecting the sample. If the researcher knew he had access to 100 children with cerebral palsy but wanted a sample of only 25 for study, the systematic sampling method would be appropriate. The population (100) is divided by the size of the sample (25) to obtain a quotient of 4 (100 ÷ 25 = 4). The researcher would place the names of the first four children into a hat and select the name of one randomly. Thereafter, every 4th name appearing on the list would be selected until 25 children were selected into the sample. In practice, some researchers arbitarily establish a systematic procedure other than the one discussed; for example, every other child with cerebral palsy appearing in the clinic where the researcher is employed is selected for study.

The Sample of Convenience. Researchers often accept volunteers or subjects into the study because the subjects are available to the researchers. In the hospital the sample might consist of 20 patients having fractures of the humerus; in the university it might consist of 30 volunteer students or the 50 rats purchased because these members of the sample were conveniently available or willing to participate. This method permits little choice about which subject will be chosen.[26]

Some statisticians have reservations about this technique, in spite of its frequent use in research. The procedure is subject to biases.[23] If you wanted to determine whether a new approach to increasing muscular strength was effective, a hidden bias might be that all volunteers are highly conditioned athletes and strength gains would normally be slow with this group of subjects. The effects of the new approach to exercise might be overlooked or not be evident in this group because of the bias caused by conditioning. Defining the population as being composed only of subjects conditioned similarly to those included in the samples has been suggested as an acceptable solution.[29]

The Cluster Sample. Another method of sampling that saves time and money, and is convenient, is cluster sampling. The population is defined and then non-overlapping regions of sub-groups (clusters) are formed. The cluster method seeks heterogeneity in the cluster. Clusters may be composed of geographical or census units. Once the clusters are identified, several are selected randomly. When the randomly selected clusters are formed, samples from each of these clusters are selected randomly, and combined to form the desired sample size.

Suppose a researcher is interested in seeking information about a sample of patients having had the Neer shoulder prosthesis during a particular period of time. Fifty hospitals where the type of shoulder surgery was performed during the designated period are identified. Ten hospitals are selected randomly from the 50 hospitals and then two cases are chosen randomly from each selected hospital to compose a sample of 20 patients.

CHARACTERISTICS OF THE SAMPLING METHODS

Random Sampling

The random sampling method is used when a population is defined so that any individual may be drawn independently for inclusion in the sample. Usually, individuals are selected from intact groups. An intact group might be students of a particular school, all patients in a particular hospital on a given day, or all therapists assigned to a particular state chapter of the American Physical Therapy Association. It is a good technique for survey research. Random sampling has certain advantages: no prior knowledge of the traits or characteristics of the population are necessary, the larger the sample size the more representative the sample becomes because it approaches the population size, and most statistical analyses are appropriate.[30] Use of random sampling is difficult if the study requires patients having a particular condition because the type of patient is not generally a member of an intact group. The intact group might, however, be possible if time and money are available for studying patients over widely dispersed geographical areas. Random sampling requires that all individuals in the defined population be labeled or numbered; this may also be costly and time consuming. Other sampling methods which are available can gather the same information but much more economically than the random sampling method.

Stratified Sampling

This method of sampling is used when representativeness of a defined population is essential to the study. It identifies sub-group characteristics within the defined population and permits random sampling of individuals within the sub-groups (strata). Stratified sampling increases in precision when the characteristic being observed has some relationship with the characteristic by which the sub-groups are defined. Since the weight of subjects is related to their height, precision is gained for estimating height if the population is subdivided by weight. If the individuals within the strata are listed separately, the proportional samples are easily obtained. Although large numbers of individuals are required in the population, fewer numbers in the population are required than for random sampling. Stratified random sampling requires elaborate methods for estimating the population's parameters.

Systematic Sampling

The systematic sampling method is used to replace the random sample technique because of similarities or in conjunction with other methods (e.g., stratified). The method is generally inexpensive and rapid to complete. The procedures are easy to grasp. It differs from random sampling because each member of the population is not selected independently. Members of the sample are automatically selected once the first subject has been chosen. The procedure requires a list of individuals in the defined population which can restrict its use because of the inability to list all members. Arrangements of individuals on the lists can cause trends or periodic variations rather than random selection of samples. Systematic sampling is an acceptable replacement for random sampling if the list of individuals is in random order. The estimation of the population parameters is difficult.[30]

Cluster Sampling

Cluster sampling is used to reduce the large numbers of individuals needed for the random and stratified methods. It is well suited for use in studying intact groups; for example, students in classes of a school. It is used when it is either impossible or impractical to obtain a list of all members of a defined population. Clusters are relatively representative of a population and save sizable cost and time required by most other methods. The parts of a cluster are considerably more homogeneous than in random samples. Statistical analyses are difficult and the homogeneity of clusters results in some loss of precision. Individuals are not selected randomly but are drawn in bunches (clusters).

Convenience Sampling

This method is used when other procedures of sampling are not practical. Convenience sampling is used more and more in health related research because legal and ethical constraints require the researcher to obtain informed consent from human subjects prior to their participation in the study. Although research has revealed that volunteers display distinguishing characteristics that may or may not require consideration when planning a study,[31] it is virtually impossible to obtain informed consent of all individuals when selected randomly. Once volunteers have consented to participate in the research study, they can be assigned randomly to a

Table 5.7
Cumulative Summary of the Research Processes Presented

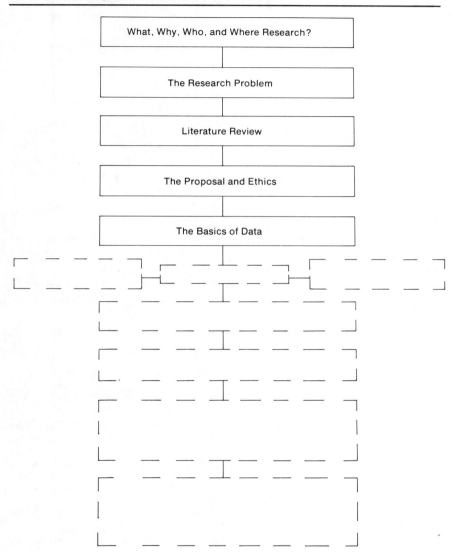

control group or to different experimental modes. Considerable savings in time and costs result from using a sample of convenience. It, however, affords little choice about which individual will be chosen and this may cause biasing. This sampling method may permit selection of individuals in such a manner that random selection is not assured.[26] Although a sample of convenience does not meet the requirements of random sampling, it is acceptable providing that the researcher infers that the study results only apply to populations resembling the sample.[28] The population should be defined so that individuals drawn from samples compose a larger collection of subjects having similar characteristics.[26]

The student should be aware of the uses and shortcomings of the various sampling methods before engaging in research.

SUMMARY

Research involves the process of observing and measuring phenomena. When measured phenomena are quantified, mathematics can be applied to simplify interpretation. Quantitative measurements increase efficiency of research enormously, but before an investigation begins the researcher must have a clear understanding of the basics of data. Probability theory is an important concept in research and is the base of statistics that enable researchers to analyze data.

Data gathering or samping is important to the researcher in order to avoid making incorrect conclusions and predictions. Several methods of sampling have been presented.

This chapter has introduced the reader to the concept of quantitation in research. Table 5.7 provides a summary of what research processes have been presented thus far.

REFERENCES

1. Random House Dictionary of the English Language, unabridged ed. New York, Random House, 1967
2. Meyers LS, Grossen NE: Behavioral Research Theory, Procedure, and Design. ed 2. San Francisco, WH Freeman and Co, 1978
3. Curwen MP: Statistics in clinical research. Physiotherapy 56: 116–118, 1970
4. Wandelt M: Guide for the Beginning Researcher. New York, Appleton-Century-Crofts, 1970
5. Alder HL, Roessler EB: Introduction to Probability and Statistics, ed 6. San Francisco, WH Freeman and Co, 1977
6. Morehouse CA, Stull GA: Statistical Principles and Procedures with Applications for Physical Education. Philadelphia, Lea & Febiger, 1975
7. Ferguson GA: Statistical Analyses in Psychology and Education, ed 5. New York, McGraw-Hill Book Co., 1981
8. Sokal RR, Rohlf FJ: Introduction to Biostatistics. San Francisco, WH Freeman and Co, 1973
9. Inman VT, Ralston HJ, Saunders JB de Cm, et al: Relation of human electromyogram to muscular tension. Electroencephalogr Clin Neurophysiol 4: 187–194, 1952
10. Michels E: Measurement in physical therapy: on the rules for assigning numerals to observations. Phys Ther 63: 209–215, 1983
11. Peat M, Campbell G: Measurement in physical therapy. Physiother Canada 31: 132–136, 1979
12. Stevens SS: Mathematics, Measurement, and Psychophysics. In Stevens SS (ed): Handbook of Experimental Psychology. New York, John Wiley & Sons, Inc, 1951

13. Brown FG: Principles of Educational and Psychological Testing, ed 2. Hinsdale, IL, The Dryden Press Inc, 1976
14. Bolton B, Lawlis GF, Brown RH: Scores and Norms. In Bolton B (ed): Measurements and Evaluation in Rehabilitation. Baltimore, University Park Press, 1976
15. Style Manual, ed 4. Washington, American Physical Therapy Association, 1976
16. Schor SS: Fundamentals of Biostatistics. New York, GP Putnam's Sons, 1968
17. Edwards AL: Statistical Analysis, ed 4. New York, Holt, Rinehart and Winston, Inc, 1974
18. Weinberg GH, Schumaker JA: Statistics: An Intuitive Approach, ed 4. Belmont, CA, Brooks/Cole Publishing Co, 1980
19. Guilford JP, Fruchter B: Fundamental Statistics in Psychology and Education, ed 6. New York, McGraw-Hill Book Co, 1977
20. Horowitz, LM: Elements of Statistics for Psychology and Education. New York, McGraw-Hill Book Co, 1974
21. Huntsberger DV, Leaverton PE: Statistical Inference in the Biomedical Sciences. Boston, Allyn and Bacon, Inc, 1970
22. Currier DP: Placement of recording electrode in median and peroneal nerve conduction studies. Phys Ther 55: 365–370, 1975
23. Remington RD, Schork MA: Statistics with Applications to the Biological and Health Sciences. Englewood Cliffs, NJ, Prentice-Hall, Inc, 1970
24. Kerlinger FN: Foundations of Behavioral Research, ed 2. New York, Holt, Rinehart and Winston, Inc, 1973
25. Wilson EB Jr: An Introduction to Scientific Research. New York, McGraw-Hill Book Co, 1952
26. Daniel WW, Coogler CE: Sampling in physical therapy research. Phys Ther 55: 1326–1331, 1975
27. Crocker LM: Let's reduce the communication gap. Guidelines for preparing a research article. Phys Ther 54: 971–976, 1974
28. Makrides L, Richman J: Research methodology and applied statistics, Part 5: experimental design. Physiother Canada 33: 6–14, 1981
29. Dunn OJ: Basic Statistics: A Primer for the Biomedical Sciences, ed 2. New York, John Wiley & Sons, Inc, 1977
30. Montoye HJ: Collecting Data. In Hubbard AW (ed): Research Methods in Health, Physical Education, and Recreation, ed 3. Washington, Am Assoc Health Phys Educ Rec, 1973
31. Rosenthal R, Rosnow RL: The Volunteer Subject. New York, John Wiley & Sons, Inc, 1975

6

Non-Experimental Research

Research is a great adventure of the mind.
Gen. Dwight D. Eisenhower

Non-experimental research is an endeavor which depicts and portrays traits and abilities of subjects; shows the status of a group or organization; or reveals trends or changes in characteristics of people. It may describe conditions as they occur without the influence of the research.[1] Descriptive studies are called behavioral research if used to study the behavior or reactions of human beings,[2] or they are referred to as survey research if used to answer a question or depict opinions of subjects.[3] Non-experimental research may satisfy curiosity, may solve a problem, and may be considered as any investigation not involving experimentation.[4] The data gathering procedures of non-experimental research enable the investigator to determine how facts relate to the problem being studied. Non-experimental research may be considered as a process of systematic data collection.

Non-experimental research is used in this book as an "umbrella" term to include techniques that permit collection of data without rigid controls, that do not involve experimentation, that measure behavioral characteristics by means of software instruments, and that may be descriptive. Instruments used in non-experimental research methods are generally less precise than instruments used in experimental investigation because of the often evasive nature of the substance observed and studied. Software or paper instruments are the data gathering tools of non-experimental research.[5] Statistical analyses can be applied to data gathered by software instruments because numerical values can be assigned to behaviors. A criticism of descriptive procedures is that they depend heavily on verbal behavior of respondents[6] and judgment of the observer.

Although non-experimental procedures are commonly used in social sciences, psychology, education, and the humanities, they are also used widely in business and health fields. In health and medical research non-experimental methods are used to study the nature and extent of illness, attitudes about use and receipt of health services, socioeconomic problems, growth and development processes, and harmful factors in the physical environment.[7]

Non-experimental research uses techniques of obtaining information directly or indirectly from the people being studied. Some specific instruments used in the direct technique are the oral interview, observations of behavior, rating scales, checklists, photographs, oral or practical test, and case reports. The indirect technique employs the questionnaire, attitude scale, classroom tests, and examinations of records. Depending on their use, some instruments may be used for direct and indirect techniques. If the instrument is administered and recorded by an observer, the technique is direct. On the other hand, an instrument may be self-administered and recorded by the individual being studied indirectly. Rating scales, checklists, questionnaires, and diaries could be interpreted as being direct and indirect techniques of non-experimental research.

Instruments are used in non-experimental research to obtain standardized information from sampled individuals or groups. The same instrument must be administered to all members of the sample, as well as the maintenance of similar conditions of administration. Information gathered from the sampling must be quantified (forced or multiple choice questions) or codified (open-ended questions) so that it can be analyzed and reported quantitatively. If the information is collected from a sample selected from a predetermined population and is gathered at one point or period of time, it is a cross-sectional survey. If the entire defined population is querried, the survey is called a census. When the data are gathered at different points or periods of time to study time-ordered relationships, the process may be referred as a longitudinal survey.[8]

Discussion in this chapter will concentrate only on certain procedures and instruments used in non-experimental research. These procedures and instruments represent direct and indirect approaches to data collection. The various instruments presented can operate in and outside of laboratory situations. That is, instruments such as rating scales, checklists, and questionnaires can be used in experimental research. An investigator may wish to compare behaviors of a group of subjects on two different occasions using rating scales. Whenever a method of comparison involving two or more groups, events, or quantities is used in a study, the process may be an experiment. The experimental methods of research are discussed later in this book. The historical method is also discussed briefly. This method is performed outside of the conventional laboratory setting. Although informative studies are descriptive and exploratory, they establish norms or baseline data.

DIRECT METHODS

Oral Interview

The oral interview is a way of involving the investigator or his assistants face-to-face with the subject for the purpose of obtaining information through conversation.

Types of Oral Interviews. The interview can be classified into one of two types which are functions of their classification.

1. Informal. This type of interview is used in reviewing applicants for employment or college admissions, or in counseling employees. Questions are usually devised during the actual process of the interview in accord with the spontaneous needs of the interviewer and direction of the conversation. The responses are free (open-ended); that is, the interviewee responds spontaneously to questions or flow of conversation between the individuals involved in the interview. The informal interview is very flexible in the directions of conversation. The informality enables the respondent to relax and react as if the situation were taking place in a natural and commonplace fashion, an everyday type of situation. The informal interview can be held with the respondent and several interviewers; for example, while dining or during the process of group dialogue.

Since the purpose of interviewing is to gather information that cannot be obtained in another manner, the interviewer forms impressions and following the interviewing session, puts the impressions into some narrative form. A record of the conversation is made for later recall and as a source for comparing other respondents. The informal interview is not often used, however, for research because of its lack of organization of specific and similar questions asked of all interviewees. In other words, the informal interview is not structured in advance and can change directions many times during the course of conversation in regard to needs, personalities, and responses of the interviewees. This form is unlikely to be consistent when repeated. Occasionally the informal interview is used in pilot research where the researcher wants to determine the feasibility of a content area or to ascertain appropriateness of questions in advance of an actual study. As questions become more directed and organized in specific content areas, the informal interview loses some of its informality and approaches the formal type of interview.

2. Formal. The formal interview is used in research because questions are organized in advance of the interview, the questions concern only specific content areas, and the responses are controlled. In controlled responses the respondent is given specific choices of responses to each question and must select one of the choices provided by the interviewer.

For example, the patient might be questioned about how many physical therapy treatments she received for a low back strain, but the choices of response may be: "less than five," "five to ten," or "more than ten" treatments. The respondent would then select one of the choices as the controlled response to the question (forced choice). The formal interview possesses better uniformity and comparability than that of the informal interview because of its controlled structure. Responses to the formal interview can be consistent; and therefore, may be used as a research instrument. Only the formal interview is discussed in detail.

Planning the Formal Interview. Questions are planned in some coordinated pattern before the interview is administered. Several questions may have to be devised in order to obtain the desired information about one content area. Various changes of wording may be necessary when asking questions in sensitive areas. Respondents of the interview must understand the questions completely before correct or satisfactory responses can be expected. The questions must be structured in language that ensures effective communication between the interviewer and the respondent. The entire interview sequence (guide or schedule) should be planned and organized in advance of the actual interviewing of subjects. In preparation of the interview, questions should be written and rewritten several times to obtain full information and to avoid ambiguity. The informal interview can be used to test questions among friends, experts in the content areas, or a few patients for whom the interview will be intended. This pilot (exploratory) approach can provide the researcher with valuable information about appropriateness of questions, reactions to questions, levels of understanding of questions, and length of time needed for the interviews. Questions must be planned carefully and worded precisely.

Requirements for Successful Interviewing. Planning the questions carefully has been mentioned. Selection and training of interviewers are very important and will be discussed separately. The order of questioning is important; questions that seek priority information must be asked early in the interview in case the respondent becomes disinterested and refuses to answer any more questions. Controversial or sensitive type questions should be saved until the end of the interview to avoid abrupt termination of interviews before the most important information has been obtained. Using several interviewers with each having small numbers of subjects to interview reduces fatigue of the interviewer, interviewer bias, and length of time for the study.[9] A preface outlining the need, purpose, and use of the interview information is very helpful in setting the tone of the interview and relieving any apprehension of the respondent. Assurance of anonymity of the respondent is important. If a tape recorder is used, the respondent must be aware of and agree fully to its use. Taping or note taking is advisable when the respondent provides non-confidential factual and statistical information but not if he is giving confidential matter.[10] Taping and note-taking may threaten the respondent in the latter situation. Nevertheless, the interviewer must choose one of these methods. The exact recording of responses as well as the exact questioning must be followed during interviews for preservation of the information.[11]

Job of the Interviewer. Once the interview plan has been determined, the interviewer must locate members of the sample. Sometimes locating members might mean traveling to different locations within or outside a city. Going from house to house, or interviewing physical therapists while working may be examples of the traveling needs of a study. The interviewer must obtain the interview after locating a member of the sample.

The interviewer must gain acceptance of the respondent and gain access to the interview by being polite, friendly, and having consideration of the respondent's available time. The interviewer must ask questions with an acceptable tone of voice, interpret responses, and proportion the time of the interview but allowed enough time for the respondent to respond in the manner he wishes. The interviewer's job has been estimated as one-third interviewing and two-thirds traveling, locating respondents, editing interviews, and performing required clerical tasks.[9]

Interviewer Training. Training each interviewer on interview proceedings will generally improve the quality of the study. Interviewers must have training, even for highly structured interviews, if dependable and objective information is to be gathered. The amount of training required rises as the extent of the interview increases and its structure decreases.[8] The interviewer(s) must be aware of what information is relevant to the study and what information is not essential and the difference between factual, opinion, and knowledge responses. Procedures for recording interviews and editing their content should be known to every interviewer. Some instruction on how to remain neutral to responses is essential. Training should consist of familiarization with the interview structure, conditions, logistics, and controls. Once these factors are learned, interviewers should conduct practice interviews and receive corrective feedback for improving their performances. When researchers and students work alone in studies using the interview training, tapes or films should be used for training. Videotape recordings of practice sessions are effective as corrective feedback.[8]

Sources of Error. Errors are ever present in research, and interviewing is no exception. Several sources can contribute to errors; for example:

1. Errors of Interviewer. In spite of the training given to each interviewer, errors will occur. Interviewers might not ask particular questions with the same voice inflections and this might cause different interpretations by respondents. The interviewer might probe differently using different questions with the same voice inflections and this might cause different interpretations by respondents.[11] The interviewer might probe differently using a variety of questions with different respondents which could result in errors of response. Errors may result from transforming responses of respondents to records of the interview, or in coding information. Interviewers can bias the results by interjecting opinions or making subtle remarks about questions or responses. If the interviewer does not understand the language or colloquial expressions of the respondents, wrong interpretations could be made.

2. *Errors of Respondents.* Lack of understanding of the requirements of the question or lack of knowledge to answer the question might lead respondents to lie or give fictitious responses. Respondents may not wish to cooperate once the interview begins or may give replies without thought in order to terminate the interview. Of course the accuracy of the interview depends on the success of getting honest responses. The tendency of the respondent to give inaccurate responses is called the response effect.[12]

Sources of Refusals and Discrepancies. Interviewers who are trained poorly, faulty interviews,[13] and the process of the interview[14] are major contributors to refusals in interviews. Rates for refusal in interviews can vary between ethnic groups and ages. Older people are more reluctant to give interviews than people 45 years of age and younger; no distinct personality type has been found associated with refusals.[15]

Inconsistencies among respondents seem to occur more often among men, older respondents, and people having less education than among people who have had some college education. Age of respondents is usually reported more reliably than education levels of respondents. Women provide more inconsistencies about their real age than do men. Reduction in content error is attained when questions on the respondent's actual education attainment are preceded by questions of opinion on whether the respondent had sufficient opportunity to obtain all the desired education.[16] No difference in the reporting of psychiatric symptoms to men or women interviewers was found by Colombotos and co-workers.[17]

Inconsistencies might be caused when interviewers are embarrassed by certain topics in the interview; such topics include: why women cannot have babies, income, whether families are receiving welfare, religious affiliations, and who are friends.[18]

Advantages of the Interview. Each survey instrument has its own uniqueness for gathering particular types of information. As a result of its uniqueness, each instrument has certain advantages. Some advantages of the interview are:

1. *Collects Distinctive Information.* The interview is used to gather information about opinions, attitudes, and beliefs on certain issues. People are less likely to reveal information of a confidential nature in other methods of data collection than they are in the interview where they are face-to-face with the interviewer. The interview tends to be a device for asking very general or specific questions. The respondents can react freely to its questions or can be given a choice of several responses to each

question. The interview is used in seeking information which cannot be obtained by other data-gathering instruments.

2. Enables Instant Interpretation of Responses. The interviewer can interpret a response to a question and then ask other questions to supplement replies or can alter the line of questioning to other topics. Most other instruments cannot redirect questioning according to responses given. If a respondent does not understand a question within the accepted predetermined guidelines for alternative wording, the interviewer can reword the question. Alternative wording may introduce a source of variance.

3. Establishes Rapport with Respondent. The personal contact with the respondent affords an opportunity for the respondent to obtain a clear understanding of the research. Although subjects are given some information about a study before participating, they are not often given an opportunity to pursue questions about a project to any great extent. The interview permits the "personal touch" to be present during the data-gathering process.

Disadvantages of the Interview:

1. Honesty. The interviewer must assume that the responses are given honestly. Respondents may respond to a question in the manner which they think the interviewer would like to hear, or they might not wish to divulge exact or real personal information in response to certain questions; for example, income, religious beliefs, marital relations, whether they followed a therapist's recommendations for home care, or tax returns.

2. Interviewer Bias. The interviewer very often interjects personal influence into the conversation which causes the respondents to react to specific questioning that may be contrary to their own true beliefs or opinions. The interviewer may interpret responses in a manner that supports his wishes for the outcome of the study.

3. Expensive. Oral interviews requiring large numbers of interviewers and many respondents can be very costly. Each interview may require only 30 minutes, but traveling and locating the same respondent may have required an additional 30 to 60 minutes. Overhead expenses include labor, travel, and clerical costs.

Observations

Observations of an individual, groups of people, or events are a direct method of gathering information. Although some degree of observation is an essential ingredient in all reserach, various types of observations are used in descriptive approaches to research. Observation techniques are used to a large extent in educational and psychological research where behaviors of children are being studied. It is used in physical therapy during functional analyses where the therapist wants an impression of how the patient performs specific activities. Observational approaches to research are preferred over self-report data (indirect method) when prejudice or bias reporting of information by subjects might occur. Observational methods usually yield more accurate quantitative data than that which could be gathered from indirect or self-reporting methods.[8] The presence of the observer during a behavioral situation may alter the real situation, thus placing a constraint on the information collected. Repeated observations are time consuming but several sessions of a sufficiently large sampling of subjects are necessary for dependable information. Also, two or more independent observers of a single event greatly improves the consistency of the data.

The major types of observations are participant, non-participant, and ethnography.[19] Participant observation is the direct witnessing of some behavior and then recording that behavior on some software instrument for later interpretation. Non-participant observation might include simulations and case studies. Not all observations are done in naturalistic settings. Occasionally the researcher prefers simulated situations where some aspects of the activity are controlled or manipulated. In simulation observation the situation is created by the researcher. Although the behavior exhibited by the subjects is not natural, the technique permits observations of behaviors or situations that are uncommon or complex. Role playing is an example of simulated observation. This approach has been used to determine the consistency of rating scales in assessing the clinical performance of students.

Ethnography is a "shot gun" approach in observational studies. It may involve participant or non-participant observations, or both. The researcher uses a variety of data-gathering instruments or strategies along with observation. Data-gathering instruments might include interviews, questionnaires, and attitude scales. Ethnography involves intensive information-gathering of several variables over an extended period of time and in a natural setting.[19]

Observational data could be recorded by using a diary, checklist, rating scale, or by the case study procedure. Each will be discussed briefly.

Diary

The diary is an instrument that requires recording information in narrative form at predetermined intervals. The intervals might be specific times during the day, daily, weekly, bi-weekly, or some other designated period. The researcher sets the times for observing the behavior, events, or items. For example a physical therapist may wish to study movements of a child having multiple handicaps and may make observations in the morning and evening for a period of days. (A study of patients' behavioral activities or reactions to treatment sequences is another example.) The events of each observation are recorded as a chronology or diary. A case study may be a product of this instrument. The diary is often a narrative summary of occurrences during the designated interval; anecdotes may be kept on the sequence of observations. Progress notes, a patient's record covering the course of hospitalization, or records of a series of treatments could be considered as forms of the diary. Also, logs and journals are forms of a diary; the diary is a nominal level of measurement. The diary could be an instrument of the indirect method of non-experimental research if it was self-reported.

Checklists

This instrument is usually a listing of specific behaviors, events, or traits which the observer then tallies as having or not having occurred during the period of observation. The numbers or types of responses are recorded in appropriate categories by the observer. If a therapist wanted to research occurrences or presence of symptoms associated with a specific condition (low back strain) through assessment, a checklist could be used to record the presence or absence of symptoms. The list of activities to be observed is preplanned before the observation. The researcher usually is interested in certain criteria or occurrences and so prepares a list of those things that are of interest to the study. Depending upon how quantities are recorded, data may be analyzed by statistical methods; computation of means, percentages, relationships, and comparisons can be made.

Although numbers are assigned and statistical methods can be used, the underlying information is subjective, the result of the observer's judgment. Checklists are crude instruments when converted to quantitative values. Over interpretation of data is a danger which must be carefully guarded against. The researcher must constantly ask whether the checklist items are representative measures of what is being assessed. The value of the checklist can be increased by performing pilot studies to ensure that terms included on the checklist are really similar to those the respondents would use in daily behavior. This device is suited to test hypotheses and operates at the conscious and overt levels of the user. The checklist is a direct method of non-experimental research if used by an observer to list behaviors of others, but becomes an indirect method if the respondent uses the instrument for self-assessment. Using the checklist as an indirect method of survey permits responses from the respondent without his having to write lengthy narratives (checking choices) or give a long verbal discourse (free responses). The checklist is suitable for a mail type instrument for self-assessment or as a "door-to-door" type instrument for evaluation by an interviewer.[20] A profile or outline form may also be considered as a form of a checklist.

Rating Scales

A rating scale enables the researcher to observe the actual behavior or event and record what is observed or make judgment about interactions between events, traits, or behaviors. The observer may record the occurrences by checking off items on a list or may rate the object or behavior according to categories on a numbered scale. The scale measures a subject's behavior and permits an element of intensity of the responses.[9] Scaling is a procedure that attempts to determine quantitative measures of subjective abstract concepts.

Types of Scales. The kinds of scales used for recording occurrences may differ slightly.

1. Category. This form of rating scale is categorized into several behaviors which are then subdivided into levels of responses. The observer or judge checks an appropriate level of a particular category when the subject's behavior has been observed. The manual muscle test conforms to the category type scale when the grading system uses "Normal," "Good," "Fair," "Poor," and "Trace," A rating scale variant for assessing the frequency of pain among patients having low back strains is illustrated:

How often do you have pain in your low back?
——Always present
——Often present
——Sometimes present
——Seldom present
——Never present

This example is ordinally scaled because it provides a relative position or level of the patient's condition. Other examples of ordinal level evaluation forms are Disability Rating Scale, Physical Rehabilitation for Daily Living, and Maryland Disability Index.[21]

2. Numerical. Numbers are assigned to the levels of a category rather than or in addition to descriptive phrases. The numbers form a scale and permit equal appearing intervals.

Appropriate statistics can be used in describing or analyzing numerical scales.[22] In the above example the frequency of pain among low back strains can be evaluated by using a scale formed with numbered values:

5	4	3	2	1
Always Present	Often Present	Sometimes Present	Seldom Present	Never Present

The activities of daily living scale of rehabilitation of nursing-home residents is an example of a numerical rating scale.[23]

The psychological factors associated with prolonged work are of interest to researchers studying physiological stress. The psychological factors of stress (prolonged work) can be studied by subjectively rating the intensity of the physical work and is called perceived exertion. Physical work brings about certain sensory inputs (joint pain, muscular effort, breathing patterns, and sweat) that permits the participant to perceive exertion. Borg has developed a psychophysical numerical, ratio scale for rating perceived exertion (RPE). His scale ranges from values of 6 to 20 which allows a 15-point scale. The scale is both valid and reliable for many physiological variables as perceived exertion and in particular heart rate and work intensity ratings are a linear function.[24,25]

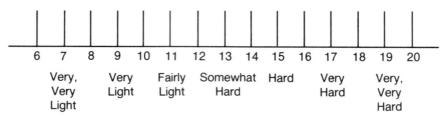

3. *Graphical.* This instrument combines the category and scale traits by forming equal appearing intervals over descriptive phrases. The graphical instrument forms a continuum of equal intervals in the mind of the observer, but does not assign numbers to the scale.[26] The example would then appear as:

Always Present	Often Present	Sometimes Present	Seldom Present	Never Present

Advantages of Rating Scales. Rating scales are an easy method for recording information. These scales provide a vivid concept of what is being judged and are quick and easy to interpret. The scales offer variety in measuring data and because intervals and numbers can be assigned, statistical analyses are possible. Additional advantages of the rating scales are that they require little time to use, are generally interesting, and have a wide range of use.[26]

Rating scales can also be constructed for use as an indirect method (self-assessment) of surveying subjects. The instrument is more sensitive and informative than merely answers of "yes" or "no."[9] Scales actually encourage guessing on the part of the respondent, so impressions are projected.

Disadvantages of Rating Scales. These instruments are often abused because they are so easy to construct and use. People sometimes treat the information from scales as being absolute or real whereas the information is really subjective by nature and indicative of where a respondent wishes to judge on a continuum.

Raters may rate hard or easy depending on the circumstances or questions of the scale. People have the tendency to rate persons whom they like higher than those they dislike. The tendency to rate hard or easy can be prevented by designing asymmetrical scales which have only one unfavorable descriptive terms and four favorable terms (poor, fair, good, very good, and excellent).[6]

The categories of a rating scale are subjective, and this can cause rater bias. Whenever a rater carries over a generalized impression of the scale's topic from question to question, a systematic bias occurs. Raters may systematically rate half or more of the questions above average, average, or below average.[4] This effect of bias can be thwarted by rating one trait at a time for all topics, or by having one trait at a time for all topics, or by having one trait on a page rather than having one topic on a page.[6]

Construction of Rating Scales. In construction of scales consideration should be given to the number of intervals along the scale. If a scale is divided into a large number of intervals, the selection becomes so finely divided that the observer has difficulty in choosing a level and rating the event quickly. If a scale has only a small number of intervals the scale will be coarse and will not differentiate between levels. Three to seven intervals are the numbers most often preferred,[6] while occasionally four to ten will be used.[9] If an odd number of intervals are used, the middle interval serves as a "neutral" zone which forces ratings to either side of the neutral zone. Some observers do not like to use the neutral level; errors of central tendency can be avoided somewhat by using the odd numbered intervals. Changing the position of the extreme favorable and unfavorable words can prevent systematic ratings, for example:

| painful | _____ | pleasant |
| well | _____ | sick |

Another concern about scales is that the two or three intervals between the extreme points are not identified as easily as the polar end points.[21]

The Case Report

The case study or report is usually a comprehensive account about an individual or a particular disease or condition. The details of the report are concerned with the unique or exceptional characteristics of a course of physical therapy or aspects of a rare condition. The case report may also focus on a family, unit of equipment, a community, or a hospital function with data being gathered over a period of time (weeks to years) making it longitudinal by design.[27] The purpose of a case report is to determine the logical interrelations of its components.[11] That is, the details may provide valuable data for formulating tentative generalizations about patients who may have similarities.

The case report is a kind of survey or profile because it encompasses observation, is a record of behavioral responses, or shows various patterns of traits. The study may involve test scales for a number of traits or characteristics. The report must be presented in a clear, concise, narrative manner.[28] Medicine, rehabilitation, law, clinical psychology, phsyiology, and education are fields that have made great use of the case, study, while it has received condemnation in physical education.[29]

Components of the Case Report. The report should have a title that briefly reveals what the study is about. The title should identify the disease, condition, or the treatment approach. Historical data covering the period of time leading to the presenting of the patient are considered important for providing background information as well as demographic data (age, sex, occupation, and race).[28] This information could be obtained from records (files) or from the patient or a member of the family, and includes details of onset and prior treatment. Complete and accurate medical and physical therapy procedures should be included in the report. A summary of diagnostic measures and physical therapy assessments, pertinent physiological and pathological findings, and unique devices yielding particular measurements are also included in the report. If follow-up information was not available when the case was reported, then statements about the prognosis are desirable. An appraisal of the effectiveness of recommendations is also helpful to readers.

Value and Limitations of the Case Report. The case report is "almost synonymous" with non-experimental research because it describes in great detail the events, characteristics, and traits of an individual.[30] The case report may also be effective in studying organizations, educational programs, or communities.[3] Since a case report relates the uniqueness of a treatment approach or a disease, the information supplied may sometimes be generalized to provide increased understanding of a number of essential qualities.[29] The report may provide insight into the factors associated with the unusual condition or treatment approach and lead to further research. It permits the researcher the chance to see a patient in his total relationship to therapy, to the institution, or to the health care system. Both subjective and objective information is acceptable in the case report as well as the study of variables that are troublesome to quantify. The case report allows the researcher freedom in amount of data to be collected and disseminated; the researcher may begin or end it whenever he has sufficient data or when time becomes a critical factor.[4] Case reports can provide readers a source for hypothesis (proposition) testing. It is particularly amenable to clinicians who do not wish to engage in experimental research but who desire to make valuable contributions to the physical therapy literature by reporting detailed descriptions of unique cases.

Because the case report does represent a single and unique situation, caution must be exercised in making generalizations about a single individual. A datum may not be representative of a population or provide a firm basis for scientific prediction or inference. Randomization, replication, and control procedures are characteristics of research that make findings generalizable but are not typically used in case reports. The information supplied in the report may not be objective but may be selectively described and may include the researcher's prejudice from working closely with the individual studied.[4] Also, since the conclusions are based on a single and unique case, the conclusions of the report are difficult to verify without undertaking a controlled study.

Occasionally the single case or subject is used in experimental research when a variable is manipulated. The single subject (time series) experiment includes the collection of baseline data before and after replications of treatment. This approach to using a single subject is presented in Chapter 9 dealing with experimental designs.

INDIRECT METHODS

Questionnaire

The questionnaire, like the formal interview, is an instrument that uses a set of predetermined and prearranged questions given to respondents for obtaining standardized, quantifiable data. The same questions are asked of all respondents so that comparable information can be gathered. Two types of questionnaires are used commonly, the self-administered and the group-administered questionnaires. The self-administered questionnaire is one which the respondent is asked to complete and return to the researcher. The mail questionnaire is the best example of this type and will be the instrument discussed in most detail in this section. The group-administered questionnaire is given to a collection of subjects assembled for answering all the questions before being dismissed. An example might be a group of physical therapists who are attending a meeting and who are given a questionnaire to complete; upon completion, the members of the group depart.

Preparation. Theoretical guides for planning the questionnaire are generally lacking. The researcher using this instrument must rely on experiences, logical reasoning, and some general rules for assisting in its development. Defining the problem is again the first step in planning research. Once the problem (question) is defined, aims and objectives are formed. Literature must be reviewed to aid in asking pertinent questions and assisting the researcher in planning the scope of questions. The researcher must decide whether a hypothesis will be tested or whether gathering general information will answer the question. If a hypothesis is to be tested, quantitative information will probably be asked for in the questionnaire (factual questions) and the method may be experimental rather than descriptive. Counts or values may be obtained so that statistical analysis can be administered, or, if general information (opinion) is asked for, the data will be qualities. Statistics to be considered might be tallies, percentages, or correlation (Chapters 7 and 10).

Careful planning of the design will help in obtaining meaningful answers to the questions. Whatever the problem or objective in sampling considerations must enter into the design. People who will be able to supply the information desired must be selected as respondents (the sample). Certain problems require a representative sample of subjects to answer the questions. For example, if the problem is concerned about a particular hospital issue then physical therapists, nurses, social service workers, administrators and procurement personnel, housekeepers, physicians, and others will have to be included in the sample to fulfill the requirements of a cross-sectional design. Some problems are very complex and require careful selection of subjects for the sample in order to disentangle complex interrelationships among variables (factorial design). Perhaps a physical therapist wishes to study the functional problems resulting from a specific type of hip surgery on patients having arthritis of the hip joint. The therapist may want to design a series of questionnaires and follow-ups over a period of years. The longitudinal design will enable the therapist to determine cause-and-effect relationships occurring over a long period of time.[18] (See designs, Chapter 9).

The design selected will help decide the type of questions to ask. The open and forced-choice questions are used commonly in questionnaires. In the open question or free response question, the respondent is free to provide the amount of detail he wishes to any or all questions of the type. The respondent is also free to determine the form of answers, short answer or narrative discussions, to the questions. The forced-choice questions provide several answers to the questions, and the respondent chooses the most appropriate answer. The question might ask: "How many classroom hours does your program devote to research instruction?"

—— less than 10, —— 10 to 20, —— 21 to 30, —— 31 to 40, —— over 40 hours

Writing Questions. The actual composing or wording of questions must be given great attention. Questions must be appropriate to the problem and aims of the study; they must provide the information necessary to test the hypothesis or provide information relevant to the general subject. Some of the common concerns about writing questions are discussed briefly.

1. Direct and General. If factual information is desired, the question must be worded so that the specific information is obtained. "How many licensed physical therapists are working full time in your department?" A general question can be constructed from the example by asking for information of a more general nature. "How many people do you have working in the department?" The two approaches should not be confused because responses will be mixed when respondents interpret a question having different meanings. The second question could be interpreted by some respondents as meaning licensed physical therapists or it could be asking for therapists, therapist assistants, aides, and clerical personnel. Ambiguity can be avoided by structuring questions in simple, easily understood forms. Avoid words that may have more than one meaning to the respondent when asking for specific information.

2. *Complex and Simple.* Questions that are very long or complex should be avoided. A respondent may be confused or may not wish to answer a complex question. "Have you treated many patients having brain damage over a long period of time, how were these patients handled, and were you successful in achieving desired treatment goals?" This particular question is vague, long, asks for too much detail, and is complex because of its ambiguity. Questions must be kept simple in construction and easy for the respondent to answer. If multiple answers are sought from questions, or if questions involve several variables, then several questions should be asked in such a fashion that no overlap of information is being requested. Questions should be mutually exclusive:

"How many children having cerebral palsy and displaying spasticity of one limb did you treat in May?"

"Was passive exercise used as part of their treatment regimen?"

"Was the Bruiminks-Oseretsky Test of Motor Proficiency used to assess effects of treatment?"

Perhaps more questions could be asked to obtain the information being requested in the original question. Questions must be sensitive to wording and emphasis. Leading questions or questions about memory are considered poor questions.[9]

3. *Examine Questions.* After writing questions, put them side for a few days and then reread and rework them to improve quality and to eliminate ambiguity. When questions have been constructed to your satisfaction, administer them to friends or colleagues who are knowledgeable in the content area. Ask your colleagues to critique the style, wording, and meanings of the questions. You will be surprised to learn how many questions will still need rewriting. Different people will have different frames of references and will offer good ideas for improving the questions. Pilot work (pretesting) is a good idea in non-experimental research for the improvement of the data-gathering instrument and method. Pretesting the questionnaire helps in identifying instrument deficiencies as well as help from respondents making suggestions for improvement. Pilot work can assist the researcher in determining the accuracy of the responses. Some responses can be checked for accuracy (e.g., income) and if found to be inaccurate, questions can be reworded or forced-choice questions can replace free-response questions. The researcher can determine which questions will be most successful, which questions are weak and vague. Additional questions may be suggested to the researcher by the pretest results.

Ordering Questions. The questions requiring the least thought or reasoning should occur first on the list. If the respondent is put at ease and thinks the questions are simple and not requiring much effort, then chances for completing the questionnaire are improved greatly. The more provocative questions should follow in a logical sequence if interrelated. The respondent will not mind having to put a little thought into the answers and as he gets into the "swing of things" he will want to finish. Questions which are of sensitive or are of an embarrassing nature should occur last, if important enough to use, and be few in number to assure completion of the questionnaire.

Length of Questionnaire. Setting the length of a questionnaire is a difficult decision but one which everyone constructing the instrument must make. If the researcher knows the sample members being queried, then longer questionnaires might have a good chance of success; but if the researcher is unknown to the sample members, the success rate of the questionnaire will probably be low. People have a tendency of ignoring questionnaires which are lengthy and appear to require large amounts of time and effort to complete. If the questionnaire is of a timely and interesting nature, the success rate will, of course, be high. Students wishing to use the mail questionnaire for class projects or for investigative studies should keep the length of the questionnaire short, thirty questions or less. Sometimes just identifying the questionnaire as belonging to a student will "turn people off."

Uses of Questionnaires. The mail questionnaire is used to gather information about issues, opinions, or views. The executive body of an association might send questionnaires to a representative sample of its voting members to determine their wishes or beliefs, or the feasibility of the study before deciding to take a stance on certain policies or political matters. A physical therapist might pool chapter members before introducing a motion at the annual business meeting to change the name of the chapter's newsletter. The questionnaire is used to determine status of an issue. A politician may sample constituents concerning their views of a particular piece of pending legislation before he returns to his legislative body to vote on the issue. The politician is determining the status of the problem before commiting himself on the issue.

Questionnaires are used in research to obtain facts and knowledge about a specific subject. They are used to determine how strongly held are the views on an issue, to determine reasons for a course of action, to determine general feelings on an issue, and to determine respondents' awareness of an issue.[9] The McGill pain questionnaire has been designed for clinical assessment of pain and can be analyzed statistically. It measures pain by means of a pain-rating index, number of words chosen, and intensity.[31]

Reasons for Rejecton by Respondents. Responses to mail questionnaires are frequently meager with returns of 40% to 50% or less being common,[32] while a response rate of 60% is good and 70% is very good.[11] If questions are poor, complex, long, or ambiguous, the respondent will become discouraged because of confusion, or lack of understanding of what is expected of him. Lengthy demands made of the respondent may prevent the questionnaire from being returned to the sender. Often questions are embarrassing or too personal for the respondent. If there is no relationship between respondent and researcher and they are strangers, then chances of completing a lengthy questionnaire are extremely poor. Timing the questionnaire mailing is important. A teacher who receives a questionnaire just prior to examination periods is not likely to respond; an administrator who receives a questionnaire at the time he is working on the annual report or budget may not respond; or the physical therapist who is just returning from vacation and having to get caught up in clinical work will also not respond to a questionnaire. Perhaps you can think of many other reasons; if so, consider those reasons when planning a survey. Responses may be extremely poor if respondents must incur personal costs for the return of the questionnaire, or if budget considerations dictate questionnaire information or mailings. The Readership Survey Results—1972 of PHYSICAL THERAPY may be a good example in which only 5% of readers responded to the questionnaire.[33] The researcher must decide whether anonymity on the questionnaire is important. Some questions, particularly of personal nature, may be threatening to respondents if they are asked to identify themselves. However, anonymity probably increases the honesty of responses and the number of returned questionnaires. Follow-ups are difficult and inefficient when the researcher does not know who did and did not respond.[19]

Aids for Improving Returns. All questionnaires must be accompanied by a self-addressed stamped envelope. Respondents refuse to cooperate when they must spend their own money to assure the success of someone else's research. The questionnaire must be constructed for the convenience of the respondent: not too many questions, questions must be clear and not ambiguous, the questionnaire must be easy to respond to by way of answer (forced choices are good), and questions should be impersonal. The questionnaire must be neat and organized, and not contain too much reading. A letter must accompany the questionnaire explaining the purpose and use, and providing clear instructions for its completion. Authoritarian or excessively polite letters may be ignored. People forget, misplace, or need persuasion for completing and returning questionnaires so follow-up mailings are recommended. Follow-up mailings increase return rates. Two to 4 weeks between mailings are a reasonable lapse of time. Follow-up mailings can be improved by rewording the cover letter and sending another questionnaire along with another self-addressed stamped envelope. A mere reminder to complete and return the questionnaire is worthless if the original questionnaire has been destroyed (filed). Persistance often pays dividends. If the return rate is low enough to jeopardize the study, a second or third follow-up may be necessary, but the researcher must decide when the returns no longer justify the expense of sending out more questionnaires. Members of a sample who are not interested, have little education, or represent an economically poor social class may contribute to poor response rates.[8] Sample selection is important for assuring responses.

The Cover Letter. A cover letter must accompany all mailed questionnaires. It briefly explains the purpose and significance of the study and helps to motivate the individual to complete and return the questionnaire. Cover letters should be addressed specifically to the potential respondent (Dear Ms. (name), not Dear Ms. or Sir). The "personal touch" helps to improve the percentage of returns. If possible, some reference to association (professional) ties is desirable. Endorsement by a respected, well-known member of the association (group, institution) improves responses, particularly if the researcher is a student. Respondents should be given a deadline date for returning the completed questionnaire (2 to 4 weeks). Neatness and composition of the letter and questionnaire are important. Duplication by the offset process on letterhead paper improves appearance of material as well as the image and value of the responses. A sample letter is shown in Figure 6.1.

Presenting Results. The total sample size, the percentage of returns, and the rate of response for each question should be presented in the results of a questionnaire survey. Presenting the percentage of respondents choosing alternatives to each question is one approach to reporting results.

Advantages of Questionnaires. The mail questionnaire has several advantages to the researcher. Some of these advantages are its:

1. Low Cost. When compared with the interview, the mail questionnaire is inexpensive. Costs involve supplies, postage fees, and clerical assistance, and are dependent upon the size of the sample and the number of follow-up mailings.

2. Sampling Representation. If time to complete the study is unimportant, a good representation of a sample can be obtained. Follow-ups can be continued or additional subjects can be sampled until a good sized sample is reached. The questionnaires can be mailed and additional work or research can take place during the interim between mailings and returns. This type of survey often requires months to complete.

3. Low Personal Error. Errors which occur when repeating a question many times in an interview are nonexistent since exact copies of the questionnaire are mailed to all members of the sample. The data are computed easily because tallies and simple statistical methods are used in analysis. Since the respondents do not have access to results of the survey or interviewers, they cannot influence answers recorded by an observer.

4. Data Verification. Sometimes factual information can be verified by comparing data supplied by respondents with that of other known sources.

Letterhead paper	Program of Physical Therapy University of Null Blackbird, PA 17261
	March 14, 1984
Use sample matching → in cutting offset stencil	Miss Mary Doe Department of Physical Therapy Null Hospital Blackbird, PA 17261
Use offset process for appearance of individually typed → letter when duplicating	Dear Miss Doe:
Purpose →	The enclosed questionnaire concerned with procedures used in selecting physical therapy students is part of a statewide study being conducted by the Program of Physical Therapy at the University of Null. The results of this study will help to provide criteria to be used for improving present selection procedures and determining the administrative status of the selection process. The selection process affects the caliber of students that you receive for clerkship.
Importance →	
Reasonable time → limit	Your cooperation in completing the enclosed questionnaire by April 5 will be greatly appreciated. Each return ensures a more accurate assessment of the selection process. Your comments concerning any aspect of the present selection process not covered in the questionnaire would be welcomed. A copy summarizing the survey results will be mailed if you desire. Thank you for your cooperation.
Offer results →	
Thank respondent →	
	Sincerely yours,
Different color → to appear personally signed	I. M. Smith, Dean

Figure 6.1. Sample cover letter for questionnaires.

Respondents' ages or positions may be verified by obtaining files or records if they are members of an organization, employees of a hospital, or students enrolled in a university. This advantage is important because researchers want to be able to defend the accuracy of their data.

Disadvantages of Questionnaires:

1. Ambiguity of Questions. In spite of rewriting questions several times and subjecting them to pilot work, ambiguity may creep into the questionnaire. Ambiguity may occur in the technical detail of the question if the respondent's level of understanding is less than expected.

2. Finality of Responses. Once the questionnaire is returned, the responses are final. The researcher cannot ask the respondent what was meant by a certain reply. No rechecking, further probing, or asking of additional questions is possible after the questionnaire has been mailed.

3. Alteration of Questions. Even when forced-choice answers are supplied along with questions, respondents often alter the answers to suit their convenience. The questions may not fit the respondents' situation exactly so they may alter the question or the response. Respondents see the entire questionnaire before responding to the first question, therefore, responses to one question are not always independent of responses to other questions.[9]

4. Identity of Respondent. Questions are usually designed for a particular group of people by virtue of occupation, membership, patronage, or experience. The researcher, however, is never sure that the respondent was actually the person for whom the questions were intended. A physical therapy administrator might be asked about administrative procedures used in his clinic, but a secretary may be asked to complete the questionnaire. The researcher has somewhat limited control over who the respondents actually are.

Attitude Scales

An attitude is a state of mind in regard to some event or person. The mind may be in a quiescent state or in an active state concerning an attitude which is expressed through behavior. Attitudes may have cognitive components (beliefs), emotional components (feelings), and action components (behavior). Attitudes can be weak (no identified conviction), strong (firm conviction), abstract (theoretical), intense (tender, violent), and enduring or transient (exist over a long or short period of time).[11,20] A scale is a collection of phrases or numbers placed on a continuum (linear sequence) for the purpose of weighing or measuring values. Thus, an attitude scale is a device for assessing the predisposition toward an event or person.

An attitude scale consists of a series of statements to reflect the cognitive, emotional, and action components of attitude. The subject is given a series of statements and is asked to respond to them by agreeing or disagreeing with the assertions. Since statements are structured to represent various levels or degrees of a particular component, the subject's response will be dependent upon the wording of the statement. The device is a crude measuring instrument but of all the survey instruments the attitude scale is probably the most sophisticated. The attitude scale has acquired the greatest amount of technical development among non-experimental research instruments.[20]

The purpose of the attitude scale is to divide people into broad categories (partitions) based on their attitudes toward some stated object or situation. The scale may be designed to determine physical therapists' attitudes toward their job or professional scope, practices, or opportunities. Patients may be assessed to determine their attitudes about their physical therapy. Attitude scales have been used to a great extent in sociological, educational, and psychological studies. Searches of the physical therapy literature have not revealed the use of attitude scales with much frequency. These devices might yield important information about public or professional reaction to physical therapy, or physical therapists' satisfaction with academic preparation for meeting the demands of clinical work, or physical therapists' reactions toward their associations' activities. Many relevant questions could be asked about any one of these suggested topics. In practice, more statements can be made about a topic than can actually be used in the scale form.

Although attitude scales have received much technical attention (outside of physical therapy), the contents of measurement are subjective and are not inclusive. As stated earlier about rating scales, the device is subject to error and really indicates the numbers of subjects expressing certain states of mind toward a situation or person. Analysis of scale values of data can, however, yield considerable information about attitudes. The information can serve as an indicator or guide in establishing policies or procedures, approaches to treatment, curricular changes, and many other applied interests. A single statement or reaction to a single statement cannot be regarded with much authenticity. Reactions to many statements must be averaged before meaning can be extracted from the scaling devices. The device is valuable if administered to a group of subjects or administered to a single subject when normative values are available for comparison.

Those planning to measure how an individual or group of individuals feel about a specific topic should first search the literature to ascertain whether an attitude scale has been constructed that might meet their needs. Most likely an attitude scale that has been published and found suitable for the student's or clinician's purpose measures what it was developed to measure and the results that it obtains are repeatable if measured on another occasion. These assurances of a scale can save the researcher a tremendous amount of time and effort. If a suitable scale is not available, it will be necessary to develop one.

Careful attention must be given to the construction of the scale so that the respondent's choices are presented to the respondent in a fashion that indicates neutrality of the researcher. Moser has cited three steps for assuring success of an attitude scale: (1) identify statements which are appropriate and logically related to the attitude dimension being considered, (2) put the statements together in a meaningful fashion so that there is representativeness of the attitude dimension, and (3) perform pilot work on the device to establish baselines for assisting interpretations of the responses.[9]

Considerations of Measurement. Certain features of the scale must be built into the instrument to assure its success. These features must be considered when preparing the scale and when modifying the instrument following a pilot test.

1. Homogeneity. All statements in the scale must relate to a single topic or attitude component. If beliefs toward a particular issue are to be assessed, then statements involving emotional aspects of the topic should be excluded. For example, if the instrument is to measure the patients' beliefs about the benefits of physical therapy, then statements about difficulties concerning transportation to the clinic should be excluded.

2. Equal Intervals. Although units of value and intervals are assigned arbitrarily, the units should maintain equality or at least appear to be equally distant between intervals. Equal-appearing distances on the scale make the data easier to handle than if the scale was not linear. Linearity relates to a bi-variate distribution which means that as the quantity of one variable increases (or decreases) the quantity of the other variable increases also. One variable can decrease as the other variable increases and still be linearly related. In an attitude scale, the most favorable statements should hold the highest weights to maintain linearity or be constructed so that a straight line relationship is maintained. For example, if three statements are made, they should be graduated in value so that the stronger statements have more (or less) value than the weaker statements.

"Physical therapists make good citizens."	0.15
"I find physical therapists are vigorous people."	0.48
"I think physical therapists are conceited."	0.50

The difficulty is equating the proper weights to the particular attitude, but techniques have been devised to measure different aspects of attitudes and take into account the problems of linearity.

3. Repeatability. Scales should be designed so that if a particular attitude scale is administered to a group of subjects today, it should have similar values or scores if administered tomorrow. The difficulty with attitude measurements is that people do change their attitudes about conditions frequently. For example, the boss may reprimand you about a certain administrative error you committed yesterday. You may believe that the boss was unfair or that the reprimand was unnecessary; and therefore your attitude may be guarded or negative toward the boss. If the boss takes you to dinner the following week and the event is very satisfying, you may then believe that the boss is not such a rotten egg after all; your attitude has changed. The outcome of the attitude scale may change between two administrations because of the occurrences taking place between measurements (temporal effect of internal difficulty). Repeatability of attitude scales is quite high. The illustration is an isolated instance of an attitude change in a transient issue, but repeatability is more lasting on many issues: political, religious, professional, and educational views. A graduated scale or continuum where higher values (6 and 5) are equated in size to differences occurring elsewhere on the scale (2 and 1) will assist greatly in the repeatability of the instrument.

Types of Attitude Scales. Only the two most commonly used scales will be presented, but these will provide differences in approaches to measuring different components of attitudes; these scales represent equal-appearing (Thurstone), and summated (Likert) scales.

1. Thurstone Scale. Thurstone was a pioneer in attitude scaling and his scale is one of the best known methods of measuring attitudes. The scale is an attempt to assess the strength of an attitude by an agreement-disagreement continuum in which each item is assigned a scale value. The scale value indicates the strength of the attitude and differentiates strength by means of equal-appearing intervals.[32] Thurstone attempted to assess people's attitudes by comparing statements in pairs and then judging which statement was more positive (or more negative) than the other statement. His work in experimental psychophysics led to the method of equal-appearing intervals.[20]

The procedure begins by forming a large pool of graduated statements ranging from least to most favorable. The pool of statements is written on separate strips of paper and then edited for ambiguity, duplication, grammar, and sentence structure. Editing has the effect of reducing the numbers of statements in the pool. A group of people are selected as judges to assess each item in the pool by its degree of favorableness. Judges are ideally people who are knowledgeable in the content area of the attitude under consideration. Careful instructions must be given to the judges so that each has a complete understanding of how to rank and judge the statements. Groups of judges differing widely in views usually have good agreement when assessing attitude statements.[20] The judges assess each statement and place the statement in a pile according to its degree of favorableness. Judging is performed independently. The number of piles are predetermined as 7, 9, or 11. Odd numbers of intervals provide a "neutral" position or value of the statements. Each statement receives a ranking given by each judge in accord with the pile it was placed.

The median and interquartile deviation for each statement are then determined. The interquartile deviation and median measure the variation and central tendency, respectively.[5] These statistics now enable the researcher to further reduce the pool. Statements in each pile are now examined for their interquartile deviations. Those statements having the highest deviations indicate ambiguity and are eliminated. Next, the medians for each statement pile are examined; the medians may be unevenly distributed along the scale, but represent distinguishable differences among statements resulting from the judging. The medians, for example, may be 9.0, 8.4, 8.1, 7.5. 6.9, 6.7, and so forth.

The desired number of statements, 20 to 30, is selected for the instrument. In the Thurstone method the higher the scale value, the less positive the attitude toward a situation or person.[34] The mean of the scores obtained from an administration of the instrument indicates the respondents' attitude grouping. That is, the mean computed for a group of respondents will determine the attitude for a particular group, class, or organization of people. For example, an attitude scale administered to physical therapists attending an annual conference will indicate the group's attitude toward increasing the membership fees of the Association. The attitude of an individual can be compared to a group's attitude by comparing means obtained from the group and individual. Some criticisms of the Thurstone scale have been the characteristics and attitudes of the judges such as ages, sex, and skill. The Thurstone scaling process is laborious.[9] Table 6.1 provides a partial example of a Thurstone scale.

2. Likert Scale. The Likert scale is a summated rating scale or set of statements that are considered to be of equal value in describing the attitude. Respondents choose between the degrees of agreement or disagreement associated with each statement. The sum of the scores represents his attitude.

Construction of the Likert scale is less laborious than construction of the Thurstone scale, but the results of the two scales agree well.[20] The Likert scale is concerned mostly with homogeneity, making sure all statements center on one topic or attitude. No judges are needed in its construction.

Five levels or degrees of agreement-disagreement are used for each statement. The levels are "strongly agree," "agree," "neutral," "disagree," and "strongly disagree." Weights are assigned to each level (numerical

Table 6.1
Example of a Partial Attitude Scale: Attitudes Toward Physical Therapy*

Check (   ) every statement below that expresses your feeling toward physical therapy. Interpret the statements in accordance with your own experience.

1. When I receive physical therapy I enjoy the atmosphere of the clinic.	(4.0)
2. I believe in what the physical therapist tells me, but I have some reservations.	(4.5)
3. Sometimes I feel that physical therapy and the therapist are necessary and sometimes I doubt them.	(5.6)
4. I believe in physical therapy and its benefits because I have been accustomed to good treatment.	(4.0)
5. I believe physical therapy is losing ground as a science.	(7.4)
6. Physical therapy is needed in health care; it has always provided benefits and good feelings.	(1.4)
7. I like physical therapy, but do not miss it much when I miss a treatment.	(5.1)
8. I believe physical therapy is a powerful form of medicine for rehabilitating the sick and injured.	(1.2)

* Respondent's attitude grouping is the mean. $\bar{X} = 33.2 \div 8 = 4.2$ on a 9-point scale.

rating scale) for the purpose of scoring and analysis. The ordering of weights may have to be reversed according to whether the statement is stated positively or negatively; scores may be 5, 4, 3, 2, and 1, respectively. In the process of score reversal, "neutral" level is always number three.

The writing and collection of statements form the initial process of constructing a Likert scale. Statements are composed for the "agree" and "disagree" levels only because people have a tendency to respond to extreme statements in similar fashion; that is, very little disagreement to extreme statements. Experience has shown that statements of neutrality do not function well.[9] Since only two levels are aimed for when writing statements, an equal number of "agree" and "disagree" type statements can be constructed. All statements are scored from 1 to 5 arbitrarily and then all scores are summed to determine the range. If 100 statements have been written and scored, the lowest sum in the range would be 100 and the highest sum possible in the range would be 500. The scale is administered to a selected sample of subjects.

Agreement about scoring the statements must be made before administration of the instrument. If a positive attitude toward the job means a high score, then agreement with statements like "The chance to do research" or "The association with good people" should be scored as 4 or 5.

In the example given in Table 6.2, suppose two statements were scored as 3, three statements as 2, three statements as 4, and two as 5. A cursory inspection of Table 6.2 might give the impression that the exemplary respondent neither enjoyed nor disliked his job.

When scores are summed the total is 34.

Statement	Score (x)
1	5
2	2
3	3
4	4
5	2
6	4
7	2
8	4
9	3
10	5
	$\Sigma x = 34$

The maximum score possible on the ten statements would be 50 ($10 \times 5 = 50$) and the neutral position would total ($10 \times 3 = 30$). The score of 34 is slightly above the neutral attitude and in the direction of a positive attitude toward job satisfaction, since agreement before administering the scale was to label positive statements with values of 5 and 4. Further inspection of Table 6.2 shows that the respondent has a somewhat negative

Table 6.2

Example of a Physical Therapy Job Satisfaction Scale

Read each statement carefully; decide how satisfied you feel about that particular aspect of your present job described by each statement; be honest; check the appropriate score that best describes your feelings. Check (   ) all statements.

	Strongly Agree 5	Agree 4	Neutral 3	Disagree 2	Strongly Disagree 1
1. An opportunity to help the sick and disabled.					
2. My job offers variety.					
3. The job offers few opportunities to grow.					
4. The opportunity to be responsible for the outcome of treatment.					
5. The chance to do research.					
6. The routine in my job.					
7. The status which my job offers.					
8. An opportunity to meet important people.					
9. The challenge of the work.					
10. The association of good people.					

attitude about the opportunities the job has to offer, since five responses were in the "neutral" or "disagree" levels (statements 2, 3, 5, 7, and 9). The respondent seems to enjoy working with and having the association with patients and hospital employees but does not believe that the type of work she is doing offers a challenge or provides status. Caution in over interpretation of the responses must, however, be exercised.

No conclusions can be made about the meaning of distances between scale positions, since the instrument is not an interval scale. The Likert scale is an ordinal type of measuring device. Repeatability is good for the Likert scale; the number of statements is arbitrary but should number at least 20. One problem with this scale is that the total score can be obtained in a number of different ways. That is, scores checked for each statement could change between 1 and 5 on varied administrations, yet the total scores of the scale could be exactly the same or similar in value. When large numbers of subjects are administered, the Likert attitude scale, percentiles, and standard deviations can be computed.

HISTORICAL METHOD

Historical research is critical investigation of accounts of the past, the careful weighing of the validity of accounts and their sources, and the interpretation of the accounts after their weighing.[32] Some early historians preserved tales and accounts of the past for purposes of entertaining or provoking readers, but most used historical information to praise the state or church, or to promote an issue.[35] Modern historians attempted to bring historical methods in line with scientific methods by establishing procedures for investigation.

Historical research differs somewhat from the scientific method by necessity because of its elusive subject matter. The historian uncovers data through a search of accounts of the past such as documents, relics, and diaries while the researcher in science creates data by making observations and measurements in order to describe events and performance.[8] Modern historians contend that, within limits, the historical method is scientific.[35] The method does enable the historian to investigate subject matter and source materials critically and objectively.[4] Suppositions are established and then data which will confirm or contradict the suppositions are collected; historians, however, cannot employ controlled observations nor repeat measurements.[29]

Identifying the problems to be investigated, locating sources of past facts, evaluating these sources, and summarizing and interpreting the gathered historical information are basic steps in the conduct of historical research. Each step is discussed briefly.

Identifying a Problem

Like other types of research, one of the first considerations in historical research is to identify the problem to be investigated. As outlined in Chapter 2, a thorough review of the literature is of paramount importance in identifying a problem. Discussing the problem, topic, or hypothesis with experienced historians is also useful for initiating the research process. Since the purpose of historical research is to discover new knowledge, explain, or predict, the availability of resources to study a well-defined problem must be known prior to beginning the investigation.

Source of Investigation

In their attempt to collect information and increase their understanding about the past, historians search for historical roots. The two sources of materials used in historical research are primary and secondary sources.

Primary Sources. The historian locates and examines original materials of the past. Primary sources may be located at repositories of historical information, or may still be in existence at their original location, or may be owned and maintained by individuals, groups, and organizations. Primary sources may consist of official (state, church, minutes of organizations) or personal (letters, speeches, articles, diaries, diplomas) records, eye or ear witnesses, photographs or illustrations (drawings, paintings), published or printed materials (textbooks, certificates, contracts, accounts, articles), physical remains (ruins, equipment, relics, clothing, artifacts), and mechanical records (tapes or video recordings of interviews, meetings and speeches). Once the historian has located and collected data, he must validate the data. Although the data may be original, the historical researcher must then verify and be assured that the data are trustworthy and representative of the true account. Sometimes the process of validating primary sources is not an easy task and sometimes gaps must be filled in by the researcher or the sources accepted without being verified.[29,35]

Secondary Sources. A secondary source is an account, description, or reproduction of the original by persons who did not see, hear, or live the past accounts or experiences.

Information contained by secondary sources may have been changed or distorted through transmission from person to person. Primary sources are always best and must be sought by the researcher for obvious reasons. Secondary sources do have definite value to the researcher for obvious reasons. Secondary sources do have definite value to the researcher because: (1) primary sources are not always available, (2) they help as an introduction to the subject area, (3) they may provide an overview of the subject, and (4) they might help the researcher to form suppositions. Secondary sources of historical information may include: abstracts, newspapers, encyclopedias, periodicals or interviews, and historical accounts based on secondhand information.[29,35]

Evaluation of Sources

The existence or collection of data from primary or secondary sources does not guarantee the researcher of their validity, authenticity, or accuracy.[35] Historians have established two standards for evaluating materials collected before the research is reported.

External Criticism. This form of evaluation is preoccupied with the genuineness or validity of the source. The source might be in existence and be original, but the historian must verify whether the data are the real things; the intent or frame of reference in which the account took place, was written, or was given. Perhaps the author's original statement is located and verified as being the statement made by the author, but the researcher must determine whether the author was competent when making the statement.[29,35]

Internal Criticism. This form of evaluation is concerned mostly with the content of the source or statement and its meaning. The researcher may verify that the statement can be attributed to a certain author and that the author was competent, but the statement must still remain suspect until the seriousness or truth of the statement is determined.[32] Thus, the evaluation of the source is transferred from the genuineness or authenticity of the statement to the trustworthiness of its contents.[35]

The historical research method, unlike the scientific method, does not contain precise technical vocabulary and so terms may often have different meanings. In spite of the established procedures historical research has apparently declined somewhat in some disciplines. The decline has been attributed to the universal acceptance of the scientific method.[32]

Physical therapists could use this method to preserve the rich history of their profession.

Interpretation

Summarization and interpretation are integral parts of historical research. These activities involve logical analysis, therefore the researcher must be as objective as possible. The researcher cannot confirm that one event in the past caused another but must make assumptions or inferences that assign causality to historical events. The researcher must be careful by the choice of language used in the interpretation so as not to convey the wrong interpretation. The more information uncovered about a historical event, the more likely the cause of the event will be known or at least be defensible.

Like other forms of research, the researcher cannot study or examine the entire population of events or phenomena. The researcher, therefore, usually samples a portion of events or is limited by the availability of past documents and relics, but makes generalizations based on the sample of information. The researcher's findings are always strengthened by increasing the sample size or the amount of available data on which inferences are based. As many primary and secondary sources relating to the event as possible are needed to make correct interpretations. The researcher is cautioned to restrict interpretations about causes and generalizability of interpretations according to the evidence gathered.

SUMMARY

Descriptive or survey methods are logical and specific approaches to non-experimental research, and can provide considerable understanding from a small number of variables.[11] Non-experimental research can provide information about what respondents are thinking and feeling, and how they are reacting toward some stimulus. Information gathered can be broad, detailed, and specific. Because of the elusive nature of types of data

Table 6.3
Cumulative Summary of the Research Processes Presented

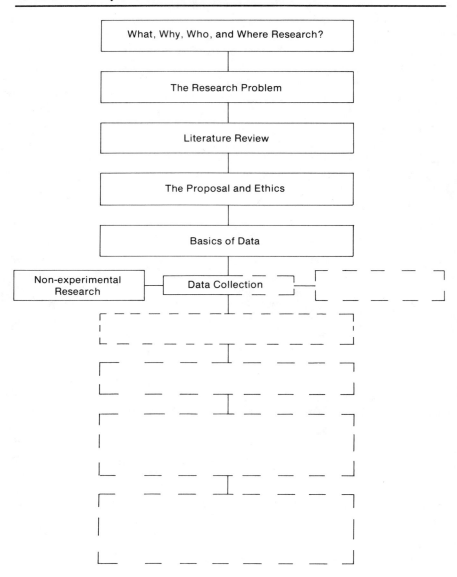

gathered, non-experimental research exerts little control over variables involved in an investigation.[4] Lack of controls in research may lead to its inconsistency. Software instruments used to collect data may not be as accurate and precise as hardward instruments used in experimentation. In spite of its weaknesses non-experimental research does enable an investigator to study areas in which controlled experimentation may be impossible.

The historical method is performed outside of the conventional laboratory and is quasi-scientific in technique. This non-experimental method can, however, make valuable contributions to physical therapy. However important, it has seldom been used in studies reported in the physical therapy literature. Using this method, physical therapists could preserve the history and examine questions vital to the well-being of the profession. Table 6.3 summarizes the research processes presented thus far.

REFERENCES

1. Ethridge DA, McSweeney M: Research in occupational therapy. 1. Introduction. Am J Occup Ther 24: 490–494, 1970
2. Meyers LS, Grossen NE: Behavioral Research: Theory, Procedure, and Design, ed 2. San Francisco, WH Freeman and Co, 1978
3. Espenschade AS, Rarick GL: Descriptive Research. In Hubbard AW (ed): Research Methods in Health, Physical Education, and Recreation, ed 3. Washington, Am Assoc Health Phys Educ Rec 1973
4. Treece EW, Treece JW Jr: Elements of Research in Nursing, ed 3. St. Louis, The CV Mosby Co, 1982
5. Scott MG: Instrumentation: Software. In Hubbard AW (ed): Research Methods in Health, Physical Education, and Recreation, ed 3. Washington, Am Assoc Health Phys Educ Rec 1973
6. Emory CW: Business Research Methods. Homewood, IL, Richard D Irwin, Inc, 1980
7. Suchman EA: The Survey Method Applied to Public Health and Medicine. In Glock CY (ed): Survey Research in the Social Sciences. New York, Russell Sage Foundation, 1967
8. Borg WR, Gall MD: Educational Research: an Introduction, ed 3. New York, Longman, 1979
9. Moser CA, Kalton G: Survey Methods in Social Investigation, ed 2. London, Heinemann Educational Books, 1972
10. Gordon RL: Interviewing Strategy, Techniques and Factors, ed 2. Homewood IL, Dorsey Press, 1975
11. Babbie ER: Survey Research Methods. Belmont, CA, Wadsworth Publishing Co, Inc, 1973
12. Sundman S, Bradburn NM: Response Effects of Surveys. Chicago, Aldine, 1974
13. Pomeroy WB: The reluctant respondent. Public Opinion Quarterly 27: 287–293, 1963
14. Schwartz A: Interviewing and the public Public Opinion Quarterly 28: 135–142, 1964
15. Dohrenwend BS, Dohrenwend BP: Sources of Refusals in Surveys. In McKinlay JB (ed): Research Methods in Health Care. New York, Prodist, 1973
16. Haberman PW, Scheenberg J: Education Reported in Interviews. In McKinlay JB (ed): Research Methods in Health Care. New York, Prodist, 1973
17. Colombotos J, Elison J, Loewenstein R: Effect of interviewers sex on interview responses. Public Health Rep 83: 685–690, 1968
18. Dohrenwend BS, Colombotos J, Dohrenwend BP: Social Distance and Interviewer Effects. In McKinlay JB (ed): Research Methods in Health Care. New York, Prodist, 1973.
19. Gay LR: Educational Research: Competencies for Analysis and Application, ed 2. Columbus OH, Charles E Merrill, 1981
20. Oppenheim AN: Questionnaire Design and Attitude Measurement, London, Heinemann Educational Books, Inc, 1966

21. Bruett TL, Overs RP: A critical review of 12 ADL scales. Phys Ther 49: 857–862, 1969
22. Gaito J: Measurement scales and statistics: Resurgence of an old misconception. Psychol Bull 8: 564–567, 1980
23. Sokolow J, Silson JE, Taylor EG, et al: A new approach to the objective evaluation of physical disability. J Chronic Dis 15: 105–112, 1962
24. Borg G: Perceived exertion: a note on history and methods. Med Sci Sports 5: 90–93, 1973.
25. Borg GA: Psychological bases of perceived exertion. Med Sci Sports Exer 14: 377–381, 1982
26. Guilford J: Psychometric Methods, ed 2. New York, McGraw-Hill Book Co, 1954
27. Cox RC, West WL: Fundamentals of Research for Health Professionals. Laurel MD, RAMSCO Pub Co, 1982
28. Style Manual, ed 3. Washington, Am Phys Ther Assoc, 1970
29. Clarke DH, Clarke HH: Research Processes in Physical Education, Recreation, and Health. Englewood Cliffs, NJ, Prentice-Hall, Inc, 1970
30. Simon JL: Basic Research Methods in Social Science. ed 2. New York, Random House, Inc, 1978
31. Melzack R: The McGill pain questionnaire: Major properties and scoring methods. Pain 1: 277–299, 1975
32. Kerlinger TN: Foundations of Behavioral Research, ed 2. New York, Holt, Rinehart, and Winston, Inc, 1973
33. Readership survey results—1972. Phys Ther 53: 293–299, 1973
34. Thurstone LL, Chave EJ: The Measurement of Attitude. Chicago, University of Chicago Press, 1929
35. Van Dalen DB: The Historical Method. In Hubbard AW (ed): Research Methods in Health, Physical Education, and Recreation, ed 3. Washington, Am Assoc Health Phys Educ Rec 1973

7

Confidence in Research and Instruments

For what a man had rather were true;
he more readily believes.
Francis Bacon

Research is undertaken to determine relationships or differences between two or more variables, and to seek good scientific results. Good scientific results are not necessarily supportive of the researcher's desired outcome, but imply freedom from errors and prejudices. The research process includes measurement which in turn involves instruments, procedures, and people. Measurements are subject to many kinds of error that may limit the effectiveness of the research findings and destroy the confidence of the consumer. The consumer may be a reader of a research report, a practitioner attempting to implement research findings, or a teacher conveying new theories to students. Accuracy and consistency of instruments, procedures, and people involved with research are of paramount importance for instilling confidence and giving credibility in research. Confidence is the assurance or certainty placed in the theory of a profession and the capabilities of its practitioners as well as in the findings of a particular clinical investigation. "It ain't so much the things we don't know that get us in trouble. It's the things we know that ain't so."[1] We must have confidence in what we do and know that the way it is being done is correct.

Earlier the concepts of sampling technique and variation were discussed. Subjects in our study samples exhibit a variety of individual differences; for example, age, sex, color of hair, body weight, height, skills, personality, and interest. Consequently, the researcher can expect different probabilities of outcome on individual scores or measures. The consistency of the final score or measure depends on the freedom of errors and biases. Errors are fallacies, untruths, and inaccuracies which may occur in the research process unless they are recognized and prevented by the investigator. Biases are prejudices or influences introduced by the researcher, technique, and instrumentation. The design, statistical analyses, or the statistician can assist in eliminating conditions which introduce error and bias into sam-

145

pling and measurement, but only the researcher can perceive how many and how varied the conditions can really be in any given study. An instrument may be highly accurate and dependable, but if the researcher has not identified the problem specifically, has not designed the study well, and has not taken appropriate steps to prevent, control, or correct for errors in measurements, the study may be worthless.

The degree of accuracy that an instrument has will be referred to later as validity, while the degree of consistency or dependability of an instrument is called reliability. Both research and measuring instruments must possess validity and reliability.

Accuracy and consistency in measurement are not faultless. Measuring devices are contrived to measure what we think is being measured and humans must take, read, and interpret the measurements. The true quantity or dimension of a characteristic is rarely, if ever, known in perfect (absolute) terms or values. The difference between a true measurement (X_T) and an observed measurement (X) is called error, and can be formulated, $X_E = X_T - X$,[2-4] where X is the combined score (recorded score), T is the true proportion of the combined score, and E is the error component or proportion of the recorded score. Measurements taken over the skin of some biological organ or structure are estimates, since more accurate measurements could be taken if the organ or structure was removed and measured. Social customs sometimes insist upon estimates of the phenomenon. An awareness of the limitations of the method of obtaining the information must be given consideration when planning research studies. Some of the more common classes of error are discussed.

ERRORS

Sampling, random, and systematic errors are inaccuracies that occur by chance during the study or experiment and are often synonymous in their meaning. A common definition of these kinds of errors is the deviation of a sample result from its expected outcome.

Sampling Errors

If we treated a group of patients having similar (severity, location) soft tissue injuries of the ankle by appropriate methods of physical therapy (ICERS—ice, compression, elevation, rest, support), we would expect the patients to show some definite improvement within 3 or 4 days. If a few of our patients did not respond favorably in the expected time, the deviations may be considered as due to chance and are called sampling error. We should not be surprised that not all of our patients reacted favorably to our treatment because different humans exposed to similar conditions will behave differently. The differences might be explained in terms of physiological differences of protoplasm or age differences. Variation plays a heavy role in the theory of scientific inquiry and measurement; variability is the central theme of research. The researcher is faced with the surmountable task of controlling the events in the research process so that the outcome of the experiment will be interpretable. Since error is forever present in the life and behavioral sciences, the researcher must be willing to take risks and accept some error. In the formula, $X = X_T + X_E$, the measured score is assumed to be a function of the true quantity related to the population trait and of the experimental error. The true quantity (X_T) of the overall observed score is related to the population trait through the design of the study.

Sampling error might be the difference between a parameter (true value) and a statistic. In the concept of error, a statistic is an estimate of a parameter and may depart at times from the true value.

Random Errors

Random errors are the inconsistent discrepancies that occur by chance. Random errors do not exhibit any trend to be above or below the mean which assumes the value of zero if a large number of repeated measurements are taken of the same quantity or trait. Random errors are not related to the individual observations or to the true score. In statistical theory the true value is the boundary approached by the arithmetic mean as the number of measurements are repeated an infinite number of times. An infinite number of measurements is not usually possible when dealing with humans because of tolerance, fatigue, time, and availability. The researcher takes consolation by assuming control over as many factors as possible in the research process and assuming that measurement errors are slight and distributed randomly. Such random errors do not form a bias but do increase the value of the computed variance or standard deviation which then becomes compounded with effect and error. The researcher has the difficulty of deciding whether the recorded values suffice for making conclusions.

Equivocal decisions where the observer was not quite sure of the value or the event lead to random error. In some studies multiple readings or duplicate responses can be made so that the mean of the recorded scores is used as the true value. The lack of practice or standardization of testing procedures before the research data are collected may induce error at the beginning of the data collecting process, but disappear once the observer acquires experience and finesse in measuring the trait. If different equipment is used to record values, some of the differences occurring between values may be attributed to the idiosyncrasies of the different equipment. In the study by Stewart and co-workers, inconsistencies were found in the timers, in the dosages per unit displayed on the meters, and leakages in the electrode cables of different ultrasound units.[5] Like people, different units of equipment performing the same function fluctuate according to the unit or in other words, have their own personalities.

If you have ever had the pleasure of measuring the width of a closet in order to construct shelving, you no doubt found your measurement was either slightly less or slightly more than the actual width after you cut the wood. The slight difference may not have caused any practical difficulty and the shelf may have fit into place. The board was not precise in measurement. If you measured the width of the closet several times you might notice that each measurement differed slightly (depending somewhat on the precision of the tape measure) such as: 60.8, 61.2, 61.1, and 60.9 centimeters. The lack of a precise measurement is a random error. If you were recording the isokinetic strength of the elbow extensors on a subject and then asked the subject to repeat the effort several times after adequate periods of rest, you would notice that each recorded value differed somewhat (30.5, 30.7, 30.4, 30.6, and 30.5 cm-kg) at a particular point of measurement. Several factors might influence the measurements and this only complicates the situation. The subject could have become somewhat fatigued, may not have given maximum effort each time, may have altered the position of the body between measurements, or the researcher may not have read the recording instrument correctly each time. These kinds of situations detract from the precision of the measurement or study. On the other hand, the researcher could have taken several measurements of the event in question, and then found the mean of the distribution of measurements; the mean would have been an accurate indicator of the true measurement because events, traits, or variations of the event would be distributed uniformly above and below the mean. Random errors are distributed similarly to naturally occurring phenomena in accordance with the normal curve.

Error can be computational, such as the misplacement of a decimal point in recording numbers or calculating results, the transposition of digits, recording the wrong number, or even using the wrong scale in conversion or reading a meter. If personal judgment must enter into reading a scale, then different observers may obtain different readings or the same individual might be inconsistent in rendering judgments. In nerve conduction measurements the greatest error is that of the examiner reading the values from the oscilloscope or photograph, or making measurements of the length of the nerve segment under study.[6] A method has been devised to exclude judgment in nerve conduction measurements by having the value recorded and readout electronically.[7]

Systematic Errors

Systematic errors are constant errors that persist until discovered and corrected. If the tape measure used to measure the width of the closet was inaccurate because of the marked units, or if the tap measure had some spacing before the first unit began (metal tip) and this space was inadvertently ignored, then all subsequent measurements would be incorrect by the amount of built-in error. The errors would be systematic errors.

If the researcher perceives the pointer on the dial of a meter as a whole for every measurement read, when in fact, the pointer is indicating a value slightly less than the whole unit, the errors will be systematic. Systematic errors are the same for each observation, procedure, or quantity being measured. If the errors are consistent and of the same magnitude, the standard deviation remains unchanged because the error becomes a constant and is added to all observations. If, however, the constant error is somehow multiplied by each measurement, the standard deviation will become multiplied by the magnitude of the constant error.[2]

Biases of various types can contribute to systematic error. A bias is a systematic deviation of the expected outcome of a measurement or of a study and is caused by factors other than those caused by the effects of the manipulated variable (treatment).[8] The researcher can systematically bias data by rounding off scores. Anytime a raw number is changed to meet the convenience of the researcher (rounding), some systematic error is introduced. The error will be greater when tenths are rounded to whole numbers than when thousandths are rounded to hundredths, for example. Bias can be present in selecting subjects, instruments, and treatment methods. In Chapter 5 several methods of sampling were presented; any deviation from a random selection of subjects can cause bias because prejudice is introduced when one item of the population has a greater chance of being selected than do other items. This type of selection occurs when selecting different methods of treatment or subjects. Suppose you are interested in studying the effects of exercise on subjects. If well trained subjects (for example, athletes) are selected for conditioning with an experimental exercise, the gains will be less than if sedentary subjects were selected for the conditioning program. If the researcher is aware of these differences between subjects before beginning and decides to select only sedentary subjects because they will show greater gains than athletes, then bias is introduced through selection. If the effects of physical therapy on edematous soft tissue injuries are to be studied and heat and cold types of therapy are selected for treating patients having acute ankle sprains, then bias is introduced because heat is known to cause increased edema if used earlier then 2 or 3 days following the injury. Again, this is an example of selection bias or systematic error.

Perhaps motivation is being studied as a factor in the therapy of patients having meniscectomies. If football players are selected as one sample and soldiers and government employees are selected as other samples, bias may have been introduced because differences in motivating factors may be evident before the study has begun. Similar differences might occur between private patients and ward patients. If a researcher elects to study only patients having minimum involvement rather than severely involved patients so improvement can be demonstrated, bias may also be introduced.

By this time the reader is probably weary and thinks that errors can never be overcome in research. On the contrary, well planned and thought out studies can prevent or control variables sufficiently so that errors are not present or are reduced to a minimum so that the researcher might sleep well at night. Very often biases are introduced purposefully so that differences can be demonstrated for specific reasons. If the researcher is aware of and can defend biases in the study, the critics are usually tolerant and will accept the biases if properly selected, controlled, and designed into the study. Defining a sample and particular characteristics of the sample, as opposed to other characteristics, could be considered as a form of desired bias.

In research that requires humans to perform while being measured for data, the outcome can be influenced by the subject's cooperation, willingness and interest in participating, and knowledge of the research. If the subject must repeat the performance several times, the results or values should be withheld from the subject until completion of the testing. The subject could place more or less skill or effort into the performance once knowledge of the values is known.

Researchers usually possess some internal feelings about the outcome of the study. They hope the results will verify some hunch, opinion, belief, or hypothesis, and they may exert some influence when taking measurements. The recorded values could be rounded off systematically to the next highest value on all measures greater than the whole unit, thereby making the statistical values larger. The researcher might even encourage the performances of the subjects more in one task than in another.

Researcher Errors

Other types of errors of analytical nature may relate to the researcher who employs inappropriate statistical analyses of the data: using the median when the mean is appropriate, using the t test for multiple comparisons of several variables when analysis of variance would be appropriate, or comparing standard deviations of several samples having dissimilar test conditions. Even the selection of the wrong instrument or of the wrong method for measuring data could contribute error to the outcome of the study. If for some reason we were interested in measuring accurately the reaction time of a group of children having cerebral palsy before and after teaching a particular motor skill and we used a wrist watch instead of a chronometer, the instrument selected may have been inappropriate. Some colleagues have advocated clinical research by using simple, unsophisticated equipment for research. The results obtained from this approach would be suspect according to the theory of measurement because of the amount of error induced by the measuring instrument. Since scientific inquiry seeks truth, the question arises as to whether a physical therapist is justified in using crude devices for measuring an existing phenomenon when refined devices might provide more accurate information and be available to the researcher if a little effort in communication was exercised. Different treatments may have specific effects and intercomparisons might be hazardous. Isometric exercise is specific to the point (position) in the range of motion for developing strength. That is, if the patient exercises only in full elbow extension, the triceps will be strongest in full extension, and will not exhibit proportional increments of strength in other points along the range of motion unless also exercised at those specific points. The initial effects of heat and cold on the skin are different and cannot be readily compared if initial effects are what are being studied. The problem and aim of the study should indicate an awareness of the specificity of different methods. The examples cited may not have any influence on the outcome of your particular study but you must be aware of their possible influence on your data and take appropriate precautions.

Errors are increased if the reader must read into the data the meaning or must interpret each reading during the occurrence of the data. In clinical electromyography the examiner must make visual measurements and interpretations of the data as the data traverse the screen of the oscilloscope. Non-numerical recordings or data can lead to faulty observations and interpretations.

Eliminating observer error is important for assuring accuracy and dependability of the study. Unless practice and standardization of the test procedure are enforced before the data are collected, observers can improve in competency with practice and if maximum competency is not obtained for each datum collected, then scores will fluctuate throughout the testing procedure. Delays in collecting data can contribute to error because of learning (experience), environment (seasons), or aging (children) effects influencing scores taken at different times during, say, 1 year. Handling of subjects, data, or equipment by the observer may possibly contribute to error. Having several therapists collect data for a collaborative study and having the data collected with different instruments at different facilities can jinx a well planned study because of too many uncontrolled variables (too many fingers in the pie).

Another situation of personal error which might occur when taking non-numerical recordings from an oscilloscope or meter is called paralax. Paralax is the apparent displacement of an object, line, or figure by change in the observer's position (random). The errors may be subconscious. Unless the person reading the information appearing on the screen of the oscilloscope is facing and looking directly (straight line) at the images appearing on the screen, the information contained in the images can be distorted, thus causing erroneous values. Angles of eye focus other than a straight line will cause this distortion. Figure 7.1 illustrates this situation.

SAMPLE SIZE

Ideal accuracy in research is achieved when all members of a population are tested under controlled conditions. Because of cost, inaccessibility, and limited time, all members of a population usually cannot be tested. Samples are therefore drawn from the population and are tested, and computed statistics estimate the values of the population. An estimate of how many subjects or observations will be acceptable in a study is of interest to researchers when accuracy is considered. If variation of a characteristic exists, the accuracy of any estimate of the parameter will be reduced as the size of the sample is decreased. This relationship will be clearly shown in this chapter's discussion of reliability and also in Chapters 10 and 11.

The student beginning to conduct a research project for the first time frequently asks his advisor, "How many subjects must I have?" or "How many places must I survey?" The answer is to use the largest sample possible. Since a researcher is interested in learning about a population, the larger the sample studied, the more likely the measured findings will be representative of the population parameters. The researcher is less likely to obtain negative results or to make incorrect inferences about the collected data when samples are large rather than small. In research studying relationships (correlation), at least 30 subjects are advisable, while in experimental studies involving comparisons of groups, a minimum of 15 is desirable. These numbers are arbitrary and not well-founded since each study should be considered on its own merit and the decision becomes a judgment of yours and the advisor's or that of an advisory committee. Several factors should be considered in making the decision about size of the sample:

1. Definition of Variable. If the trait and method of gathering data are so well-defined that each datum will possess the same value or trait as the next datum being measured, the answer is one datum. In physical therapy no variable seems to be such that every member in the population possesses

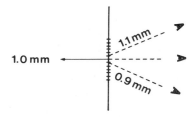

Figure 7.1.   Paralax resulting from different sightings of an object or scale.

the same amount of the variable. Humans and animals seem to have considerable variation among their members and study of the variations involves the theory of probability. Information is available for estimating sample sizes when responses are qualitative,[9] and when responses to treatments are quantitative.[10]

Researchers may elect to use the same sample size that was used in a closely related study that has been published. Knowledge about the standard deviations from previously reported studies can also be used in estimating your sample size. For example, suppose you located two reported studies in which standard deviations were cited for the dependent variable. The mean of the two standard deviations or data gathered from your pilot work can be used for estimating the sample size. Borg and Gall have offered the formula $N = (2s^2 \times t^2)/D^2$ for estimating the sample size (N) for two groups. They assume that the groups are of equal size and that the standard deviations are similar.[11]

N = number of cases needed in each group to achieve a significant difference at the 0.05 level (Table C, Appendix)

s = hypothetical mean standard deviation, 12

t = t test value, 2-tailed, for 0.05 significance level for 20 cases, 2.086

D = half of the mean standard deviation which is estimated difference between means of the two groups, 6

$$\text{e.g., } N = \frac{(2 \times 12^2) \times 2.086^2}{6^2} = \frac{288 \times 4.35}{36} = 35$$

The formula estimates that 35 cases will be needed in each of the two groups.

2. Assurance of Representation. Because of sampling variations the researcher cannot be absolutely sure that the data of the sample are representative of the population. This difficulty may be increased when samples of convenience are used, but variations occur with other types of sampling, also. The population must be defined clearly so that no doubt exists about who or what is represented. If a population is sampled, data must provide the most representative information for answering the question. Defining the problem will provide answers and insight for selecting the sample most representative of the population, but in the end the defined population determines the size of the sample. If therapists in San Francisco are defined as a population, measuring each therapist would not be too difficult and the question about representation is solved.

3. Time and Costs. Meeting the needs of the pocketbook probably determines the size of the sample quicker than most other factors. If the researcher has unlimited time and funds, great pains can be taken to assure a representative sample. Assistance can be obtained for a price and reduces time in gathering data. The sample of convenience is most often used in

practice because of constraints imposed by time and costs. The general rule of thumb is to include as many numbers in a sample as is practical for answering the question.

Some beginning researchers think that a very large number of subjects must be obtained in research to convince readers or critics of the outcome of the study, yes and no. Yes, if statistical analyses are not being used to analyze the data and only counts or percentages are used as the best representation of the parameters. No, if parametric statistical tests are used to analyze interval or ratio level measurements. Statistical tests of significance are rugged and take into account the number of data in a sample and will assist you in making the appropriate conclusion based on the number of data you have collected. Small numbers of data obtained from a well-planned and controlled study and analyzed properly will usually yield more accurate information than will large numbers of data handled and analyzed poorly. A rule of thumb is that if expected differences between treatments are large, small numbers of subjects are appropriate, but if differences are expected to be small or are unknown, then large numbers of subjects are needed.

4. Criterion for Publication. Research is never complete until the results have been published. Referees of some journals may be impressed by large sample sizes but statistics applied properly may negate use of large samples. Of course, statistics are based on sets of standards and norms which take into account the size of the sample, but surveys or relationship type studies do not have similarly established standards. The latter types of research usually contain large numbers in the selected samples since the closer the sample size is to the true size of the population the more accurate the conclusions. Statistics are not needed when the entire population has been measured; since no probability is present, the values are true.

Some colleagues maintain that more than 30 data constitute a large sample in experimental studies while others state that more than 50 constitute a large sample. Alder has defined a small sample as being less than 30 variates and a large sample as more than 30 variates.[12] Small sample sizes are used in research involving animals because of their costs and their having to be sacrificed.

5. Large samples are needed when:

a. Many variables are uncontrolled. If the researcher cannot control many of the important variables in the study, large samples are needed to achieve confidence in the results.

b. Small changes are expected. Sometimes differences between group means or associations between groups will be small because of the nature of the measurement. Large samples are desirable in these situations.

c. Groups are subdivided. Occasionally the researcher must subdivide cases into small groups because of the design of the study. To prevent very small numbers of cases appearing in each subgroup, increased numbers are desirable.

d. Dependable scores on the dependent variable are not available. If data are inconsistent because of the elusive nature of the dependent variable, a greater number of cases or measurements should be included in the study. This situation may apply more in research using software instruments for measurement.[11]

RELIABILITY

Suppose a physical therapist determined the heart rate of a subject by counting the pulses of the radial artery in a unit of time. The same procedure of palpating the artery, counting the pulses, and measuring the time with a stopwatch was repeated several times. The closeness of the measured outcomes would then indicate the dependability of the procedure. Reliability is the dependability, repeatability, or reproducibility of research or a measuring instrument. Whenever close agreement exists among several measurements of the same phenomenon, the reliability of the procedure, instrument, or research will be high. Under conditions of minimal error, the researcher and consumer may interpret the results of a single study with considerable faith or confidence.[13]

Several instruments used in non-experimental research were discussed in Chapter 6 while instruments of experimental research are discussed in Chapter 8. The concept of reliability applies to both methods of research and is presented so that the reader can develop an awareness of the importance of precision in research.

Definitions of Reliability

Several synonyms for reliability have been used earlier. Some additional synonyms used commonly to define reliability are stability, consistency, and predictability.[14] An instrument is reliable if it consistently measures similar values upon repeated application of the instrument for measuring the same quantities or qualities. Reliability might refer to the extent to which an instrument agrees with itself, an index of relationship.[15] A reliable instrument should be capable of displaying similar scores when the same instrument is used for a second administration of the same quantity; the instrument should give constant values for a constant quantity being measured. In measuring muscular strength of a group of individuals, random errors may be present because of transient effects of fatigue, motivation, paralax from reading of the instrument's indicator, learning, or any other factors that are temporary or changeable. An instrument may be reliable, but the study is not because of errors. Precision also describes reliability. High values of reliability are indicative of the relative absence of errors of experimentation and sampling.

Theory of Reliability

We know that measures of values (scores) are confounded with errors. The theory of measurement takes into account that all scores of human behavior contain amounts of the variable being measured in addition to the error component. The true amount of the variable or person's trait is reflected by measured values and that amount of the trait should be constant when measured repeatedly under similar conditions. We know that variation occurs between individuals and we know that the amounts of the trait (dependent variable) will vary when conditions are varied. Suppose we assess the amount of injured soft tissue of a patient by measuring the heat emission of the injured area. We assume that the measure (degrees Celcius) will remain constant until healing begins and when healing begins the recorded temperatures will change in proportion to the graduation of healing. We must also assume that part of the recorded temperature is due to error (measuring) and that part is due to the amount of soft tissue injury (true value). Since measuring errors are random or occur by chance in different directions (e.g., self-compensating),[14] each occurrence of an error is independent or disassociated with all other errors of measurement.[15] Random errors follow the probability curve of distribution.

Let us examine the reliability of the mean which we accord with high respect in research and science; this examination of the concept of reliability from a theoretical approach will increase your understanding of measurement and the concepts of central tendency.

Reliability of the Mean. We know that in order to study the heat produced by injured soft tissues, we cannot measure all patients in the world having injured soft tissues of a specified area. We must take a sample that is sufficiently large and representative of patients having injured soft tissues of the type we wish to study. To be representative we must select patients from wide and varied sources. The computed mean of our sample data will depend upon the number of patients in the sample and the variability of the measures being recorded (degrees Celcius for electromagnetic radiation). Examination of any number of data will clearly show that the addition of one or more datum to the sample will alter the original mean. The additional datum will affect change more in a sample with 16 data than in a sample with 64 data. The reliability of a statistic increases in proportion to the square root of the number of additional data. The mean obtained from 16 data is four times more reliable than a single datum ($\sqrt{16} = 4$). The mean obtained from 64 data is eight times more reliable than a single additional datum ($\sqrt{64} \div \sqrt{1} = 8$), but only twice as reliable as the mean from 16 data ($\sqrt{64} \div \sqrt{16} = 2$). We also know that if the variance or standard deviation of a sample of data is large, the individual data tend to scatter widely. The opposite effect of scatter is noted among data when the measure of variation is small. Scatter of data influences the mean (extreme scores).

The reliability of the mean is measured by its standard error. The standard error of the mean (SEM) is the standard deviation of a distribution of means taken from all possible samples of a population. If a variable, X, is distributed in a population with a mean, μ, and standard deviation, σ, and if all possible samples are taken from the population, then the sample mean, $\bar{X}$, will be distributed so that as the sample size increases in numbers, the standard deviation (standard error) of the mean will be $s_{\bar{x}}$.[16] The formula for the SEM

$$s_{\bar{x}} = \frac{s}{\sqrt{n}}$$

where s is the standard deviation and $\sqrt{n}$ is the square root of the number of subjects in the sample. The SEM is influenced then by the standard deviation and the square of the size of the sample. A decrease in the standard deviation or an increase in the sample size will result in a small SEM or an increased reliability of the mean.[17] Sample size is an important consideration in planning research.

If we wanted to measure the functional lung capacity of a patient having emphysema before beginning a therapeutic program to increase the functional expiratory capacity, we could ask the patient to breathe into a respirometer. The value recorded would give us an indication of the patient's functional lung capacity for that particular effort. The score recorded, remember, is combined with the true measure (capacity) and error. If we ask the patient to repeat the effort, rest, repeat, rest, repeat, and continue many more times without causing fatigue, the recorded scores will not be exact. With repeated efforts and recordings, we must assume that the range of capacities have been recorded, and that the mean of all the scores is the best estimate of the patient's true capacity and can be used to predict the patient's next score. If the recordings are repeated many times, the distribution of scores should also form a normal distribution when frequency and magnitude of scores are plotted. The first value recorded is not as reliable a measure of the patient's true capacity as is the mean of scores from many repeated efforts.

Each recorded measure of capacity contained a true value and an error value. The situation is represented by the formula:

$$X = X_T + X_E.$$

If the mean is the true score of the patient's capacity, then the variation in scores can be represented by the standard deviation of the mean (SEM).

Reliability of the Variance. Scores can also be discussed in terms of variance (standard deviation squared) by using a formula similar to the one above; that is, $S_x^2 = S_T^2 + S_E^2$ where S_x^2 is the variance of the observed scores, S_T^2 is the true proportion, and S_E^2 is the error proportion. In practice we cannot separate the true proportion and error proportion from a recorded score. The theory of measurement gets around this dilemma nicely by assuming that two equivalent measures of the same trait can be measured and their relationships studied (correlation).[18] The reliability of a measuring instrument can then be stated as the proportion of the true variance to the combined variance of the recorded scores.

Factors Influencing Reliability of Instruments for Non-Experimental Research

Since most of the instruments used in the methods of non-experimental research are paper instruments (questionnaire, scales, written tests, and checklists), certain factors can influence the dependability of the measured scores. These factors are not necessarily unique to the paper instruments but also influence some of the mechanical and electronic instruments when the subjects must cooperate in the execution of the measuring process.

In taking measurements with paper instruments, errors or variations can result if subjects do not understand or cannot follow the instructions or directions for performance. Personality characteristics may interfere with the scores or responses provided on the instruments. Attitudes or degrees of motivation may be influencing factors present on one instrument but not on another. Presence of these factors depends on the instrument and the subject's behavior toward and reaction to the particular instrument or to specific items or questions on the instrument. A subject's ability to respond to certain questions or items will vary according to skill or knowledge of the topic. An individual may respond truthfully to some questions because he knows the correct response or true situation whereas at other times he will create responses to appease the examiner or to complete the questions on the instrument. Physical or mental conditions of any individual at a given time may vary according to moods, health, fatigue, interests, or feelings. The person administering the measurement operation could be another influencing factor. Different administrators or researchers collecting the data can influence responses through their degree of enthusiasm; delivery of instructions or directions; voice; personality; and ability in handling the situation or environment of the area where data are being collected. Environmental fluctuations can influence outcomes or information gathered by paper instruments. Distractions can disturb respondents when concentrating on answers or responses to the instruments. Distractions may include noises and interruptions.

Determining Reliability of Software Instruments

Standard error of measurement can provide an index of the stability of a score. The reliability (correlation) coefficient is the most frequently used index for determining the internal consistency of instruments but it is a measure of relative stability.[15] Several varieties of designs for obtaining reliability are available, some are suited for paper instruments only.

Split-Half Method. This method is also referred to as an immediately equivalent form method.[15] The split-half method is used when construction of an alternate or equivalent form of the instrument is not feasible; that is, the administration of the instrument twice is unwise. In the split-half method, questions or items on the instrument are divided (split) into two equivalent parts (halves); the single form of the instrument is then treated as two. The division into two groups can be made before the instrument is administered, or the instrument can be scored after administration with scores of odd numbered items going to one group and scores of even numbered items going to the other group. This method is likely to be used when testing the reliability of certain questionnaires measuring personality traits, attitude scales, and performance tests (written or skilled types) such as motor or dexterity tests given to children having developmental disabilities. Repeated measurements using these kinds of instruments may be difficult because familiarity of content increases one's skill of performance. The split-half method reduces the necessity of repeating the administration of the instrument because all data essential for computing the reliability are gathered during the one administration. Chance errors may affect the scores on both halves of the instrument in a similar fashion which causes a trend for inflation of the reliability coefficient. The instrument designed for use with this method of determining reliability should be longer than other instruments (numbers of items) so that relatively few items on each half becomes a problem of influencing reliability. When an instrument is split in half, the correlation between scores tends to underestimate the reliability. The Spearman-Brown formula can be used to correct for the reduction in length of an instrument and for the lowered correlation coefficient.[19]

$$r_D = \frac{N r_{12}}{1 + (N - 1) r_{12}}$$

where r_D is the correction correlation coefficient to be estimated, r_{12} is the split-half correlation coefficient computed on data, and N is the proportional increase and is always 2 for split-half. Using data for the Attitude Toward Physical Therapy, Table 6.1 of Chapter 6, the split-half correlation was found to be 0.75. Substituting values into the Spearman-Brown formula, we have:

$$r_D = \frac{2(0.75)}{1 + (2 - 1)0.75} = \frac{1.50}{1.75} = 0.86$$

The correlation coefficient for the instrument if it was full length is estimated to be 0.86, a reliable attitude scale. (Discussion of the theory and computation of the correlation coefficient will follow later in this chapter.)

When planning an attitude scale, for example, the statements are generally distributed randomly rather than according to their weighted value on a scale. The reason for doing this is to prevent the respondent from responding systematically to only a cluster or a group of statements in one portion of the instrument. When testing the instrument for reliability, the odd-even arrangement will be a mixture of weighted values unless statements are arranged according to their level of difficulty or are of similar weights. No rule exists for arrangements or approaches to obtaining two equivalent halves and, therefore, the reliability of the split-half can vary according to the researcher's arrangement of the odd and even statements. In the example cited and computed for split-half ($r_D = 0.75$), the reliability can be as high as 0.97 when the right items are arranged in a certain way (e.g., odd = 1, 2, 5, and 6; even = 3, 4, 7, and 8). An r_D value of 0.11 is a big difference (0.86 vs 0.97) in reliability and the researcher must decide whether this method is the best approach for testing the reliability of this instrument.

Alternate Forms Method. This approach is also known as parallel forms method. The amount of agreement between two separate forms of an instrument is used by many psychologists to test reliability. The idea is to compose two separate instruments measuring the same content but yet not be so identical as to be revealing, and to administer them on separate occasions. A difficulty arises, however, if the instruments are administered too close together in time because respondents may remember items. Alternatively, when two different froms are administered, the danger of respondent's memory is eliminated because respondents have not seen the second form previously. Because alternate forms are different in appearance, they are often administered immediately after the first form is administered. Thus, the instrument can be administered without any effects from learning entering into the responses, and since little time intervenes between administrations of the instrument, a measure of stability is reflected in the coefficient.[20] Reliability coefficients will be inflated if the forms are identical and underestimated if the forms are too dissimilar.[17] The product moment method of correlation can be used to determine the reliability coefficient of alternate forms. Alternate forms can be easily constructed from the Thurstone scale since items are worded similarly and have similar weightings. Reliability is also good on the Likert scale because range of answers permits variation for the respondent. A reliability of 0.85 is common on Likert scales.[21]

Test-Retest Method. Repeating the administration of a test to measure the same quantity under similar conditions is an easy method of determining dependability of the instrument. Repetition of measurement must be made on the same group of subjects and under similar testing conditions to assure duplication. Test-retest reliability is the degree to which scores are stable or consistent over time. This approach provides evidence that a score measured at one time will be the same or be a very similar recorded score if the instrument was used to measure the quality or quantity at another time. Analysis of variance is used to determine the index of reliability (intraclass correlation).

Using this method for determining reliability of paper instruments can cause some difficulty if the tests are administered too close to each other. If sufficient time has not elapsed to erase memory and reduce recall, then respondents mark quickly the responses they recognize or made previously. Respondents concentrate on the areas of the instrument which they had difficulty with or were unable to complete earlier. Concentrating most of the test time on a small area of content can result in increased score values or altered responses which might then cause a lowered coefficient of reliability for the instrument. Thus, a sufficient lapse in time between the first and repeated administrations of the instrument is essential to reduce or prevent the effects of memory, practice, and transfer effects of contact with other respondents. If sufficient time does take place between administrations of the instrument, a reliable index of consistency can be obtained.

This approach is used in checking reliability of paper instruments because it negates the need for an alternate measuring instrument or splitting a group of measures into halves for the purpose of comparison. The alternate form and split-half methods are, however, preferred to the test-retest method for determining reliability of paper instruments because of the uncertainty of memory effects on the retest form.[17]

Determining Reliability of Hardware Instruments

The test-retest method is an excellent approach to assessing the reliability of mechanical or electronic instruments used in experimental research. The interval of time between measurements is usually not as important a factor with hardware instruments as with paper instruments because the subject does not apply memory. What is of importance, however, is that the measurements using hardware instruments be recorded at similar times during the day if physiological traits are being recorded to avoid influence of diurnal and circadian rhythm effects. Physiological traits can change in the same individual at different periods of the same day, month, or year because of influences of activity (wakefulness, fatigue, experiences, postures), environment (climatic factors of temperature; humidity; terrain; lightness and darkness; seasons), and menstruation in women. Most body systems are affected in some fashion and to a certain degree by factors or events throughout the day. The alterations in measures or scores of these physiological changes may or may not affect the outcome of your experiment but they certainly must be taken into consideration when planning the procedures used in the study and in the interpretation of the data collected.

Suppose you were interested in checking the consistency of an electrogoniometer. You could measure a series of specified angles along a range of motion in random fashion and note the markings on the recording paper. Another series of angles along a range of motion can be measured and recorded with the same electrogoniometer, again measuring each specified angle at random so that no systematic arrangement of angles is selected. The two sets of scores constitute a bivariate distribution and can be compared for their degree of consistency by the product moment method of correlation.

The researcher must decide what level of reliability is required of the instrument or measurement method to be used in the measurement of the dependent variable. No universally accepted correlation values have been established for reliability coefficients; however, two schemes for consideration are offered.

A[19]		B[22]	
0.90 to 0.99	High reliability	0.80 to 1.0	Very reliable
0.80 to 0.89	Good reliability	0.60 to 0.79	Moderately reliable
0.70 to 0.79	Fair reliability	0.60 and below	Questionable reliability
0.69 and below	Poor reliability		

Inter-Rater Reliability

We have been discussing reliability of a research study and of an instrument used in research for gathering data. Another concern of the measurement process is that of obtaining consistent results or readings from an instrument when read by different individuals. When two or more observers or examiners are measuring some quantity, the consistency of their recorded values should be similar. Different individuals should be able to record the same value but this is not always the case. The amount or degree of agreement between observers is called inter-rater reliability. Earlier, the term paralax was discussed. If observers are positioned differently from an oscilloscope or meter, they could perceive the quantities being displayed differently which would then detract from the consistency, dependability, or reliability of the readings.

The common approach to assessing inter-rater reliability is to test and retest and calculate the reliability coefficient for the two distributions of scores. Inter-rater reliability must be high or else the instrument is ineffective. Sometimes personnel must be trained to read a particular instrument. If the observers are familiar with the instrument and units of measurement and measuring techniques are standardized, then the correlation coefficient between scores observed by different observers is usually high. The researcher must be aware of inter-rater reliability if the task of gathering data is delegated to collaborators or assistants. The collected data and results of the study could be erroneous if high agreement between observers does not exist. Inter-rater reliability may be poor when many individuals are involved in gathering data (reading instruments); for example, several therapists gathering data at different facilities and on different instruments.

Calculating the Reliability Coefficient

Many statistical techniques for estimating reliability such as the Spearman-Brown formula, the standard error of measurement, Pearson's product-moment correlation, and analysis of variance have been used.

The test-retest method has been used extensively for estimating the consistency with which a measure assesses a given trait or characteristic or the amount of error attributable to two observers performing the measurements. The Pearson product-moment correlation method (presented in Chapter 10) has been commonly used to determine the degree of agreement in each situation. This method calculates an interclass coefficient and has several limitations.[22,23]

Testing subjects or making observations on two different days or occasions is a common procedure with the test-retest approach. Two sets of scores are obtained with this approach; however, only one variable is measured which requires a univariate statistic, not a bivariate statistic. The product-moment correlation is limited to two scores per subject (univariate situation) and cannot differentiate among several possible sources of error. The product-moment correlation coefficient (r) could be high when scores are inconsistent; systematic increases or decreases in one set of scores may occur while the scores of the other set do not vary similarly. The product-moment correlation method is unable to identify portions of the variance that are attributable to systematic and random influences.[23] Systematic increases and decreases are then treated as reliability, when in effect these changes may reflect familiarization, learning, fatigue, or disinterest among subjects.[24]

Because reliability is concerned with consistency over time, several remeasurements should be considered a better index of stability than two measurements. Analysis of variance (ANOVA) procedures are appropriate for determining reliability involving several trials,[23] and when one variable is measured on two occasions (inter-rater reliability). Although computational and theoretical details of one-way ANOVA are covered in Chapter 10, a brief discussion of ANOVA as it relates to reliability is included in this chapter.

ANOVA has an advantage over the product-moment correlation method by examining the sources of variability between and within scores. The symbol for the reliability coefficient is R when ANOVA is used in its estimation. The coefficient is a ratio representing specific components of score variation and can offer separate estimates of the relative size of each component. The ANOVA and R coefficient are considered more accurate than the product-moment method.[25]

Since the test-retest approach to reliability examines variability of measurements on repeated trials, it measures one variable. The coefficent R examines a single variable and is appropriate when used with ANOVA. R is an index of the relative homogeneity of scores within the groups or trials in relation to the total variation among all scores. Thus, the computed R decreases in magnitude as the heterogeneity of the intraclass scores increases and R increases as all intraclass scores become more homogeneous.[24] Interpretation of the R coefficient is similar to that of r, product-moment correlation. Maximum negative association with R occurs when the heterogeneity of the intraclass scores is maximum and trial means are similar.

The R coefficient is determined from variance scores in ANOVA but the variance terms (mean square) used in the calculation of R will vary with the different ANOVA designs. For example in the one-way ANOVA design, R is determined by using between-subjects and within-subjects variation. The more complex ANOVA designs, in addition to the variances used for the one-way ANOVA, will use subject-by-trial interaction as a source of variation to compute R. Between-subjects variation is considered true score variance so interaction or within-subject variance is considered a measurement error. Reliability using ANOVA can, therefore, be estimated by the formula:

$$R = \frac{MS \text{ between-}MS \text{ within or } MS \text{ interaction}}{MS \text{ between}}$$

where R is the reliability coefficient, MS between is the ratio of sum of squares between trials (SS_B) divided by degrees of freedom (df) between, and MS within (or MS interaction, depending on ANOVA design) is the ratio of sum of squares within trials (SS_W) divided by df within.

Using the theory and the computation for one-way ANOVA of Chapter 10, an example can be given. Let us assume that we want to determine the reliability of a method of manually holding a Doppler flow meter probe to measure blood flow velocity effects of electrical stimulation to a particular muscle. Six subjects are selected and three measurements are taken from each subject undergoing similar test conditions on the same day. Summary of the measurements and computation are shown in Table 7.1. A one-way ANOVA, random design, is applied to the data as if each score was randomly obtained rather than as a repeated measurement. The ANOVA computation of Table 7.1 follows that illustrated in Table 10.5. The obtained R coefficient is 0.84 which is interpreted as good reliability for the method of measuring blood flow. For a more complex ANOVA design, for example a two-way ANOVA, the MS interaction term for determining

Table 7.1
Computation of the R Coefficient of Intraclass Correlation as an Estimate of Reliability
(Fictitious Data in Cm/Sec)

Subjects	Trials			ΣX	$(\Sigma X)^2$	ΣX^2
A	36	35	38	109	11881	3965
B	35	35	37	107	11449	3819
C	36	36	36	108	11664	3888
D	33	32	34	99	9801	3269
E	37	36	38	111	12321	4109
	Totals $(\Sigma\Sigma)$			534	57116	19050

$$n = \text{number of subjects} = 5 \quad N = \text{subjects} \times \text{trials} = 15$$

$$SS \text{ total} = \Sigma\Sigma X^2 - \frac{(\Sigma\Sigma X)^2}{N} = 19050 - \frac{534^2}{15} = 39.60$$

$$SS \text{ between trials} = \Sigma \text{ samples} \frac{(\Sigma X)^2}{n} - \frac{(\Sigma X)^2}{N} = \frac{57116}{3} - \frac{534^2}{15} = 28.27$$

$$MS \text{ between} = \frac{SS \text{ within}}{\text{subjects} - 1} = \frac{28.27}{4} = 7.07$$

$$MS \text{ within} = \frac{SS \text{ within}}{N - n} = \frac{11.33}{10} = 1.33$$

$$R = \frac{MS \text{ between} - MS \text{ within}}{MS \text{ between}} = \frac{7.07 - 1.33}{7.07} = 0.84$$

the F ratio is used as the source of measurement error in the numerator of the formula for finding R (designs are discussed in Chapter 9).

The interclass correlation coefficient is often used for determining reliability of dichotomous data and two raters but is most appropriate for polychotomous data and more than two raters or one rater over several trials.[25] The calculation of the intraclass correlation coefficient (R) is preferred over the product-moment correlation coefficient (r) for estimating reliability.[25-28]

VALIDITY

Suppose a physical therapist repeated an experiment several times in which the heart rate of subjects was measured by counting pulses of the radial artey in a unit of time. If the mean heart rate from experiments did not agree closely with the mean heart rate recorded simultaneously by a cardiac catheterization method, then their relationship is suspect. Assuming that the cardiac catheterization measure (criterion) is the more accurate method, the amount of agreement between the two constitutes the degree of validity of the palpation technique. The criterion measure is considered a standard by being the most accurate method for measuring heart rate; all other methods are compared with it for accuracy determination. If errors or biases are nonexistent or minimal in research, the accuracy of the investigation will be high.

The accuracy of an instrument or of a research study is essential for reasons which should now be obvious. Systematic error was discussed as contributing to the inaccuracy of an instrument or study, and the lack of systematic error helps to increase accuracy. Validity then constitutes the degree to which an instrument measures what it is purported to measure; the extent to which it fulfills its purpose. This definition limits the scope of an instrument to measuring only that unit which it is supposed to measure; validity is specific to each instrument or to each study. Validity of one type of strength-measuring instrument does not guarantee or include validity of a similar appearing instrument. That is, a tensiometer may be valid for assessing forces but a strain gauge which appears to be very expensive, sophisticated, and valid looking may not necessarily be a valid instrument. Certainly the instrument may be capable of measuring kilograms but if checked with known forces and found to be measuring values higher or lower than the known forces, the instrument is not accurate (valid). Sometimes the instrument can be adjusted or corrected for this systematic error and then it becomes more valid than before the corrections. We must have some assurance that we are indeed measuring what we are supposed to be measuring. Validity is less of a problem in the physical sciences than in the behavioral sciences when measuring instruments are involved. When the measure or quantity is relatively stable or constant, the quantities can be measured easily by mechanical and electronic instruments designed especially for measuring the particular quantity. For example, many instruments have been designed simply to measure accurately distance, masses, electricity, and time, but measuring the behavior of a human becomes more complex and difficult because of the elusiveness of behavior. More methods are available for assessing the validity of paper instruments than are available for assessing hardware instruments; the need is greater for assessing paper instruments than the mechanical or electronic instruments. This discussion will cover concerns of validity for instruments of experimental and non-experimental research.

Validity of Software Instruments

In Chapter 6 several instruments for measuring qualities and quantities directly or indirectly were discussed. How do we know that an instrument will measure what we think it will when we design it for our research? Survey instruments are designed for the purpose and use of the user, and therefore, the type of validity is dependent upon the intended use of the instrument. Specific types of validity assessments must be available to determine the degree to which an instrument measures what it is purported to measure. The American Psychological Association has identified three types of validity (content, criterion-related, and construct) for tests and survey instruments.[24]

Content Validity. Content validity is a measure of how well an instrument measures the content of a particular trait or body of knowledge. Content validity is the representativeness of the subject by the items selected to measure a trait or characteristic; it is how well the instrument reflects the information about a particular phenomenon in the universe or about a population.[14] If a therapist wished to study the attitudes of patients toward a specific form of mobilization, a pool of items or statements would be compiled. When the instrument has been constructed and the 20 or 30 items have been selected, the researcher might want to assess the content validity of the instrument.

Content validation is essentially judgmental. The statements in the attitude scale are examined individually for their representativeness of the attitude to be measured. The relevance of each statement to the attitude must be considered as well as the assigned weighted values. The researcher could ask colleagues who are knowledgeable about the process or about the attitude to be measured to evaluate the appropriateness of the statements for representing the content. In essence, the Thurstone scaling method does this somewhat when judges are asked to order items. Of course, if the judges do not comment on the representativeness of the statements, but only order them according to the continuum, then content validation is not provided. When the particular trait or attitude to be measured is clearly defined by the researcher, then the associated content of the trait or attitude can be established. Judges associating or relating the statements to the defined trait have a good grasp of the contents to be included in the instrument, and make good judgments. The statements are judged for representativeness of the identified content. The process of using judgments to determine representativeness is, of course, subjective or qualitative. Use of several different judges helps to determine which statements are consistently rated high or low. The instrument must be reliable to be valid. The split-half method of reliability can be used to determine the internal consistency of the instrument and is more objective than judgments. A high correlation coefficient would tell the researcher that the statements are measuring the same variable. If an instrument measures one variable or factor and if it is identified as being representative of a certain content area, then the instrument has content validity.

Criterion-Related Validity. If an instrument demonstrates a close relationship to another instrument (criterion) when measuring some known quantity or quality, the instrument is said to be valid. The criterion is an instrument which is well established, well accepted, or considered the best instrument of its kind. Because of this high degree of acceptance or authoritative figure, new instruments can be compared with it for determining criterion-related validity.

Suppose a therapist wishes to measure the job satisfaction of colleagues working in general hospitals in Dallas. A new instrument is designed and constructed. The instrument could be tested in pilot work by being administered to a group of therapists. The Minneosta Satisfaction Questionnaire (a normative instrument) could be administered to the same group of therapists. The scores obtained on the two instruments form a bivariate distribution and can be analyzed for their degree of association by the product-moment method of correlation. If the correlation coefficient is high, the new instrument is valid for measuring job satisfaction because it agrees with the criterion. If the two instruments are administered at the same time, the validity is concurrent. That is, concurrent validity is a type of criterion-related validity and is measured when the predictor instrument (the one being tested) and the criterion instrument are administered concomitantly (concurrently). The extent of the relationship of the two instruments or the degree in which the two instruments measure the same trait or quantity of a variable reflects accuracy. Predictve validity is another type of criterion-related validity and is measured when the criterion measurement is made some time after the predictor instrument (new) has measured data. If the personnel director of a large hospital administered a job satisfaction questionnaire (new instrument) to all new physical therapy employees after 1 or 2 months of employment and then administered the questionnaire 1 year later, the first set of scores administered can predict the employee's satisfaction. If the two sets of scores are closely related after the second administration of the questionnaire, then the instrument has good predictive validity.

The two types of validity are similar, time is the only real difference. Instruments possessing predictive validity are often used to solve problems. In education, an aptitude test is used to predict success in college or some vocation. Intelligence tests in psychology predict a person's ability to learn or to cope with technology. Faculty of programs in physical therapy are greatly concerned about admitting those students who will make the best therapists. If "best therapists" could be defined and then an instrument developed to measure the desired traits, perhaps the instrument could be predictive of candidates who will make good therapists. The instrument could be tested for its predictive qualities by measuring a group of successful therapists who had been measured before admission to the program and had graduated; scores for determining predictive validity could then be compared. A validated instrument of this nature would be helpful in selecting future students; perhaps research ability could be one content measure.

The degree of association or difference between two variables provides evidence to support criterion-related validity. Statistical methods can be used to provide a relative measure of association (correlational) and difference (mean differences between groups). In the correlational approach

the students could be grouped into categories—"successful" or "un
ful." The coeffecent is computed to predict from a test score to a measureu
criterion of success on a job sometime later. The measurements taken later
can then be compared with those obtained earlier to determine relationships by means of the product moment method of correlation. Degrees of
job success could be determined. Correlation does not imply causation or
effect; that is, the reason for the outcomes. Relationship studies only
measure the degree variables vary together. A positive correlation implies
that variables tend to vary in the same direction, higher scores on one
variable tend to relate or vary with higher scores on the other variable.
Low correlation values indicate that there is little association between the
variables. Small sample findings can lead to false information because
coefficients obtained from small samples often tend to be inflated.

Another way of establishing criterion-related validity is to test the
differences between means obtained from different samples. If the difference between means is great, the instrument differentiates between groups.
If the admissions instrument discriminated between good and unsatisfactory candidates for becoming physical therapy students or on the job
success, the instrument could predict accurately and would be a desirable
instrument for basing student selection.

Construct Validity. Construct validity is concerned with identifying the
concept (construct) that accounts for the variance of the survey or test, or
explaining the differences in the measured scores by the instrument. In
addition, validation of the theory behind an instrument is a concern of
construct validity. When concepts are identified for explaining the variance, then hypotheses can be formed for testing the construct. The results
derived from testing hypotheses determined the acceptance of the identified
concept. This particular procedure then places the determination process
on a high level of scientific inquiry (hypothesis testing) and enables the
research and instrument to gain acceptance in the scientific community.

Validity of Hardware Instruments

Error is not often a problem to physical scientists as it is to scientists of
the behavioral and life sciences. In the physical sciences, error is minimal
or if error exists it is corrected or eliminated. If a device does not measure
what it is supposed to measure, it is eliminated, reconstructed, or adjusted
and the experiment goes forward. No matter what scientists do in the
behavioral and life sciences, error or variation exists. Validity is less of a
problem than is reliability when using mechanical or electronic instruments. When test instruments are new or are new approaches to old
instruments, the researcher or manufacturer wants to know to what degree
the instruments measure what they are purported to measure. Often the
researcher is faced with defending the validity of the instrument which is

to be used or was used in a research study. Three approaches for determining validity of hardware instruments are discussed.

Face Validity. Some instruments are one of a kind, the only instrument that measures the phenomenon. Face validity is used because it merely defends the extent to which the instrument appears to measure what it is supposed to measure. This validity approach merely provides a narrative or verbal defense of the instrument. A manufacturer markets a measuring device to measure speed of electrons and it is the only instrument capable of measuring electrons, the only one of its kind. If the particular instrument is the only one of its kind, then it cannot be compared to another measure; it is defended on faith or face value. The instrument measures what the manufacturer states that it measures. Face validity is determined or judged to be an accurate device for measuring what it is supposed to measure after the device is constructed.[25] Face validity is used in the physical sciences and does not become a major concern. In experimental research where comparison type studies are performed, the researcher may or may not be concerned with the validity as far as determining that the instrument actually measures what it does. The validity of an instrument may be accepted on face value and used appropriately for measuring the data. Experimental research often involves the custom construction of instruments that are not available commercially, and therefore, will be one of a kind for measuring a defined measure.

Criterion-Related Validity. This approach is similar to that of instruments of non-experimental research. If a newly contrived instrument or a new approach to measuring a known phenomenon is improved, but another measuring device is available and accurate, the researcher can use the criterion-related approach for determining validity of the new tool. The older established instrument is used as the criterion measure and the degree of agreement with the new instrument is determined by the correlation method. Each instrument measures several quantities of the known unit, and the bivariate distribution formed by the scores obtained by each instrument is determined for degrees of relationships. An example of this is the Scholander apparatus used to measure quantities of P_{CO_2} and P_{O_2} from expired air of subjects exercising. The Scholander apparatus is simply constructed, accurate, and inexpensive, but it is tedious to operate. Electronic devices, which are available commercially, measure the quantities easily and rapidly. Researchers who wish to know to what degree a commercial apparatus agrees with the standard Scholander unit often determine the criterion-related validity of the commercial unit to be used in exercise research.

Another form of criterion-related validity which is used more commonly than that used in the previous example is calibration. Calibration is the determination of accuracy of an instrument to a known scale or standard unit. An oscilloscope is calibrated by comparing a deflected unit of voltage with the grid on the face and if perfect agreement is not obtained, the oscilloscope is "trimmed" until the displayed quantity corresponds with the standard scale or unit. Calibration is a relative approach or an approximation to the unit believed to be real. The irony of calibration (criterion-related validity) is that determinations are occasionally objective for subjective values. That is, if interval level measurements are being performed and the instrument is calibrated, the zero point on the interval scale is arbitrary, not absolute as in ratio measurements. However, since good research results are dependent upon minimizing error, great efforts are made to calibrate instruments for accuracy before gathering data. This procedure of validating instruments instills in readers and the researcher confidence in the outcome of the study.

The instrument's measuring ability may drift from accuracy because of constant use, age, handling and abuse of the instruments by users, maintenance given the instrument during its life-span, and environmental conditions surrounding the instrument during its operations.

Calculating the Validity Coefficient. Criterion-related validity is the degree to which scores on one instrument are related to those on another. The coefficient is determined by establishing relationship. The Pearson product-moment correlation technique (Chapter 10) is appropriate for determining relationship or association because a single variable is being assessed. Measurements are taken from a defined group of subjects by administering the new instrument and then the established instrument (criterion measure). The two sets of scores are then correlated.

The resulting coefficient indicates the criterion-related validity of the new instrument. The scheme for comparing reliability coefficients of instruments is similar for interpreting the validity index.

The paired t test (Chapter 10) would also be appropriate for testing two groups of scores on a single variable. The t test would determine whether there were additive effects or bias present between the two groups of scores. The coefficient of variation (Chapter 5) could be used to show the relative degree of variability for the two groups but this approach is less desirable than the other two suggested approaches for determining validity.

SUMMARY

Sampling, random, systematic, and researcher errors are inaccuracies that can occur during an investigation. Research must be consistent and accurate if it is to be useful to the practitioner.

Error affects both reliability and validity. Reliability is the degree that research or an instrument is consistent or dependable, while validity is the degree that research or an instrument does what it is supposed to do. The test-retest method is a common means of determining reliability and

Table 7.2
Cumulative Summary of the Research Processes Presented

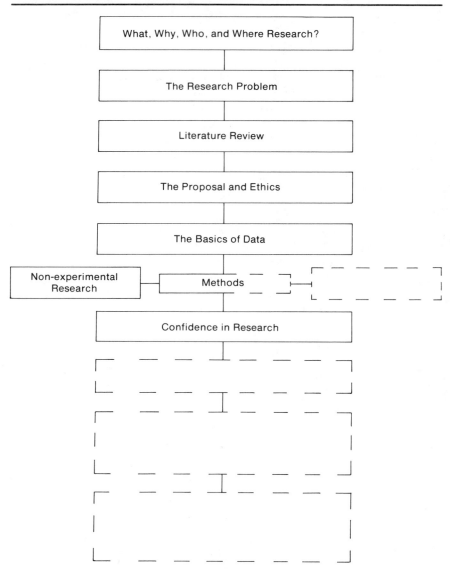

requires that a project or measurement be adminstered two or more times to the same subjects. The criterion-related method of determining validity requires that measurements taken with a new or unestablished instrument be compared with those gathered from an established (criterion) instrument.

Calculation of ANOVA and R can provide an index for reliability and validity. Table 7.2 provides a summary of research processes presented thus far.

REFERENCES

1. Cox KR: Planning Clinical Experiments. Springfield, Charles C Thomas Pub, 1968
2. Ferguson GA: Statistical Analysis in Psychology and Education, ed 5. New York, McGraw-Hill Book Co, 1981
3. Wilson EB Jr: An Introduction to Scientific Research. New York, McGraw-Hill Book Co, 1952
4. Guilford JP, Fruchter B: Fundamental Statistics in Psychology and Education, ed 6. New York, McGraw-Hill Book Co, 1977
5. Stewart HF, Harris GR, Herman BA, et al: Survey of use and performance of ultrasonic therapy equipment in Pinellas County, Florida. Phys Ther 54: 707–715, 1974
6. Honet JC, Jebsen RH, Perrin EB: Variability of nerve conduction velocity determinations in normal persons. Arch Phys Med Rehabil 49: 650–654, 1968
7. Nelson RM, Brooks R, Currier DP: An automated method to determine the conduction time of peripheral motor nerves. Proc World Confed Phys Ther 7: 140–146, 1974
8. Cain RB: Elementary Statistical Concepts. Philadelphia, WB Saunders Co, 1972
9. Cochrran WG, Cox GM: Experimental Designs, ed 2. New York, Wiley, 1957
10. Cochran WG, Snedecor GW: Statistical Methods, ed 6, Ames, Iowa, Iowa State University, 1967
11. Borg WR, Gall MD: Educational Research: An Introduction, ed. 3. New Hork, Longman, 1979
12. Alder HL, Roessler EB: Introduction to Probability and Statistics, ed 6. San Francisco, WH Freeman and Co, 1977
13. Schor S: Fundamentals of Biostatistics. New York, BP Putnam's Sons, 1968
14. Kerlinger FN: Foundations of Behavioral Research, ed 2. New York. Holt Rinehart and Winston, Inc, 1973
15. Thorndike RM: Reliability. In Bolton B (ed): Handbook of Measurement and Evaluation in Rehabilitation. Baltimore, University Park Press, 1976
16. Morehouse CA, Stull GA: Statistical Principles and Procedures with Applications for Physical Education. Philadelphia, Lea & Febiger, 1975
17. Garrett HE: Statistics in Psychology and Education, ed 5. New York, Longmans, Green and Co, 1958
18. Gulliksen H: Theory of Mental Tests. New York, Wiley & Sons, 1950
19. Blesh TE: Measurement in Physical Education, ed 2. New York, The Ronald Pres Co, 1974
20. Moser CA, Kalton G: Survey Methods in Social Investigation, ed 2. London, Heinemann, 1972
21. Oppenheim AN: Questionnaire Design and Attitude Measurement. London, Heinemann, 1966
22. Richman J, Madrides L, Prince B: Research methodology and applied statistics, Part 3: Measurement procedures in research. Physiother Canada 32: 253–257, 1980
23. Roscoe JT: Fundamental Research Statistics for the Behavioral Sciences, ed 2. New York, Holt, Rinehart and Winston, Inc, 1975
24. Standards for Educational and Psychological Tests. Washington, Am Psych Assoc, 1974
25. Bartko JJ, Carpenter WT: On the methods and theory of reliability. J Nerv Ment Dis 163: 307–317, 1976
26. Safrit MJ (ed): Reliability Theory. Washington (DC), Am Alliance Health Phys Educ Rec, 1976

27. Kroll W: A note on the coefficient of intraclass correlation as an estimate of reliability. Res Q Am Assoc Health Phys Educ 33: 313–316, 1962
28. Safrit MJ: Evaluation in Physical Education: Assessing Motor Behavior. Englewood Cliffs (NJ), Prentice-Hall, 1973
29. Makrides L, Richman J: Research methodology and applied statistics, Part 6: Ethics in human research. Physiother Canada 33: 89–94, 1981

8

Experimental Research

I have formerly lived by hearsay, and faith,
but now I go where I shall live by sight. . .
John Bunyan

The ultimate in scientific inquiry is experimentation. Through experimentation, testing hypotheses are possible, authority can be questioned, and traits or variables can be classified and differentiated. An experiment is the manipulation of some variable or variables (independent) under rigidly controlled conditions for the purpose of observing the effects of the manipulation. Experimentation enables the researcher to compare two or more variables to determine whether the effects (dependent variables) are equal, unequal, larger, or smaller than the other variables. The unique feature of experiments and comparative type research is hypothesis testing. The experimental method is the only approach of truly testing hypotheses as they concern cause and effect relationships. Testing hypotheses in research experiments is characterized by measuring, recording, analyzing, and interpreting data as a result of manipulating at least one variable under investigation. Experimental and comparative research are synonymous in meaning and, therefore, are used interchangeably in this book.

Hardware instruments are metal implements, devices, equipment, or machines used in the research process and will consume a proportion of the discussion in this chapter. Although hardware instruments are commonly associated with experimental research, software instruments, for example, may be used in experimental research to compare behaviors of a group of subjects on two different occasions. Discussion in this chapter will concentrate on the what and where of experimental research, the research process, control in research, its limitations, general considerations of instruments, and research needs in physical therapy.

DEFINITIONS AND PURPOSES

Experimental research is the process or procedure of testing a hypothesis or a principle. It involves the manipulation of a controlled variable(s) and the observation of the effect of such skilled handling on a predetermined variable.[1] Experimental research can be further defined as observation under controlled conditions in which software and hardware instruments are used to measure responses resulting from the controlled conditions. In experimental methods of research, controlled conditions are standardized procedures used as a norm, model, or baseline against which the effects of the experimental treatment or manipulation may be assessed.

In experimental research the investigator manipulates one or more independent variables, observes the effect on at least one dependent variable, while controlling other appropriate variables. The act of the researcher manipulating the independent variable is a characteristic or an action that separates experimental research from other forms of research. The independent variable is the cause that brings about the difference between variables being tested. The independent variable is also referred to as the experimental or the treatment variable. The outcome or posttest results of an experiment is the dependent variable or the experimental effect. The dependent variable is sometimes called the criterion variable and accounts for the difference or change occurring between groups or events as a result of manipulating the independent variable(s). In other words, the dependent variable is contingent on the independent variable(s); it is the measureable outcome. The dependent variable may be measured by a hardware or software instrument.

The purpose of experimental research is to observe behavioral or physiological characteristics which change with various treatments or controlled conditions and to compare observed differences. It permits researchers to make comparisons between different approaches to treatment and to establish cause and effect relationships between two or more variables.[1] In experimental research the researcher creates the cause by deliberately manipulating or making the independent variables or groups different, and then observing what effect that difference has on the dependent variable.[2] The researcher judges the effectiveness of a particular method by observing the difference occurring between pretest and posttest measurements. The pretest scores serve as the control against the outcome of the study.

Experimental research occupies the highest position of the hierarchial scale of investigative methods. It is the most demanding and the most productive of all research methods. If properly managed, it produces the best evidence concerning cause and effect relationships of hypotheses.[2] Outcomes of experimental research enable inferences and predictions. It is comprised of several operations that have been presented and processes still to be discussed. Such operations include the identifying and delimiting of the problem, the literature review, the approval of the proposal which contains the method of the study (design in Chapter 9 and analysis in Chapters 10 and 11), sampling data, controlling variables, and reporting the findings (Chapter 12). Experimental research provides the scientist with the opportunity to measure quantities, to determine causes or effects of measured quantities, and as a result of findings to question authority.

Experimentation in physical therapy uses designs which enable control of certain variables and also enable certain interpretations to be made. The experiment is a scientific way of determining cause and effect relations quantitatively. Comparative studies usually involve statistical analyses which determine differences between two or more means. The experiment is designed in such a way that the factor or factors causing the difference between means has been isolated and is identifiable. Chapters 10 and 11 will discuss statistical methods for determining differences in comparative research.

THE SETTING

Scientific research can be conducted in many settings. The setting may range from simple observations of a child's behavior during a specified activity, in a place, or for a period of time (case study of child behavior) to a complex experiment rigidly controlled (comparative study). A laboratory is often the setting for experimental studies that remove the subjects or animals from their natural environment in order to manipulate treatments or variables. Some authors make a distinction between laboratory and field settings.[3] The laboratory setting is usually considered as a room or suite where extensive equipment is available to measure and to permit controlled conditions of experiments. The laboratory could be considered as an artificial setting when taking subjects or animals away from their natural settings for observation. An example of this situation might be the energy cost studies of walking performed in a laboratory as opposed to performing the measurements in a natural environment where individuals are walking and engaging in their normal work activities. The latter situation can be considered as a field setting. The field setting is one in which the researcher goes to the natural environment to take the measurements or observe the behavior under certain conditions. No distinction between the two settings will be made hereafter, since the laboratory is defined as the environment where the researcher and subjects operate to gather data for the study. Distinction is made in this book, however, between descriptive and comparative research methods through the modes of performing the research and the levels of measurement. In non-experimental research the investigator is interested in describing the status, while in experimental research he is interested in uncovering the cause and effect relationship. The experimental methods involve both the micro and macro levels of research.

THE PROCESS

As mentioned, the steps in experimental research are similar to those used in other types of research. The researcher chooses and defines the problem, chooses subjects and measurement tools, selects the appropriate experimental design, collects data by following specific procedures, analyzes data, and makes predictions or inferences.[2] The experiment is conducted to confirm or refute the hypothesis. Experimental investigations are directed by one or more hypotheses that state the expected outcome between variables. Experimental research usually involves two or more groups, an experimental and a control group. The experimental group(s) receives a specific treatment to be tested, the control group either does not receive any treatment other than measurements or receives a form of treatment different from that received by the experimental group. The group(s) that are designated to receive the experimental forms of treatment are equated on all variables, other than the treatment variables, so as to unduly influence performance on the dependent variable. The control group serves as a comparison against the group(s) receiving different treatments.

Assuming that pretest measurements were similar among groups, the various forms of treatment are administered to the experimental group(s). Following sufficient time for the treatments to take effect (if possible), the researcher remeasures the groups on posttest. If the groups change on posttest measurements, the researcher determines whether the change or difference is significant. If the change or difference is found significant (e.g., by statistical methods), the researcher assumes that the treatment(s) or intervention was a success or a failure. The outcome is then generalizable (prediction, inference) to situations with similar conditions such that it might permit judicious approaches to patient care.

CONTROL IN EXPERIMENTATION

The concept of control is central to scientific inquiry and experimentation because control serves as a baseline for comparing the effects of the manipulated variable(s). Experimental designs sometimes require a special control group of subjects for comparison with the effects of experimentation, or sometimes each subject serves as his own control. Experimental designs incorporate controls where several variables are involved; no variable is allowed to operate in the control group. Zero values or placebos are used as baselines or controls where the characteristics under study are measured on all subjects of each group. One group's measurements are used as the baseline for later determination of the effects of the manipulated variable (difference between means may be claimed as the effects).

Controls in experiments may also relate to factors, or measures, other than the effects of a certain treatment. If two or more groups of subjects are to be used in the experiment, selection of subjects conforming to specified criteria can also serve as controls to eliminate error, to enhance precision and accuracy of the experiment, and to standardize the testing procedures. Selection of subjects based on a narrow range of ages, similar sex, similar occupational activities or physical life styles, severity of diseases, or similar body weights and heights can serve as controls. If most variables are controlled by selection of subjects, standardized testing procedures, using the same measuring instrumentation, and using the same individual to take all data measurements, error is reduced and variables are controlled so that differences in means may be attributed to treatment effects. Experiment designs may account for certain changes in the experimental variable, but the researcher must control all aspects of the experiment that are capable of being controlled. Testing must adhere to rigorous procedures to ensure proficiency; use of control groups help in instances where maturation and learning factors may influence results[4-6]

Certain experimental factors can be controlled during the experiment as routine procedures to reduce error and to permit only the effects variable to operate in the experiment.

The researcher must choose subjects or animals with care. Sampling procedures have been discussed in Chapter 5 along with their advantages and disadvantages. Other factors must be considered when selecting subjects and adherence to decisions must be controlled. Ages of subjects could be an important factor if the problem centered on a particular variable that is influenced by age. If the researcher was interested in the conduction velocities of a certain nerve, age could be considered as influencing results. Studies have been reported where the results were analyzed on the basis of velocities for certain decades of age.[7,8] On the other hand, a specific age or range of ages may be of interest such as the physical working capacity of sedentary men between the ages of 40 and 45 years. The decision must be made whether homogeneity or heterogeneity of age is an important factor to be controlled in the experiment. The sex of the subjects must be considered. In some studies a mixture of male and female subjects is not an important factor, while in others sex is important. Motivation and interest factors may be important in studies where the measured data depend upon the cooperation of the subject. Strength measurements are dependent upon the motivation and interest of the subject; whereas, nerve conduction values are independent of the subject's motivation or interest. The occupations of subjects or the physical activities of the subjects being drawn into a sample for study may be important for physiological measurements. The contention is that active subjects would be expected to achieve more desirable scores than sedentary or passive subjects in tests where conditioning factors influence the outcome of the scores.

Cox and West[9] have offered other controls for enhancing the validity of experimental research. Random assignment of subjects to groups eliminates bias by making the groups as comparable as possible prior to the administration of the treatment(s). Matching individual subjects on extraneous variables (those of no interest but those that may influence the outcome, e.g., sex, age, and handedness and then assigning one member of each pair randomly to the experimental group is a useful technique of obtaining equivalent groups prior to administering treatment. Another approach is to eliminate an influencing variable from the study by holding it constant. An example is to have one observer take all measurements so differences caused by different observers will be eliminated. Using a placebo to let subjects think that they are receiving the experimental treatment, and using analysis of covariance, a statistical method, to adjust scores on the dependent variable for pretest differences between groups are other approaches of obtaining equivalent groups to improve control in experimental research.[9]

The use of proper controls in comparative research can result in more convincing results than if controls were lacking. A convincing answer to an important research question is the basis for expanding the body of knowledge of physical therapy.

LIMITATIONS

Experimental research has limitations even though it is the best approach to conducting research. The process of randomization is an excellent way of obtaining equivalent groups and eliminating bias prior to administering experimental treatments but it may be impossible to apply. In health research, subjects are not commonly members of intact groups which is a condition required to apply the randomization process. Experimental treatments are frequently applied to subjects for a period of time insufficient for an effect to take place. For example, exercising trained subjects for 1 or 2 weeks with a new or novel approach may be an insufficient period of time for the new treatment to take effect. Likewise, the intensity or the difference of the treatments may be so subtle that any change between pretest and posttest is not measurable. If electrical stimulation is applied to a muscle with an intensity equal to 15% of maximum voluntary contraction of the muscle, the difference of 15 from 0% may be insufficient to show a treatment effect. Withholding treatment or using the placebo approach to a group of patients may be unethical and unacceptable for experimental research. Also, the control over extraneous variables or maintaining constant environment during the experiment may be impossible.[9] Researchers must be aware of such limitations and make every effort to avoid, prevent, or eliminate as many of the limitations as are possible.

HARDWARE INSTRUMENTS

Research must be objective and objectivity implies that data must be measured quantitatively (Chapter 5). A variety of instruments, old and new, are available for measuring and recording quantities which physical therapists deal with constantly. Applied research assists the practitioner by validating those things which are used in the management of the patient. The researcher measures forces, motion, temperature, light, sound, gas volumes and contents, respiratory functions, action potentials, currents, and cardiac functions.[10] The researcher must, therefore, become acquainted with instruments that are available to assist in objective measurements. Only brief and superficial coverage of instrumentation will be covered in this chapter; the student is advised to seek appropriate details about instruments through a number of possible sources: manufacturers' catalogues in purchasing departments of any hospital, university, or research center; visitation of laboratories, workshops, local, state, and national conferences; writing to authors who reported the use of particular instruments in their studies, and certain other resources such as:

MEDICAL ELECTRONICS & EQUIPMENT NEWS. A paper published semi-monthly by Reilly Publications Co., Park Ridge, IL 60068. The paper is available by subscription to physicians, clinicians, researchers, medical faculty, and hospital personnel. The aim of the paper is to report availability of instruments and scientific apparatus; electronic and electro-mechanical devices; laboratory supplies; materials and accessories used in clinical applications, diagnoses, therapy, radiology, surgery, analyses, and research.

DIRECTORY & BUYER'S GUIDE. This is usually the December issue of the MEDICAL ELECTRONICS & EQUIPMENT NEWS and contains information for equipment purchases for the forthcoming year.

Walker RB (ed): Source of Equipment for Sport Science Laboratories. Guelph, Ontario, Canada, Canadian Association of Sports Sciences.

SCIENCE GUIDE TO SCIENTIFIC INSTRUMENTS. This guide is published annually as a supplement to the journal SCIENCE. Thousands of instruments and manufacturers are listed.

Considine DM (ed): ENCYCLOPEDIA OF INSTRUMENTATION AND CONTROL. New York, McGraw-Hill Book Co, 1971. This book contains nearly 700 entries of instruments arranged alphabetically into categories of measurands, measurement systems, instrument data processing, control systems, and applications.

USES OF SCIENTIFIC INSTRUMENTS

Quantitative measurements are important in experimental (comparative) research. Much of the data gathered in comparative research is from either humans or animals. Clinical research constitutes perhaps the greatest portion of comparative research methods and deals only with humans. Instrument systems are necessary for gathering quantitative data which may encompass interactions with electrical, acoustical, chemical, thermal, mechanical, hydraulic, pneumatic, or optical phenomena. In physical therapy instruments may be used for:

1. Patient Assessment. Before treatment or management of a patient can be planned intelligently, clarifying examinations must be given. Improvement of existing tests and measurements are needed, as well as the development of new tests. Procedures are needed for accurately measuring quantitative values of strength, motion, gait, and effects of a given therapy. Instruments used for these purposes must be economical, convenient to apply or operate, safe, and able to provide information expeditiously. Once baseline data are gathered about the weaknesses and strengths of a condition or problem, the therapeutic program can be planned and executed.
2. Monitoring. Instruments are used to monitor ongoing events or treatment and to measure effects of a given treatment or procedure. Continuous or periodic information is essential to the therapist for the purpose of modifying the therapeutic program or supplying information about the status of the patient undergoing therapy.
3. Control. Sometimes instruments are used in physical therapy to control an operation or provide support to a patient.
4. Research. Instruments are needed in research for gathering information. Variables must be measured in quantitative terms to assist the researcher in analysis and interpretation of the experimental effects. Sometimes clinical and research instrumentation are the same. Generally, clinical instruments are used to assess and treat while research instruments are used primarily to gather precise information about effects of treatment, validity of treatment, and new knowledge pertaining to problems in physical therapy.

GENERAL CONSIDERATIONS OF INSTRUMENTATION

An experiment is the manipulation of independent variables under controlled conditions for the purpose of observing the effects of the manipulated variables. Instruments are necessary to assist in the measuring and gathering of data. Instruments are also used in experiments to manipulate variables (provide a specific treatment or condition and to stabilize subjects). Instruments are used in experiments to hold some variables constant and to change other variables in a fashion necessary for the conduct of the experiment.[11]

Instruments are adjunctive rather than central to physical therapy research. The study must be designed to seek certain information, while the instrument is appropriately selected to fit the design and fulfill the requirements of the study to gather quantitative data.

The laboratory provides a facility where techniques and their effects and responses to treatment may be measured and recorded with controls. Through the use of laboratory techniques, clinical assessment and treatment procedures are developed or verified. Clinical practice should place reliance on laboratory methods, instruments, and findings. While some individuals may be reluctant to accept gadgetry as a means to achieving goals of patient rehabilitation, instrumentation is recognized by most for its precision of measurement and quantitative delivery of physical phenomena. Instruments (gadgetry) of measurement are extremely important to physical therapists for measuring and assessing responses to treatment.[10]

Whatever the instrument used in research, the setup must be planned and designed with the purpose and research problem kept in mind. The researcher is advised to use established measurement instruments because they usually are valid and reliable. Imperfections are likely to have been removed from established instruments, the researcher saves important time by not developing a new instrument, and results obtained in the study using established measuring instruments can be compared with those of previous studies using the same instrument.[12]

Manufacturers

Instruments for measuring a particular phenomena may be available through several manufacturing sources. Some manufacturers provide good value for the cost of the instrument, while others provide overpriced instruments of limited value. Most manufacturers provide specifications for their product, and specifications vary between models, brands, and costs. The researcher must know specifically what specifications are needed of an instrument for measuring the phenomena under investigation. A researcher may have to accept equipment that is available, but in the event that equipment must be purchased, he must study the instruments' specifications, talk to the manufacturers' representative and even request demonstrations, examine closely the availability and policies for repair services, and then decide which brand and model to buy. Discussing equipment capabilities with colleagues is very helpful and can prevent mistakes in selection of equipment for research.

Most manufacturers offer warranties which serve as protection to buyers against failure of equipment operation within a specified period of time from purchase.

Specifications

The specifications of equipment must be known to the researcher before purchase for use in gathering data. Specifications pertain to the particular features, characteristics, and functions of an instrument. The researcher selects an instrument on the basis of its function and specifications. One does not select a steam roller to kill a fly, one uses a flyswatter. This analogy holds true for research. Instruments are selected for their capabilities and precision within the buying power of the researcher's money. Everyone should be entitled to receive the best value for his dollar and therefore, the importance of studying specifications of instruments, talking to colleagues about them, seeing them in operation, and planning thoroughly before gathering data cannot be overemphasized.

The researcher must plan or establish specifications for the instrument or equipment that will be used in the investigation. A certain type of instrument needed to measure dependent variables of the experiment may vary from source to source, qualitatively and quantitatively. The variations in specifications from different sources warrant planning and consideration by the researcher. Table 8.1 provides a list of general considerations when purchasing or custom manufacturing instruments for research.

The considerations for purchasing or custom manufacturing research instruments as shown in Table 8.1 are relatively straightforward. A few illustrations of problems which may be encountered by the researcher if the above considerations are not taken into account are presented.

A researcher may want to study exercise effects on the cardiopulmonary system of a group of subjects. An electrically operated treadmill is purchased within the allotted budget but upon delivery the door of the laboratory is found to be too narrow to accommodate the treadmill. Because of the lack of insight, additional money may be necessary to alter the doorframe. Suppose the treadmill is very heavy and mechanical assistance is required for carrying and lifting it to the laboratory located on the second floor of the building, and no elevator is available. Also, the treadmill may require 220-volt AC current but 115-volt AC current may be all that is available in the space allotted for the treadmill. Perhaps the respiratory assessing device is not appropriate for providing oxygen to the subject performing the exercise and being tested. In this case the subject may

Table 8.1
List of Considerations When Purchasing or Custom Manufacturing Research Instruments

Cost	Ease of manufacture
Size	Maintenance, repair servicing
Weight	Availability, delivery time
Material	Flexibility, adaptability
Strength	Validity, reliability, calibration
Durability	Ease of operation
Properties (chemical, electrical, mechanical)	Range, sensitivity, frequency response, noise level
Accompanying instructions	Method of recording, display (manual or automatic)
Trial loan, demonstraton	Safety

collapse shortly after beginning the exercise when his nose is blocked and his mouth is occupied with a gas-collecting piece. This situation illustrates what could happen if the researcher has not planned properly and has not studied the specifications of the instruments or facilities prior to purchasing research equipment. Suppose a tensiometer with a range between 0 and 500 kg has been purchased, but most subjects selected for a study can only exert 50 kg of force. The possibility exists that the instrument will not be sensitive in the 0- to 20-kg range because of the wide range incorporated in the design and the response of the materials used in its construction.

Cost must be a major concern to researchers. Funds may be available for purchase of the equipment but suppose the costs of operating the equipment are very expensive. Supplies may be very costly; for example, film and film processing or special recording paper.

The versatility of the instruments must also be considered. Perhaps several studies can be conducted while using the same instrument. But, limitations of an instrument may prevent its use in other applications of study or compatibility with other equipment manufactured by different firms.

The complexity of operating an instrument will be somewhat dependent upon the function of the instrument, the mode or form of the instrument (console or modular), and the knowledge of the operator about instrumentation. Researchers should read the instrument manuals that accompany instruments, and learn to operate, calibrate, and make minor adjustments upon need.[13]

Measurements form an essential part of any quantitative investigation in the life sciences, and for a measurement to be useful, the results must be understood properly by the researcher. Quantitative measurements improve our understanding of phenomena and enable us to control a process or system.[14] Certain features of any instrument should be considered, some of these considerations follow:

Accuracy. In hardware instruments accuracy is the degree of systematic error. Cromwell and co-authors[15] have suggested several errors of instruments which interfere with accuracy. These errors are: (1) attributed to operational deficiencies of the instrument because of design or materials of construction, (2) because of mechanical errors of meter movements; (3) caused by component drift or temperature variations, (4) a result of poor frequency response of an electronic instrument, and (5) attributable to reading variations of parallax, inadequate lighting, or excessively wide ink traces on a pen recording. A calibration check of an instrument before each series of measurements is important to ensure that the baseline reading (zero) is correct. Among other causes of instrument error are laxity in quality control during construction, mishandling during shipping, incorrect assembly and usage, accidental injury to the instrument, deterioration caused by wear, improper maintenance, and faulty repair.[16]

Linearity. Linearity is the degree to which output variations agree with the input variations of an instrument.[15] That is, the amount a measurement deviates from the calibration curve is of importance when taking precision recordings. The amount of deviation can be expressed by the full-scale input of the instrument. If the researcher determines the straight line relationship (linear regression in Chapter 10) for input at several calibration readings and then forms a distribution of scores from various inputted quantities (measurement readings) another regression line can be formed for comparison of slope with the line formed by scores from calibration readings (Fig. 8.1).[14]

Hysteresis. Hysteresis is a characteristic of some electrical and mechanical instruments such that when readings of known quantities are taken in descending order they deviate somewhat from the readings taken in ascending order.[14,15] In mechanical systems, hysteresis is the result of energy being absorbed by the system during the loading (ascending readings) and the energy not being recovered during the unloading (descending readings).[14] This characteristic can be illustrated (Fig. 8.2) by a cable tensiometer. If a cable and an attached weight-pan are suspended from an anchoring point on the ceiling and weights of known quantity are added in gradations and corresponding readings are taken, the observer will note deviations in readings taken when corresponding quantities are removed in a gradated fashion.

Range. Recording instruments have a span in which readings may be taken. The span or range is usually referred to as the full-scale readings of a meter. The range begins at the lowest number or point on the scale, and ends at the highest number or point on the scale. The range is sometimes

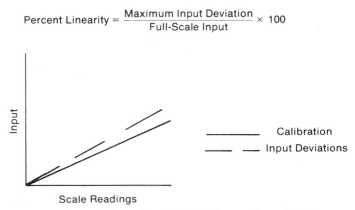

$$\text{Percent Linearity} = \frac{\text{Maximum Input Deviation}}{\text{Full-Scale Input}} \times 100$$

Figure 8.1. Hypothetical calculation lines for calibration and input deviations.

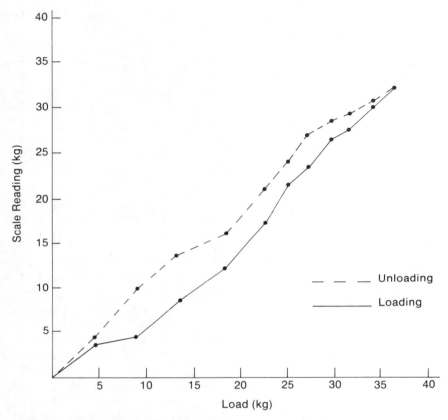

Figure 8.2. Hysteresis loop of a cable tensiometer.

referred to as full scale. An example might be the range of a cable tensiometer, 0 to 100 kg. The instrument selected for a particular investigation must be capable of measuring all quantities varying within a group of subjects or measurements.

Sensitivity. This characteristic of an instrument determines the degree or amount of variation that the device is capable of measuring. Sensitivity is considered in terms of its ability to detect the smallest variation in quantities. An amplifier for recording bioelectric potentials of muscular activity during contraction might have a sensitivity of 5.0 microvolts (μV) per millimeter of pen excursion or 5.0 μV per major division on an oscilloscope screen.

Frequency Response. This condition deals with measurement of quantities that vary with time. In an electronic amplifier the frequency response is its variation in sensitivity over its range of detecting electrical signals. An amplifier is limited to its highest frequency that can be reproduced.

The limitation of the frequency range is expressed by its bandwidth. The bandwidth is proportional to its gain (sensitivity) to handle certain frequencies,[17] for example, the frequency response of an electromyographic amplifier may be 2 to 10,000 Hz, and that of an electroencephalographic amplifier may be 0.02 to 100 Hz.[18] The instruments being used in a study must provide faithful reproduction of the original physiological signal when recorded for measurement. Therefore, it is important to anticipate the upper and lower limits of the time-course of the response you wish to record and then to use a recording system that is capable of sensing and displaying the responses faithfully.

Stability. The researcher wants instruments that provide constant baseline values, meters, or components which do not constantly drift or vary from the starting point or standard baseline during the course of an experiment.[15] A competent investigator will incorporate into the experimental protocol a regular test of baseline and calibration factor stability of all instruments used in the study.

Although this concept has been introduced in the discussion of console and modular instrument forms, all systems and instruments should be designed to be operated and controlled as simply as possible. Instrument simplicity for operator control eliminates human error. Each component of a measuring instrument or system is calibrated individually at the factory against a standard, but the researcher must calibrate the system once assembled and this should always be done by using error-free methods or devices of the simplest kind.[15]

Electronic and mechanical instruments are expected to comply with predetermined specifications of the manufacturer. The degree to which instruments consistently meet established values is of paramount importance in both research and clinical applications.[16]

MACHINE ANALYSIS OF DATA

For large studies or studies using complex statistical analyses (analysis of covariance or multivariate analysis) the computer can save the researcher's computing and rechecking time. Analysis of research data requires planning, time, and the appropriate machine selection by the researcher. If the group sizes are small, the number of variables are limited, and the statistical analyses are simple, use of a calculator should be a logical choice of the researcher.

Computer facilities which offer personnel services, instruction, and equipment are available at most universities and many large hospitals. Small hospitals or small towns may not have computer capabilities for processing research data. This situation may dictate the use of a calculator for handling data analysis.

Use of computers will require that the researcher learn about facilities, services, and equipment. In some situations these requirements will be unnecessary because all facilities and services may be available for a price. Both approaches should be investigated by the researcher prior to beginning a research project.

Preparing data for computers not only requires time but also costs money for processing. Generally, costs associated with computer analysis are for programming, keypunching, and operation or computer time. Researchers often do not have to write programs for their data analysis because programs for standard statistical analyses have been written and are available for use by the researcher. These prepared programs for standard statistical analyses are referred to as statistical packages. Each program in a particular package contains instructions for operating the program. The instructions are available at computer facilities or university book stores. Two packages that are commonly used are SPSS and BMD. SPSS includes programs for statistics frequently used in research of the social sciences, while BMD provides for a wide variety of statistical analyses used in educational research.

Data are transformed from data sheets to punched cards that are placed into the computer for processing. The process of punching data cards is called keypunching. Keypunching requires time to learn and time to perform. Personnel who are trained in keypunching and who commit few errors are often available for reasonable charges.

The actual data analysis requires little actual time on a computer, and the cost of computer time is usually reasonable. Costs for data analyses are often defrayed by grant funding, by some employers, or are often free to students.

The researcher must select the appropriate computer program for the required statistical analysis. The program chosen will indicate the format for keypunching data and the instruction cards to be used. Instruction cards give the computer directions for processing a particular statistical program. The key punched cards are then dispatched to the computer center for processing. The turnaround time for the processing of the program will vary greatly among computer centers. The completed analysis will be printed on several pages of computer paper ready for the researcher's interpretation.

AREAS AND INSTRUMENTS OF EXPERIMENTAL RESEARCH

Physical therapists use basic and applied research methods in many areas. The diversity of research interests in physical therapy is to be expected and is a healthy sign of growth. For each diversified interest in physical therapy research, a variety of conventional hardware instruments exist. An attempt to cover general areas of research interests and instruments used to measure physiological responses associated with those specified areas is made in this section.

THERAPEUTICS

Cardiovascular Studies

Peripheral Blood Flow. Muscular tissue becomes perfused with additional amounts of blood during dynamic types of exercise, while strong static muscular contractions result in temporary compression of blood vessels and reduction in blood flow. Experiments designed to study alterations in blood flow through the arms or legs of human subjects have been accomplished by using a venous occlusion plethysmograph. Plethysmography is a measurement of change in volume of a body structure and a plethysmograph is an instrument that detects the volume of blood that enters a leg or arm with each pulse. The segment of leg or arm to be studied is surrounded by an air-filled or water-filled chamber and measurements are made of the volume displacement (swelling) that occurs when the venous outflow (but not arterial inflow) of the segment is temporarily occluded. By recording the increase in pressure or volume of the chamber associated with three or four contractions of the heart, the volume of blood entering the limb segment can be calculated. The trapped blood (swelling) escapes as soon as the venous occlusion pressure (supplied by a blood pressure cuff) is released. Blood flow can be sampled intermittently and expressed as X milliliters (ml) of blood flow per 100 ml of tissue per minute.

An impedance plethysmograph can be used to measure relative changes in geometry or composition of tissues and fluid betwen two large electrodes. The heart and respiratory movements cause impedance changes between the extremities when monitored. Excitability levels of cutaneous receptors to electrical current decrease with increased electrical frequencies; frequencies between 10 and 25 kilohertz (kHz) used with 1 milliampere (mA) or less of DC current cause no discomfort and can be used to monitor impedance changes resulting from the action of the heart and breathing. Cardiac activity is a function of the resistance component and respiratory activity is a function of the capacitive component of impedance.[19] An impedance plethysmograph can be used to eliminate capacitive impedance changes so that resistance caused by blood pulsations can be displayed and recorded.[20,21] Two or four surface electrodes are placed over the skin of the limb being studied, and variations in volume of the limb are measured by the passage of a weak, high frequency current. Volume changes are supposed to be proportional to electrical impedance changes, but some question exists about whether the noted recordings are really physical changes between the skin and the recording electrodes rather than purely impedance changes.

The photoelectric plethysmograph operates on the principle of changes in optical density of a segment of tissue capable of transmitting light through it. The plethysmograph contains a photocell which senses relative changes in the intensity of light transmitted through the tissue. Red blood cells passing through capillaries in the tissue absorb some of the light. Flow of blood through the capillary bed is pulsatile; therefore, the more blood entering after a heart beat, the less light is transmitted. The output of the photocell varies in proportion to the amount of transmitted light and sends a signal to display and recording components.[20,21] A light source and the photocells are mounted over the body surface near a capillary bed. Transducers have been constructed for placement over the pad at the finger tip, aural pinna, and nasal septum. The nasal septum placement monitors terminal branches of the internal carotid artery.[22] The capillaries may lie between the photocell and light source so that as light is transmitted through the capillaries it can be detected.

The output from the photocell can be displayed on an oscilloscope and recorded by a pen writer. Since the instrument really indicates pulse rates rather than blood flow in many instances, it has been called a "pseudo-plethysmograph."[20]

Ultrasonic flow meters based on the Doppler principle are used to detect blood flowing through arteries, action of the heart or detection of movement of the fetal heart, intestinal movements, and passage of urine and gastric juices.[21] Moving objects (e.g., flow of blood) reflect sound at a frequency proportional to the velocity of the object (Doppler effect). When ultrasound is projected toward the object, some of the energy is scattered or rejected from the object if it is moving and the reflected signal is detected by the ultrasonic device. A second transducer detects the difference between the direct and the altered frequency. A hand-held probe containing the two transducers is moved over the skin to detect the location of vascular obstructions.[20,21]

Blood Pressure. Some information about the status of the cardiovascular system can be provided by measurement of the blood pressure. Indirect methods are commonly used for clinical testing. Systolic and diastolic arterial pressure can be determined by using a sphygmomanometer with an inflatable cuff and a mercury or aneroid manometer to register cuff pressure, and a stethoscope to detect Korotkoff sounds occurring during contraction and relaxation phases of the ventricles. This method of measuring blood pressure can be performed automatically and electrically with transducers and graphic recorders. Measurements obtained by indirect methods are subject to greater error than those obtained by direct methods, and they are difficult to record when the subject is active because of motion artifacts or when the subject is in circulatory shock. In addition, the recording does not provide details of the pressure wave form. However, the indirect methods are widely used and can provide useful information.

Direct methods such as percutaneous insertion, catheterization, and transducer implantation are used to provide continuous monitoring of blood pressure, records of the pressure waveform, and more accuracy than the indirect methods. The disadvantages of the direct blood pressure methods are that some trauma is involved in the procedures and the measurements on humans are limited to certain personnel.[20] Both direct and indirect methods are difficult to manage during activity of the subject.

Heart. Information about the heart is essential in certain kinds of research, particularly during work, energy cost, conditioning, and preventive programs. The shape and time-variant voltages produced by the contracting heart musculature are of interest and can be displayed on the electrocardiograph (ECG or EKG) or cardiotachometer. The ECG is a valuable instrument for detecting abnormal cardiac action potentials but not for measuring cardiac function.[23] Continuous ECG monitoring before and during multistage exercise testing must be an integral part of research. Submaximum or maximum exercise testing carries risk. Risk factors are of particular concern when testing men over the age of 35 because of their increased potential of heart disease. Heart disease is associated in such ECG abnormalities as ventricular tachycardia, atrial-ventricular blocks, bundle-branch blocks, and ST wave displacement.[24] In addition to being a source of information of heart rate and rhythm, the ECG has been used to detect ST displacement which is indicative of myocardial hypoxia. A horizontal or downward displacement of 0.1 mV or more of the ST wave constitutes the sign of myocardial hypoxia which often is revealed during exercise testing. Maximum information from the electrocardiogram can be obtained during exercise testing when the bipolar X-axis lead system is used with the positive electrode at the V_5 position (over the left fifth rib), the negative electrode over the right scapular angle, and the ground over the area of the right kidney. Frequent calibration checks of the ECG paper speed (marking paper at a 30-second run and measured by a stopwatch) and of pen deflection (10 mm = 1 mV) are necessary for proficiency.

Increased heart rate from many types of exercise is linearly related to the amount of work performed (intensity). Submaximum to maximum heart rates are better indicators of a subject's physical condition than are resting rates. The mean maximum heart rate for a given group is used in the evaluation of maximum aerobic power from the extrapolation of the heart rate at submaximum work intensities (stress tests) with known oxygen requirements.[25]

Work and Energy Cost Studies

In recent years physical therapists have become increasingly involved with the management of patients who have had myocardial infarctions as well as with assessment of the cardiovascular status of subjects enrolled in preventive medicine programs. The energy costs of patients having various physical handicaps are of considerable interest to the practitioner who is faced with rehabilitative efforts to increase function. As a result of these interests, research is being conducted to find solutions to the problems of and develop alternatives for enhancing function.

Laboratories containing treadmills and ergometers are used in the investigative studies of work physiology. These instruments provide a known workload for the exercising subject so that the effects of gradated stress can be studied. The treadmill involves all of the extremities of the subject so that distribution of body motion is somewhat uniform. The ergometer is essentially a stationary bicycle with controlled loads, but it involves mostly the lower extremities in the work. Although some ergometers can be altered to provide workloads for the upper extremities, simultaneous motion of all extremities, such as in running, is difficult unless two units are operating. Electrically operated treadmills have various speeds and inclinations for altering workloads. Speeds should be available from 0 to 16 mph, and inclinations from 0% to 20% grades. Grades are based on the percent of elevation that would be obtained from elevating one end of a horizontal plane 100 feet in length by measured amounts. Thus, a 3% grade would be an inclination created when the far end of the horizontal plane (100 feet) is elevated 3 feet. The ergometer can be operated mechanically or electrically, is compact, is reliable, and is cheaper than a treadmill.

Energy cost studies use both the treadmill and the ergometer when a laboratory setting is critical. But, the studies can be performed without these instruments when the natural working environment is preferred. Energy costs are best determined on the basis of oxygen consumed and carbon dioxide produced during a particular workload or activity. Indirect calorimetry is used in such studies and additional instruments are required for collecting and analyzing the cases involved during the work. Electronic gas analyzers are used with vacuum pumps which draw the expired air to the CO_2 and O_2 analyzer. This indirect method of assessing the CO_2 produced and O_2 consumed during an activity are reliable, accurate, and convenient. The instruments to equip a laboratory capable of handling these measurements can be quite costly; however, the instruments are durable and the information generated can be invaluable to physical therapists.

Additional information such as respiratory quotients and efficiency can be gathered in a laboratory equipped with instruments for measuring work physiology. Measurements of the volumes of CO_2 produced and O_2 consumed during an activity can be used to calculate a respiratory quotient ($RQ = CO_2/O_2$) which provides an indication of the relative preponderance of carbohydrate, fat, or protein being metabolized. The RQ of carbohydrate metabolism is 1, protein metabolism is 0.8, and fat metabolism is 0.7.

Efficiency is derived by determining the O_2 required for a particular work activity and dividing it by the net O_2 requirement. A percentage is formed by multiplying the ratio by 100.

Pulmonary Studies

Patients having chronic lung disorders are referred to physical therapy for breathing and work tolerance exercises, and postural drainage. Studies to determine the efficacy of the exercises and drainage techniques might involve the use of various pulmonary function instruments and the laboratory support for analyzing blood gases and sputum contents.

The usual measurements of respiration involve tests of the mechanics of breathing, physical characteristics of the lungs, the diffusion of gases in the lungs, and the analyses of gaseous contents. Lung volumes and capacities are indexes of the physical condition of an individual's breathing mechanism. A spirometer can be used to make most assessments of lung volumes and capacities. Dynamic measures involving forced breathing tests can also be recorded by a spirometer to provide information of muscle power associated with breathing and resistance of the air passage.

The spirometer is a cylinder containing water with a movable bell fitted inside the cylinder. Air is also contained inside the cylinder above the water line; the air is kept at atmospheric pressure by a counterbalancing weight. The subject breathes the air inside the cylinder through a flexible tube connecting to a mouthpiece. Attached to the cable is a pen that writes on a calibrated paper as the bell moves up and down. A recording is made on graph paper as the bell moves to provide a measure of the subject's lung volume and capacity. Prolonged breathing generally cannot be allowed with the spirometer unless a carbon dioxide absorber is inserted into the system. The usual spirometer has a 9- or 13.5-liter capacity.

Electronic instruments are available, and these provide instantaneous readouts of pulmonary functions such as peak flow, vital capacity, and various forced expiratory volume measurements.

Impedance plethysmographs are used to monitor changes in chest impedance. Small impedance variations can be detected and measured with respiration. Impedance measurements (15 to 50 kHz frequencies) between two chest electrodes may range between 400 and 1,000 ohms and during respiration the variations may be as small as 0.1 ohm.

A body plethysmograph is a volumetric displacement chamber in which the entire subject is placed. The chamber is closed tightly so that no gas can enter or escape except through a connection leading to the subject's mouthpiece. The connecting outlet may be attached to a spirometer, pneumotachograph, or a respiratory function unit for obtaining a variety of measurements. Some measurements may include pulmonary blood flow, minute ventilatory volume, respiratory work, oxygen uptake, and respiratory airway resistance. The chamber is designed for supine, sitting, and standing positions and so that the subject being tested does not breathe against pressures generated by the thoracic cage or abdominal muscular conditions.

The efficacy of respiratory gaseous exchange in the lungs and blood, and the gaseous exchange between the blood and the body cells is of interest in studying stresses placed on the body, techniques of drainage, and techniques of artificial gaseous exchanges. Devices for measuring gaseous content may use chemical. CO infrared, paramagnetic oxygen, sonic gas, and carbon dioxide methods.

Analyses of the partial pressures of O_2 and CO_2 in the blood, oxygenation of the hemoglobin, and the pH of the blood can also be made by blood gas analyzers.[20]

Exercise Studies

Therapeutic exercise is commonly used for maintaining or increasing joint motion and strength. Types of exercises performed for these purposes may be active, passive, assistive, and resistive. Although much research has been done in the area of therapeutic exercise, much remains to be studied. The literature has not provided convincing evidence of the reasons for selecting the number of repetitions used in exercise; of the efficacy of performing exercises at certain rates; of the efficacy of performing exercises in classical planes or patterns; or of finding a formula for converting force from static muscular contractions to dynamic forces when recommending a starting resistive load for patients having post-surgery or traumatic conditions. Another area needing further research is the enhancement of muscular force in addition to resistive exercises. Body positioning and support have been found to enhance force generated by maximum isometric muscular contractions.[26-30] The determination of optimum training regimens and techniques is still engaging the interest of researchers who attempt to improve approaches to rehabilitation and sports.

Instrumentation used for studying and measuring force have consisted of various mechanical and electrical devices. Mechanical devices include dynamometers, tensiometers, and hydraulic devices. Dynamometers are usually metal devices which contain a spring mechanism. When the spring mechanism is compressed or stretched, the displacement of the spring metal moves a needle that registers proportional amounts of relative force on a dial. Dynamometers can be used for assessing hand grip, back and leg strength, and finger pinch strength.

The pneumatic dynamometer consists of a rubber bulb connected to an air pressure gauge. The rubber bulb is squeezed and the amount or force produced by squeezing the bulb with the hand is transmitted to the gauge which provides a reading. Another version of this type of pneumatic dynamometer is the use of a sphygmomanometer and recording force in millimeters of mercury. These dynamometers could be used to study the grip strength of patients having arthritis or traumatic hand injuries and weak musculature.

The cable tensiometer is an instrument that measures tension placed on a cable. Force is determined by measuring the tension placed on a cable or by measuring the tension needed to move spring mechanisms enclosed in the unit. Force applied to an attached cable moves a riser that presses against the spring mechanism which in turn moves a dial to indicate tension proportional to the relative force applied on the riser. The tensiometer is suited for measuring isometric muscular contractions. Dynamometers are valid and reliable instruments for measuring the relative force generated by muscle groups being investigated.

Muscular forces can also be measured indirectly by a variety of displacement-type transducers connected to adaptive amplifiers and recording devices. Electronic transducers contain an appropriate elastic-restoring member, a spring. Because of the mechanical mechanisms involved with the operation of the instrument, transducers measuring force function with some hysteresis and non-linearity but usually with less than 1% combined error. Electrical devices have included the resistive potentiometer and strain gauge. The potentiometer transducer consists of a variable resistance element and a movable contact. The force imparted on the potentiometer is transmitted as an electrical signal which is proportional to the actual force applied. The force produced on the potentiometer changes the position of the electrical contact to the appropriate point of electrical resistance of displacement against the linear spring.[20,31] The strain gauge is another type of displacement transducer consisting of special wiring arrangements. An electrical wire has resistance that is proportional to its length and inversely proportional to its cross-sectional area. When force is applied to the wire in one direction, its length increases and its area decreases proportional to the force applied on the wire. If the wire is serving as one leg of a Wheatstone bridge circuit, the change in length and cross-sectional area will produce a change in the electrical resistance of the wire and the change in current flowing through the circuit is transmitted to the signal conditioner. Strain gauge readings express the percentage of resistance proportional to changes in length of wire. Meters and graphs are used to display measured units.

Dynamometers are available for measuring the force developing capacity of muscle groups while moving joints. These dynamometers can assess isokinetic muscular performance during eccentric and concentric modes of exercise. The devices offer computer-controlled exercise and testing at selected velocities, constant joint angles, constant force, and alternating reciprocal static or dynamic contractions.[32]

Electronic goniometers are available for recording joint motions in one or two planes. The potentiometer is usually an angular type varying between 0 to 10,000 ohms of resistance for 0 to 360 degrees of rotation.

One arm of the goniometer is secured to the potentiometer but free to describe an arc as the potentiometer rotates. The other arm is constructed with one or two hinges so that it will conform to the contour of body parts in which the arm is attached. The varying changes of resistance can be amplified and integrated for a displayed signal. The displayed signals can be interpreted by equating the magnitude of the recorded signal with a specific point along the range of motion of a particular joint. The electro-goniometer is a very useful instrument for research because it provides a continuous graphic readout of the variation of joint angles.

Physical Agent Studies

Many different physical agents (heat, cold, light, water, sound, and electricity) are used in the therapeutic intervention of patients having varying physical problems. Use of the agents has been based on research of several disciplines other than physical therapy. Not all agents have received thorough investigations nor have all been investigated while using modern measuring instruments. Much of the research reported was conducted when a single agent was used on a particular tissue; for example, the effects of short-wave diathermy on muscle temperature. Little investigation has been done when the physical agents have been used in tandem; for example, moist heat followed by ultrasound, electrical stimulation, massage, and exercises. Questions have been raised about the efficacy of the agents as therapeutic.[33,34]

Instruments used in the delivery of the agent must be studied for improved design according to needs of the therapist and patient rather than the convenience of the manufacturer, and the efficiency of the instruments must be studied for accuracy and reliability.[35] These instruments can be used in studies involving their effects, but monitoring and measuring instruments must also be used to quantitate effects for evaluations. Many of the instruments mentioned in this section can be used along with the application of the physical agents to investigate the efficacy of therapeutic treatments. Procedures used by physical therapists, such as those used to improve mobility of joints and facilitation of weak or nonfunctional muscles, must be studied to validate their effects. Combinations of procedures and physical agents must be studied to determine which are best for given problems at a given time or situation.

Manufacturers frequently are marketing new devices, although simulating a variety of physical agents that have not been validated for their efficacy in therapy. Physical therapists must not blindly accept new products that have not been investigated for their therapeutic effects. Electrical stimulators claimed to increase muscular strength, blood flow, reduce edema, suppress pain, and reduce subcutaneous fat; and lasers (light amplification by stimulated emission of radiation) that heal wounds and suppress pain are examples of devices being marketed prior to support of controlled research. Numerous other devices also fall into this situation. Techniques using biofeedback and TENS (transcutaneous electrical nerve stimulation) are examples of devices that have received much support by controlled study and can be used judiciously in patient management. Much research is needed to enhance the understanding of existing physical agents.

PATHOKINESIOLOGY

Kinesiology is the study of human motion and has traditionally been referred to as "normal" motion. The study of human motion disorders may be referred to as pathokinesiology and has been proposed as the clinical science of physical therapy.[36] As in any science, knowledge is built through research. Research of pathokinesiology has been conducted largely through the use of electromyography, biomechanics, and photography.

Electromyography

Electromyography (EMG) is the study of the electrical current or voltage generated by motor unit activity. It is an excellent method of studying the function of muscles in movement or stationary as prime movers, synergists, stabilizers, and co-contractors. Muscles have been studied according to their length-tension, velocity-tension, and tension-duration relationships. Electromyography, coupled with mechanical and photographic methods, can enhance sensitive analyses and interpretations about man in action.

The electromyograph is a sophisticated tool for detecting the electrical activity of muscle. The recorded electrical signals may range in size from 10 microvolts (μV) to 4 millivolts (mV). Their rates of occurrence (frequency) vary from 3 Hz to 5 kHz but components of EMG frequency responses may occur in excess of 5,000 Hz.[37] High frequencies (>250 Hz) contribute little to total voltage of the signals, since most signals occur between 20 and 200 Hz in healthy subjects.[38] Because of frequency variations, researchers using EMG should report the frequency responses employed in investigations. Although not inclusive, the electromyograph's essential components contain the transducer, signal processor, and recorder.

External recording transducers, usually called surface electrodes, consist of small discs of varying sizes (5 to 15 mm), shapes (cups, flat plates, floating cups, and clips), and modes of attachment (adhesive tape and collars, spray-on, suction, and glue). Surface recording electrodes are satisfactory for studying superficial muscles that are widely separated and for convenience.[39] Surface electrodes are vulnerable to the influence of other muscles of close proximity because their bioelectrical potentials travel by volume conduction and may be confounded with that activity of specified muscles (cross-talk). Internal recording transducers may be needles or fine wire. Fine, insulated, stainless-steel wire is preferred for studying fine movements and deep muscles because they are inserted directly into tissue being studied; they cause relatively little discomfort during muscular contraction; and they provide information that is representative of muscular functions. The diameter of the fine insulated wire ranges from 25 to 75 micra and is used in lengths of 5 to 7 cm. Preparation of fine wire electrodes has been described in detail.[39]

The signal processor consists of a differential amplifier which discriminates against unwanted electrical signals. The inputted signal consists of in-phase and out-of-phase portions. The in-phase portion of the total EMG signal arrives at the active input terminals (the third terminal is ground) with the same polarity (common mode) and is rejected as an unwanted signal (electrical noise and artifact, and distant potentials). That portion of the total EMG signal that is out-of-phase (opposite polarity) is detected and amplified by the differential amplifier. The in-phase portion of the EMG signal can be rejected at a ratio between 1,000 to 1 and 100,000 to 1. The amplifier discriminates, for example, 10,000 times more against the in-phase portion than it does against the out-of-phase portion of the signal (10,000:1). The amplifier must also be limited to low noise levels which are inherent to electrical devices and can distort wanted bioelectrical signals. The researcher is advised to consult the specifications of electromyographic equipment before purchase.[40-41]

Recording devices for electromyograms vary widely in their frequency response to inputted signals. Most pen writers are slow (80 to 120 Hz), some ink recorders will go to about 400 Hz, but optical galvanometers can provide responses up to 3 kHz. The oscilloscope and computer will record the most rapid occurring signals, while the latter has the added advantage of analyzing signals when programmed appropriately.[40,42] The electrical activity of muscles can be recorded by direct or indirect methods.

Direct Methods. The electrical activity of contracting musculature can be displayed on an oscilloscope for observation and photographing, or displayed by the movement of a pen writer over moving graph paper, or both. These methods are useful for studying the phasic activity of different contracting muscles during specific motions. If the muscular activity is recorded over a given time period, the size (amplitude) of action potential patterns may be compared.[43] Observation of the phasic activity by means of the number of potentials and their summation, amplitude, and type can also be used for interpretation of the electromyogram. Interpretation of the raw data has caused difficulties, however. Formation of an interval scale for assessing the amplitude or frequency or both of the EMG signals has been suggested. The scale ranges from no activity (0) to very marked activity (++++).[39,44] This approach to interpretation has been challenged, since zero ranges from no activity when in fact background noise is always present in EMG records. Also, the question of whether zero activity would be similar if the recording was taken from an adjacent electrode location has been asked.[40] Simple descriptions of the raw EMG data may still be an appealing approach to interpretation of kinesiological EMG. Indirect (machine-assisted) methods of quantitating raw EMG data have been developed.

Indirect Methods. By processing the raw motor unit signals using amplitude, duration, and frequency, the data over a period of time can be displayed quantitatively for the convenience of immediate readout, and requiring little manipulation for immediate interpretation by the researcher. The electrical activity associated with muscular contractions can be quantified by using electronic devices to integrate the signals detected by EMG electrodes.

The integrated signal is a measure of the total EMG activity over a varying time and its signal is proportional to the total area which occurs under the negative and positive excursions of the EMG wave forms. The integrated signal can be recorded graphically or numerically by an electronic counter. Various integrated EMG methods have been described. The raw EMG signals can be converted into continuous,[40,45] or interrupted curves,[40] spike counts,[46] turning points of changing EMG excursions,[47] and signal to frequency conversion.[48] Kaiser and Petersen[49] have described a power spectra method in which the sine wave harmonic components of the EMG signals are analyzed. The raw EMG signals are passed through four octave bandpass filters centered at 50, 200, 800, and 1,600 Hz. The filter outputs are rectified and the direct current voltages resulting are compared by using 200 Hz as the reference to provide a measure of the shape of the power spectrum. The power spectra analysis determines which muscles have the greatest concentrations of power for operating prostheses.[49]

Biotelemetry

Biotelemetry is the simultaneous recording of certain functions of a living organism by remote (distance) recording through wireless transmission linkage. Electromyographic data can be transmitted by this method, for example. The transmitter (transducer) may be implanted (intestine, mouth, bladder, or skeletal muscle) or mounted on the surface (skin) of the animal or person. Through appropriate transducers the bioelectrical signal can be transmitted, amplified, and recorded. Miniaturization of electronic transducers makes it possible to implant them in animals or humans for long term studies without adverse tissue reactions. Surface electrodes may be conventional types.

The bioelectrical signal is amplified and processed into an analogue signal and modulated for transmission. An analogue signal is a bioelectrical potential that has been converted into another form for convenience of processing; for example, EMG activity converted into a sine wave which represents the time and quantity components of wave forms. The analogue signal is then transmitted to a receiver which accepts the transmitted signal by means of a selected frequency (80 to 250 mHz). Once received, the analogue signal is separated from the carrier wave (demodulated) and displayed for interpretation.

Modulation is the process of sending radio frequencies through air in the form of electromagnetic waves. Amplitude modulation (AM) causes the transmitted wave to vary in magnitude as the mode of transmission, while frequency modulation (FM) causes the waves to vary in their frequency (88 to 108 mHz).[21] The amplitude of the carrier signals varies with the information being transmitted and can be conveyed over long distances (e.g., radio and television). The frequency of the carrier signals varies with the transmitted waves in frequency modulation and as a result electrical interferences can be removed before modulation. Because of less electrical interference during transmission, FM is the method of choice in biotelemetry.

Multichannel transmission of data (multiplexing) is possible with telemetry but difficulty arises because of cross-talk (signals from adjacent structures mix). Small amounts of cross-talk can give misleading information and pose problems with interpretation.

Biotelemetry is useful if the distances between the receiving station and the subject are relatively short, less than two kilometers. The range is a function of the power source and limits have been set by the Federal Communications Commission. A license is required to transmit signals beyond certain distances. A radio telemetry system will predictably fail if the subject goes beyond the range capabilities of a particular unit. Long range telemeter systems are not readily available through commercial sources and usually must be custom manufactured. Large and heavy batteries are required if long transmission life is desired.

Much of the knowledge and sophistication of telemetry was developed in the aerospace program. Almost any quantity that can be measured with a transducer that produces an electrical output signal can be telemetered, such as ECG, EMG, EEG, blood and gastrointestinal pressures, blood flow, temperature, and respiration signals.[20]

Biomechanics

Biomechanics is the study of mechanics and its effect on biological structures at rest and during movement. The study of biomechanics is concerned with measures of length, velocity, acceleration, mass, volume, energy, power, moment, angle, and force as they relate to human and animal bodies. Although observation by an examiner may be used to assess some movements,[50] researchers make extensive use of instrumentation to measure each particular quantity of interest. Computers, counters, electro-goniometers, cameras, electromyographs, switches, force plates, accelerometers, recorders, and walk grids are some instruments that have been used to study movement.

The measurement of mass of biological structures has been of interest from a static and dynamic approach. Whole-body mass is measured by dry weighing against a standard or scale, or by locating the mass center. Body dynamics in gait are often determined for the mass properties of body segments; for example, foot, lower leg, thigh, trunk, arms, and head.[51,52] Analyses of body compartments such as total body fat have used biochemical and underwater weighing methods.[53,54]

Biomechanical studies frequently measure quantities with respect to time such as gait frequency and steps per unit of time.[55-57] Cameras, footswitches, and grid devices are some of the instruments used to obtain information about temporal and distance quantities.

Angular measures (radians, degrees, and revolutions) are used in movement analyses. Electrogoniometers have been used to study the inclination of limb segments through their length in coordinate directions. Goniometers which are secured to body segments and measure one[58] or more planes,[59] of joint motion have been used. Non-body contacting, polarized light goniometers are now in use.[60]

The variation of ground-to-foot force during the walking cycle has been of interest to researchers. Typical components (vertical, anterior-posterior, and mediolateral) or the ground reaction force are measured by a mechanical system using a force-plate.[61] Gait deviations can be studied in patients affected with joint diseases of the lower extremities and a quantitative assessment can be made against standards.

Instruments and methods used in the laboratory to study human movement have not been used widely in clinical assessment of abnormal movement patterns. Observation continues to be the tool of choice in clinical situations because of convenience and economy. Information derived from biomechanical research, however, can and will continue to assist the practitioner in assessment and treatment of deviant movement patterns.

Photography

Photography has served as an important tool in the study of human motion because rapidly occurring events can be recorded and then analyzed at the researcher's convenience. Cinematography is the photographic technique for recording and storing information about bodies in motion.

Photographing motion must be planned in advance so that proper dimensional views are taken to gather all needed information. Three-dimensional photography is ideal for gathering maximum data about a particular motion. Cameras can be positioned in front, at the side, and above the subject being studied. The three cameras would represent the three cardinal planes. If only two cameras are available, the side and front views are usually preferred, but the side view is selected when only one camera is available.

Since cameras are one of the major pieces of instrumentation for cinematography, camera specifications are important. A 16-mm camera having film speeds of 32 to 100 frames per second is commonly used for most biomechanical studies.[40] The higher speeds of film carriage are used when running gaits are being studied. The driving mechanism of the camera is also important with spring-driven cameras being common for slower speeds but electrical driven cameras are essential if studies require moving the film at a rate of a thousand frames per second.[40]

The other major instrument is cinematography is the device used to analyze film. Film analysis involves measurements and drawings of movement taken from the developed film by the researcher or a computer in which changes of angles between lines marked on the moving object or body are compared with fixed references. A manual film reader can be used to analyze specific body parts frame by frame, but motion analysis by this method is tedious and time consuming. Such dynamic quantities as velocities, accelerations, and angular movement about joints are often computed from film. The automatic film reading units are most desirous but also more expensive than the manual type. The automatic unit is capable of feeding film into a printer or card punch for computer analysis which saves time and labor. Additional photographic equipment might include screens, analyzing projectors, strobes, tripods or trolleys for mounting and moving the cameras, and floodlights and control switches for the lighting.

Cinematography is versatile, simple, provides a permanent record, and can be performed without interference with the subject being filmed. It is not without disadvantages such as tedious computations, and expensive equipment and film processing.

SUMMARY

An introduction to experimental research has been given with emphasis placed on control, fields of study, and instruments used in experiments. Experimental research tests hypotheses of causal relationships among variables and permits the investigator to maintain rigorous control over manipulated variables. It can be conducted in a laboratory or field setting. Experimental research is considered the most powerful of all research methods.

Physical therapists have a diversity of research interests which include the broad areas of therapeutics and pathokinesiology. Hardware instruments appropriate for cardiovascular, work and energy cost, pulmonary, exercise, and physical agent studies are used to collect data of therapeutic effects. Electromyographic, biotelemetric, biomechanic, and photographic

Table 8.2
Cumulative Summary of the Research Processes Presented

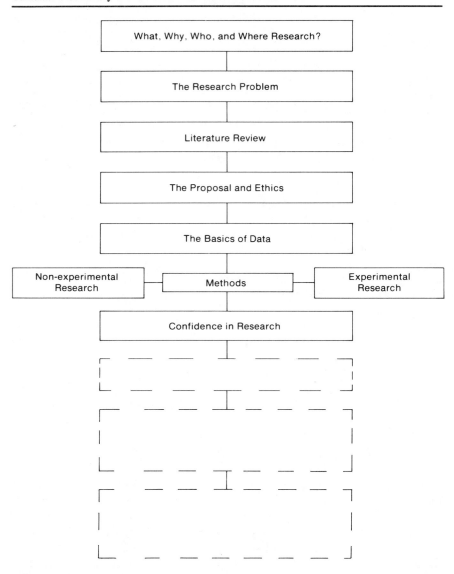

instruments are used in pathokinesiologic studies. Table 8.2 provides a summary of the research processes presented thus far.

REFERENCES

1. Makrides L, Richman J: Research methodology and applied statistics, Part 1: general principles and basic concepts. Physiother Canada 32: 135–139, 1980

2. Gay LR: Educational Research: Competencies for Analysis and Application, ed 2. Columbus OH, Charles E. Merrill Pub Co, 1981
3. Meyers LS, Grossen NE: Behavioral Research Theory, Procedure, and Design, ed 2. San Francisco, WH Freeman and Co, 1978
4. Clarke DH, Clarke HH: Research Processes in Physical Education, Recreation, and Health. Englewood Cliffs, NJ, Prentice-Hall, Inc, 1970
5. Gonnella C: Designs for clinical research. Phys Ther 53: 1276–1283, 1973
6. Lehmkuhl D: Let's reduce the understanding gap. 3: Experimental design: what and why? Phys Ther 50: 1716–1720, 1970
7. Wagman IH, Lesse H: Maximum conduction velocities of motor fibers of ulnar nerve in human subjects of various ages and sizes. N Neurophysiol 15: 235–244, 1952
8. Wagner AL, Buchthal F: Motor and sensory conduction in infancy and childhood: Reappraisal. Devel Med Child Neurol 14: 189–216, 1972
9. Cox RC, West WL: Fundamentals of Research for Health Professionals. Laurel MD, RAMSCO Pub Co, 1982
10. Hislop HJ: Modern instrumentation and its implications in physical therapy. Phys Ther 43: 257–262, 1963
11. Wilson EB Jr: An Introduction to Scientific Research. New York, McGraw-Hill Book Co, 1952
12. Richman J, Makrides L, Prince B: Research methodology and applied statistics, Part 3: measurement procedures in research. Physiother Canada 32: 253–257, 1980
13. Van Huss WD: Instrumentation Hardware. In Hubbard AW (ed): Research Methods in Health, Physical Education, and Recreation, ed 3. Washington, American Association of Health, Physical Education, Recreation, 1973
14. Cobbold RSC: Biomedical Measurement Systems. In Ray CD (ed): Medical Engineering. Chicago, Year Book Medical Publishers, Inc, 1974
15. Cromwell L, Weibell FJ, Pfeiffer EA, et al: Biomedical Instrumentation and Measurements. Englewood Cliffs, NJ, Prentice-Hall, Inc, 1973
16. Hanley TD, Peters R: The Speech and Hearing Laboratory. In Travers LE (ed): Handbook of Speech Pathology and Audiology. New York, Appleton-Century-Crofts, 1971
17. Dewhurst DJ: An Introduction to Biomedical Instrumentation. New York, Pergamon Press, 1976
18. Goodgold J, Eberstein A: Electrodiagnosis of Neuromuscular Diseases, ed 3. Baltimore, The Williams & Wilkins Co, 1983
19. Yanof HM: Biomedical Electronics, ed 2. Philadelphia, FA Davis Co, 1972
20. Cromwell L, Weibell FJ, Pfeiffer EA, et al: Biomedical Instrumentation and Measurements, ed 2. Englewood Cliffs, NJ, Prentice-Hall, Inc, 1980
21. Strong P: Biophyical Measurements. Beaverton, OR, Tektronix, Inc, 1970
22. Groveman J, Cohen DD, Dillon JB: Phinoplethysmography: Pulse monitoring at the nasal septum. Anesth Analg 45: 63–68, 1966
23. Balke B: The Measurement of Physiological Factors. In Larson LA (ed): Fitness, Health, and Work Capacity: International Standards for Assessment. New York, MacMillan Publishing Co, Inc, 1974
24. The Committee on Exercise: Exercise Testing and Training of Apparently Healthy Individuals: A Handbook for Physicians. New York, Am Heart Assoc, 1972
25. Ikai M: The Physiological Factors. In Larson LA (ed): Fitness, Health and Work Capacity: International Standards for Assessment. New York, MacMillan Publishing Co, 1974
26. Larson RF: Forearm positioning on maximal elbow-flexor force. Phys Ther 49: 748–756, 1969
27. May WW: Maximum isometric force of the hip rotator muscles. Phys Ther 46: 233–238, 1966
28. Currier DP: Positioning for knee strengthening exercise. Phys Ther 57: 148–152, 1977

29. Richard G, Currier DP: Back stabilization during knee strengthening exercise. Phys Ther 57: 1013–1015, 1977
30. Mendler HM: Effect of stabilization on maximum isometric knee extensor force. Phys Ther 47: 375–379, 1967
31. Norton HN: Biomedical Sensors: Fundamentals and Applications. Park Ridge, NJ, Noyes, 1982
32. Watkins MP, Harris BA: Evaluation of Isokinetic Muscle Performance. In Zarins B (ed): Clinics in Sports Medicine, vol 2, no 1. Philadelphia, WB Saunders Co, 1983
33. Basmajian JV: Research or retrench: The rehabilitation professions challenged. Phys Ther 55: 607–610, 1975
34. Feibel A, Fast A: Deep heating joints: A reconsideration. Arch Phys Med Rehabil 57: 513–514, 1976
35. Stewart HF, Harris GR, Herman BA, et al: Survey of use and performance of ultrasonic therapy equipment in Pinellas County, Florida. Phys Ther 54: 707–715, 1974
36. Hislop HJ: The not-so-impossible dream. Phys Ther 55: 1069–1080, 1975
37. Winter DA: Biomechanics of Human Movement. New York, John Wiley & Sons, 1979
38. Hayes K: Wave analyses of tissue and muscle action potentials. J Appl Physiol 15: 749–752, 1960
39. Basmajian JV: Muscles Alive, ed 4, Baltimore, The Williams & Wilkins Co, 1979
40. Grieve DW, Miller DI, Mitchelson D, et al: Techniques for the Analysis of Human Movement. New York, St Mutual Book & Periodical Serv, 1980
41. Reiner S, Rogoff JB: Instrumentation. In Johnson EW (ed): Practical Electromyography. Baltimore, Williams & Wilkins, 1980
42. Basmajian JV, Clifford HC, McLeod WD, et al: Computers in Electromyography. Boston, Butterworths, 1975
43. Pocock GS: Electromyographic study of the quadriceps during resistive exercise. J Am Phys Ther Assoc 43: 427–434, 1963
44. Hall EA, Long C II: Intrinsic hand muscles in power grip. Electromyography 8: 397–421, 1968
45. Tursky B: Integrators as measuring devices of bioelectric output. Clin Pharmacol Ther 5: 887–892, 1964
46. Close JR: Motor Function in the Lower Extremity: Analysis by Electronic Instrumentation. Springfield, IL, Charles C Thomas Publisher, 1964
47. Willison RG; Quantitative Electromyography. In Licht S (ed): Electrodiagnosis and Electromyography, ed 3. New Haven, Conn, Elizabeth Licht Publisher, 1971
48. deVries HA: Muscle tonus in postural muscles. Am J Phys Med 44: 275–291, 1965
49. Kaiser E, Petersen I: Muscle action potentials studied by frequency analysis and duration measurement. Acta Neurol Scand Suppl 13: 213–236, 1965
50. Smidt GL: Methods of studying gait. Phys Ther 54: 13–17, 1974
51. Drillis R, Contini R, Bluestein M: Body segment parameters: A survey of measurement techniques. Artif Limbs 8: 44–68, 1964
52. LeVeau B (ed): Williams and Lissner: Biomechanics of Human Motion, ed 2. Philadelphia, WB Saunders Co, 1977
53. Novak LP: Analysis of Body Compartments. In Larson LA (ed): Fitness, Health, and Work Capacity: International Standards for Assessment. New York, MacMillan Publishing Co, Inc 1974
54. Williams D, Anderson T, Currier DP: Underwater weighing by Hubbard tank (submitted for publication)
55. Smidt GL, Simpson CM: How fast are you walking? Phys Ther 51: 412–413, 1971
56. Gardner GM, Murray MP: Method of measuring the duration of foot-floor contact during walking. Phys Ther 55: 751–756, 1975
57. Norton BJ, Bomze HA, Sahrmann SA, et al: Correlation between gait speed and spasticity at the knee. Phys Ther 55: 355–359, 1975

58. Tipton Cm, Karpovich PV: Electrogoniometric records of knee and ankle movements in pathologic gaits. Arch Phys Med Rehabil 46: 267–272, 1965
59. Wadsworth JB, Smidt GL, Johnston RC: Gait characteristics of subjects with hip disease. Phys Ther 52: 829–838, 1972
60. Reed DJ, Reynolds PJ: A joint angle detector. J Appl Physiol 27: 745–748, 1969
61. Barany JW, Ismail AH, Manning KR: A force platform for the study of hemiplegic gait. Phys Ther 45: 693–699, 1965

9

Experimental Designs

A conclusion based upon a badly conceived
experiment is usually further from the truth
than one based on clinical observation.
Sir Robert Platt
Universities Quarterly 17: 327, 1963

The ultimate form of research design is the experiment. The experiment provides the most rigorous test of hypotheses that is available to the researcher. It determines whether the relationship between variables is one of cause-and-effect.[1]

The need for controlling variables and variable factors in research has been discussed on several occasions. Experimental designs are contrived, like instruments, to prevent or minimize the effects of bias (systematic error) and random error, and to maximize the measurement of the true quantity or quality. A proper design is supposed to enable the researcher to answer all questions without violating principles of scientific inquiry.[2] In comparative research appropriate designs will maximize efficiency, control, and validity.[3]

The design of an experiment is the planned course of action for gathering, controlling, and analyzing the data. Gonnella[4] has defined design as the assignment of subjects to different treatments, the controlling of variables, and the ordering of the testing. The design incorporates the terms defined in the experiment or study, specifies the specific treatment plan, and the way subjects will be assigned to treatment groups.[5] Design of the research procedures is given utmost consideration during the planning and writing of the research proposal. Methods of analyses appropriate for the design must be made. Statistical procedures have been created to handle data gathered by certain designs or strategies. The concepts of validity and reliability must enter into the planning of the experiment also.

In non-experimental research, designs involve the logic and technique of gathering data and making appropriate interpretations from the data. In experimental research, designs involve the selection of the appropriate statistical methods and strategies for analyzing data, and making appropriate interpretations from the data analyses. Most designs presented in this chapter are concerned with comparative research; that is, the comparison between two or more variables for determination of the difference between means of the dependent variables under investigation. Good designs will assist the researcher to eliminate systematic error, maintain precision and validity, incorporate simplicity for extraction of information from data, and help to calculate the uncertainties of treatment differences.[6]

EXPERIMENTAL VALIDITY

Earlier discussion has indicated that control of extraneous variables is of great concern in experimental research. Uncontrolled extraneous variables threaten the validity of an investigation because they may affect performance on the dependent variable. Validity is upheld if the experimental findings are due only to the manipulated independent variable(s), and if these findings are generalizable to situations removed from the research setting but with similar conditions. The concern about experimental findings or observed differences on the dependent variable being due only to the manipulated independent variable is referred to as internal validity. External validity concerns the generalizability to situations removed from the research setting.[7] Some sources of variables which could invalidate the researcher's discussion of cause and effect relationships of the collected data have been identified and discussed.[4,8-10]

Internal Sources

These sources are causes that confuse the association between independent and dependent variables.

I. History. Studies in which measurements of the dependent variable (variable measured) are recorded before and after some form of experiment or event may result in contamination of the data. The uncontrolled events occurring between measurements might influence and confuse the information contained in the data gathered from the repeated measurements. The researcher must be concerned with the influence of events occurring between measurements. If human subjects are being used, interest, motivation, and physical (injury) changes may occur to influence recorded scores on maximal muscular force. This source of contamination is prevented by methods of sampling, control of the subject's activities during the study, and methods of random testing.[4,9]

2. Maturation. This is also a time-related source of difficulty when measurements are taken between long intervals of time. The effects are directly related to the element of time rather than to the events occurring between measurements. Subjects grow, develop, or change with time. If the measurements are taken within a relatively short period of time between each other this source can cause difficulty. For example, if measurements of muscular force are recorded in sequences too short to prevent fatigue, then the data are contaminated with the effects of fatigue. On the other hand, if measurements of maximal muscular force are taken at 1-year intervals to ascertain strength retention among children from some previous program of exercise, the results may be confused because the children have grown during the interval of testing.[4,9]

3. Attrition. The best laid plans cannot always prevent the loss of subjects in a study. Ample numbers of subjects should be included in the plan of the study with allowances for attrition built into the size of the sample. Some statistical designs call for pairs of data and if one of the pair drops out of the study then the pair must be sacrificed to the study.

4. Testing. If the testing sequence affects the scores of the subjects, the values of the scores will be affected. Schenck and Forward found increased strength in subsequent single measurements of maximal isometric strength in their subjects.[11] The question could be raised concerning the learning effects that might have occurred with repeated measurements. Subjects become test wise when exposed to repeated testing or practice.

5. Instrumentation. The state of the instrument being used can influence scores. The instruments may not be calibrated properly; age, hysteresis, or sensitivity effects may influence recorded values. In paper instruments such as attitude scales or mail questionnaires cultural, racial, or intelligence factors may influence the results of the survey. Different observers may influence scores.

6. Statistical Regression. Although this threat to internal validity is only possible when subjects are selected on the basis of extreme scores (very low or very high), it, however, can account for observed gains in learning during posttest measurements. Repeated testing of a variable tends to influence the subjects' outcome. Subjects' scores tend to shift (regress) toward the mean; that is, subjects scoring higher on the pretest tend to score lower on a posttest, while the opposite is true for those scoring lower on the pretest.[8] This threat to internal validity can be avoided by not selecting subjects on the basis of extreme scores.[12]

7. Selection. Volunteer subjects are probably different from non-volunteers and, therefore, may become a source of bias. Nevertheless, required consent makes all subjects volunteers in health research. To avoid selected samples having a certain composition that may bias the results, the researcher can control for the effect of selection by using more than a single group and by randomly assigning subjects to the groups.[12]

External Sources

The researcher is concerned about threats to generalizability as well as the problems of internal validity. As more stringent controls are applied to the experiment, less realism can be achieved or be expected between the findings and situations outside the experimental setting. Thus, the researcher is faced with the choice of losing scientific rigor in his experiment so that realistic findings may not be readily transferred into clinical application. Compromise is the solution; maintain acceptable controls to make reasonable inferences.[12]

These sources of difficulty of the research method are tough to remedy, since they deal with representativeness and generalization of the data to the population. Testing subjects in a controlled environment and then making inferences about what is to be expected outside of the environment is an example. The process of measuring a patient who then believes the measuring process is a form of therapy is another example of a possible source that could invalidate the interpretation of the findings.[4,9]

The researchers in the fields of psychology and education are most concerned about these sources of difficulty in their methods of gathering data. Although these difficulties may be ever present, the physical therapy researcher can usually avoid their pitfalls by random data collection whenever possible by exerting rigid control of the independent variables, and by proper statistical design.

Bracht and Glass have cited specific sources of external validity.[13]

1. Sample to Population Effect. This concerns the extent to which the researcher can generalize from the sample results to the defined population. Does the sample being studied really represent the true population? The researcher is usually safe by generalizing the experimental results from the sample to the experimentally accessible population. Also of concern is the extent to which characteristics of the individual interact with the dependent or treatment effects. Such factors as general skills, level of ability on traits needed in the research procedure, attitudes, emotional reaction, sex, and rapport with the researcher are examples.

2. Description of the Experimental Treatment. In reporting research the author must describe the experimental treatment in sufficient detail so that other investigators can replicate the study if they choose.

3. Exposure to Multitreatments. Sometimes subjects are exposed to more than one manipulated independent variable. Because of this circumstance, the researcher cannot safely generalize his results to a situation in which variable X is administered alone. The effectiveness of any one of the variables depends on the presence of the manipulated variables.

4. Hawthorne Effect. Whenever subjects participate in research, they receive special attention. The special attention (Hawthorne or placebo effect) may alter the subjects' behavior enough that they perform better during the experimental measurements than they would otherwise.

5. Unusual Conditions. The experimental outcome may be effective because the research procedure is novel or unusual. The unusual condition may cause special effects rather than the treatment's real effectiveness. Fortunately most unusual condition effects usually wear off rapidly.

6. Researcher Effect. Subjects may react differently to the particular individual administering the experimental procedure.

7. Pretest Effects. The initial test or measurement session may serve as part of the treatment effect causing different results than if the experiment was repeated without a pretest.

8. Posttest Effect. The posttest may serve as a learning experience where subjects become "test wise" as a result of the repeated measurements.

9. Interaction of time and Experimental Effects. Experimental effects may not be generalizable beyond the time period in which the experiment took place. Attitudes and emotional responses of the researcher and the subjects may change between pretest and posttest and may effect the outcome of the measurements.

10. Measurement of the Dependent Variable. The pretest and posttest measurements may be so similar to the treatment that generalizability of the experimental findings may be limited.

11. Interaction of Treatment Effects and Time of Measurement. If a posttest is administered on two different occasions, the posttest measurements may differ. The usual custom is to measure treatment effects immediately upon cessation of the experimental procedure or training. Retention of treatment effects are usually the differences between the first posttest and a second posttest scores when some time has elapsed between measurements.

Although the outlined effects can influence the external validity of the experiment, the researcher usually reports limitations on the generalizability of the research results. Selection of appropriate experimental designs and adequate control of extraneous variables usually enables the researcher to make inferences based on valid experimentation.

The appropriate selection of an experimental design is important. The design selected should be consistent with the objectives of the study and control for various threats of invalidity, so that observed differences between pretest and posttest can be attributed with a high level of confidence to the experimental treatment. Most experiments in physical therapy use some form of a single-variable design involving the manipulation of a single treatment variable followed by observing the effects of the manipulation on one dependent variable.

Most of the designs discussed in this section can be used with statistical methods that are capable of dealing with groups of either equal or unequal sizes. The calculation procedures can take into account, groups of unequal size so that their sizes have proportional weightings. Thus, a large group cannot carry more weight than a group having a smaller number of subjects.

STATISTICAL ANALYSIS AND DESIGNS

Analysis of data is an essential part of experimental design. Descriptive and inferential statistics are the two types commonly used in analysis of experimental data.

Descriptive statistics describe, organize, and summarize data. Measures of central tendency (mean and median), measures of relationship (correlation coefficient), and measures of relative position (range, standard deviation, and coefficient of variation) are types of descriptive statistics. They permit the researcher to describe all individual scores in a sample by using one or two numbers (mean and standard deviation). Descriptive statistics are used if the recorded scores include all the observations of interest to the researcher, or if the observations are inadequately gathered or too comprehensive to be representative of a larger group. That is, descriptive statistics should be used to describe the distribution of each dependent variable, the location of central or key values in each group studied, and the variation or spread of the scores within each group.[12]

Inferential statistics enable the researcher to conclude, to speculate, to reason, and to generalize the results of the study from the sample to the population. They permit generalizations from sample statistics (small and random portion of all observations of interest) to the larger population parameters of all similar observations.[12] These types of statistics (t, F, and r) are important in experimental research, since the researcher rarely measures or studies the entire population. Inferences are probability statements that help the researcher conclude about differences between means. For example, if a difference between means is determined for two groups at the end of an experiment, the researcher infers to whether a similar difference exists in the population from which the samples were selected. Presenting both descriptive and inferential statistics in the report of a study is an effective way of representing the results.

Division is frequently made between parametric and nonparametric statistics. Parametric statistics (Chapter 10) are procedures that meet certain strict mathematical assumptions, while nonparametric statistics (Chapter 11) do not meet or approximate the rigid assumptions.

The choice of suitable statistical procedures is determined to a great extent by the design of the experiment and by the type of data to be gathered. The design and statistical procedures should be identified and described briefly in the research proposal because different designs and research objectives may require that data be gathered in different forms.

The method of data analysis is very important in the research process. Statistical procedures help make maximum use of gathered data. Familiarization of many statistical techniques enables the researcher to vary analyses in order to extract maximum amounts of information from the data. Inappropriate analyses can cause misinterpretations. In the event that the researcher is not well acquainted with a variety of statistical procedures, a friendly statistician should be consulted on the experimental design and the data analysis.

Inferential statistics and tests of significance play an important role in research designs. Tests of significance are used to test hypotheses. Their proper use is important for the success of the analysis and interpretation. Table 9.1 provides a summary of a few examples of tests of significance and their purposes.

DESIGNS FOR EXPERIMENTAL RESEARCH

Longitudinal Design

This type of design was briefly mentioned in Chapter 6. Longitudinal designs attempt to examine events or traits of a variable over a prolonged period of time.[14] Since most research is performed over time (all measurements are not made simultaneously), the amount of time between measurements is of concern. A study in which measurements are recorded during infancy and then repeated when the individual is an adult is a longitudinal study. All the influences of experience, growth, and environment are confounded into the measured scores. This type of study risks a high drop-out of subjects because of death, geographical relocations, and

Table 9.1
Tests of Significance, Inferential Statistics

Tests of Statistical Significance	Purpose
Parametric	
t test	To determine whether two means differ significantly from each other
Analysis of variance	To determine whether means on one or more factors differ or interact significantly from each other
Post hoc tests	To determine which pairwise mean comparisons are significant in analysis of variance when the F ratio is found significant
Nonparametric	
Chi-square tests	To determine whether two frequency distributions differ significantly from each other
Mann-Whitney tests	To determine whether two uncorrelated means differ significantly from each other
Kruskal-Wallis tests	To determine whether means on one factor differ significantly from each other

refusals. The information gathered is of great value when interest is centered on the changes which occur over time.

Cross-Sectional Design

This design perhaps meets the ideal sample if all possible typings or classes of a trait, event, or individuals are represented in the sample. Both the stratified random sampling technique and the systematic sampling technique can be used to provide a representative sample of a population. In random sampling the possibility exists for exclusion of certain types or classes of things, but if the types or classes are known and can be located, random proportions of the classes can be made so that no classes are unrepresented. Cross-sectional designs enable the researcher to gather information from a manageable number of subjects and to draw inferences about the population from which the sample was drawn.

Prospective Design

This design is perhaps used most frequently in research. In the prospective design the variable and sample are defined first and then data are gathered to determine incidences or magnitudes for comparing the experimental variable with other variables or known facts. This design gives the researcher the opportunity to plan the study around any factor, to study relationships between two variables, and to determine effectiveness or differences between two or more variables. This design provides great flexibility, and time factors can be established and controlled in both experimental and non-experimental research. A treatment can be given and then the effects can be observed following the manipulation or concomitant with the manipulation process.

Retrospective Design

The purpose of this approach is to uncover facts or information already existing. Historical research methods use this approach. Different treatment methods can be administered and then their efficacy can be obtained, measured, and compared. Information can be extracted from files and records and then analyzed.

Retrospective comparisons of data in clinical trials are risky. The researcher has no assurance that the outcome is not seriously affected by differences in the makeup of the samples[15] and by effects of maturation when samples are compared over varying time sequences (e.g., 1 or 2 years). Patients composing two separate samples may have been treated by different therapists, different instruments may have been involved in the treatment processes, or improved methods of treatment delivery may have succeeded those used earlier.

Blind Designs

The single-blind design tends to eliminate bias from the subject by not permitting the subject knowledge of what he is receiving. The double-blind method is an approach to prevent bias from both patient and observer. In this method, knowledge of the conditions are withheld from both the subject and the observer. In drug studies neither the subject nor the observer is told what ingredient is really in a particular capsule given to the subject. The capsules are coded for identification and recorded when given to the patient. The contents of the capsule might be the experimental drug or a placebo but the contents are only known to someone not participating in the research. The double-blind approach also prevents the observer from scheduling favorite patients at a time when he knows the elements of the treatment regimen.

Suppose a therapist wanted to study the effects of ultrasonic dosage on a certain condition using the double-blind approach; the ultrasonic generator is kept behind a screen and the controls are managed by a person behind the screen so that the therapist giving the treatment and the patient are unaware of the dosage. This situation represents one use of a double-blind design in physical therapy research.

One-Group Pretest-Posttest Design

This design uses one group of subjects. Measurements are taken before any treatment is given to a group of subjects, treatment is given to the subjects, and then measurements are again taken following the treatment or experimental procedure. Designs may be symbolized by letters where O is a measurement (pretest or posttest of the dependent variable) and X is the experimental treatment. The one-group pretest-posttest design is thus symbolized:

$$O \ X \ O$$

The differences between means of the two series of scores are compared to determine the effects of treatment. This design has been criticized[3,8,9,16] for being unstable. The arguments against the design have been based on the uncontrolled temporal effects occurring between test administrations. Temporal effects are considered uncontrolled because no comparison is made between an experimental group of subjects and an equivalent untreated or control group so that history and maturation factors are not measured or stabilized. The time occurring between pretest and posttest measurements (temporal effect) may contaminate the measurements so that the real effects of treatment are indistinguishable from the effects of passage of time. In certain studies, growth and developmental factors (maturation effect) taking place in subjects between the pretest and posttest measurements may contaminate treatment effects.[3] An example might be a study of children who exhibit growth and developmental changes in relatively short periods of time.

Cox,[17] a life scientist, has given a reasonable argument in defense of this design. If a method or treatment is tested which is already known to provide desirable effects, for example, dynamic resistance exercise increases muscular strength, then controls are not needed if the researcher is interested in determining how much of the effect is taking place.[17] A person performing dynamic exercises daily for several weeks should not demonstrate learning effects if he is measured for strength by movements similar to those performed in the strengthening program. Another example might be when ice massage and ice packs are being studied to determine which is superior for cooling muscular tissue. Both methods cool soft tissue but the researcher wants to determine if any difference exists and how much. Having a control group may not be necessary when treatment effects are known from previous research. The measurements in these situations would be taken during one setting with minimum elapse of time occurring (temporal and maturation effects are minimized). The elapsed time between pretest and posttest measurements would be the actual treatment time. Randomizing the order of pretest and posttest measurements among subjects (eliminating any set pattern) helps to eliminate contaminants due to learning, temporal, and maturation factors.[6] Reliability of pretest and posttest data can be increased when more than one measurement is taken at each point in time. The different measurements can be compared to determine difference and if no significant difference occurs statistically, the research is assured that history and maturation have not influenced the treatment effects.[18] The faults of history and maturation effects leveled at this design appear mostly in the literature of psychology, education, and sociology.

The pretest and posttest means are compared for statistical significance using the paired t test. The paired t test is appropriate because the same subjects are tested on both occasions and when a parametric test is indicated. If the rigid mathematical assumptions cannot be met for parametric statistical testing, a nonparametric test should be selected; for example, the Wilcoxon matched-pairs signed-ranks test.[1]

Two-Group Pretest-Posttest Designs

Pretest-Posttest Control Group Design:.

$$O \quad X \quad O$$

$$O \qquad\;\; O$$

This design corrects for the deficiencies of the ONE-GROUP PRETEST-POSTTEST DESIGN by using a second group of subjects for control.[9] Subjects are selected and assigned randomly to the two separate groups.

Pretest measurements are taken on each group. The experimental group is given some treatment or experimental procedure and subsequently, posttest measurements are taken. Although pretest and posttest measurements are taken on the second or control group, no experimental treatment or procedure is administered to this group.[10]

The two-group design may be varied to include paired comparisons where a number of pairs of subjects receiving different treatments are studied. Similarities (similar strength scores, blood pressures, ages, or weights) between two subjects are identified and the two subjects constitute a pair. One member of the pair is assigned randomly to a designated treatment group, while the other member of the pair is assigned to the other designated treatment group. This variation of the two-group design will provide comparisons of two treatments that are free of systematic error, sources of internal invalidity; however, it is threatened by interaction of testing and treatment invalidity.

Pretest-Posttest Control-Group Design with Matching. Matching attempts to reduce differences between the experimental and control groups on the dependent variable at pretest. The researcher may assign subjects to the experimental and control groups so that they are matched (closely comparable) on pretest scores. This design is a variation of Two-Group Pretest-Posttest designs but similar to the Pretest-Posttest Control-Group design. It is useful in studies where large mean differences between the groups are unlikely to occur and where the sample sizes are likely to be small. For example, in studies concerned with strength augmentation by electrical stimulation and the combination of isometric exercise and electrical stimulation, matching of pretest strength scores might be appropriate so that subjects begin training with parity of muscular strength. This is particularly suitable if the subjects are active physically and if they will train only for a short period of time.

The suggested matching procedure is to rank order all subjects on the basis of their pretest scores on the dependent variable. The first two subjects are randomly assigned to either the experimental or control group. This procedure is continued, taking the next two ranked subjects, until all subjects have been assigned to groups.

The best approach to analyze data of these designs is to use analysis of covariance, in which the posttest means are compared using the pretest means as the covariate. If analysis of covariance assumptions cannot be met, analysis of variance of the posttest scores is appropriate.[1]

Posttest-Only Control Group Design. Occasionally an appropriate pretest cannot be located or the pretest may have an effect on the experimental treatment. This design handles the situation by not administering pretests to the experimental and control groups. It permits the researcher to rule out any possible interaction between the two groups of subjects.

This design,

$$X \quad O$$
$$O$$

however, has the disadvantages that: (1) pretest scores are not available on the dependent variable and accordingly cannot be used to control for any differences existing between groups on pretest, (2) the researcher cannot determine whether the experimental treatment has a different effect on subjects at various levels by forming subgroups, and (3) it contains the threat of attrition to its internal validity.[1]

The independent t test is an appropriate statistical method to compare posttest scores of the two groups. The Wilcoxon matched-pairs signed-ranks test is a nonparameteric method to use if the obtained scores depart radically from the normal curve.

Solomon Four-Group Design. This design enables the researcher to combine aspects of the Pretest-Posttest Control Group and Posttest-Only Control Group designs in order to study the pretest effect on the experimental group. The random assignment of four groups, two experimental and two control groups, is involved in this design:

$$O \quad X \quad O$$
$$O \qquad O$$
$$X \quad O$$
$$O$$

One group receives the pretest and the experimental treatment; a second group is given a pretest and a posttest but no experimental treatment; the third group is not given a pretest but receives the experimental treatment and a posttest; while the fourth group receives only the posttest. This design permits testing of the difference between experimental and control groups in addition to the interaction of pretest scores and the experimental treatment. Although this design is a powerful experimental design, it requires a large number of subjects and a lot of researcher effort.

Statistical analysis of the data generated by this design is complex and requires the services of a computer and a statistician. A form of analysis of covariance is used to analyze data.[1]

Cross-Over Designs

If different treatments are applied to the same subject in random order at different times, the design is a cross-over design, also called change-over and shift designs. This design is used only when the administration of treatments applied during one period of time does not extend into or affect subsequent treatments applied during another period of time.[9] Suppose that the administration of some form of heat causes benefit (residual effect) for 30 minutes. If another form of treatment (heat or cold) is administered before the end of the residual effects of the first treatment, contamination results and the cross-over design is not being used appropriately.

This design maximizes subject performances and eliminates the influence of testing on a training process such as that of studying effects of static and dynamic exercises.[19] The authors of this study studied two groups of subjects performing static exercise and two groups of subjects performing dynamic exercise. At the end of 29 days one group performing static exercise shifted to dynamic exercise and one group performing dynamic exercise shifted to static exercise. The effects of given tasks on each other can be studied by using this design. By transferring tasks among two groups and retaining the other remaining groups as controls, the results supported the concepts that load is not important in performing exercise as long as subjects perform to the point of fatigue, and that the best training technique for a particular type of exercise is that type of exercise itself.[19]

This two-group design is used appropriately with the independent t test (when scores of each group are independent of each other) or the paired t test when scores of pretest and posttest are dependent (taken from paired subjects). If more than two groups are involved in the analysis concomitantly, then the analyses of variance would be the appropriate statistical method (Chapter 10).

Sequential Trials

The method of sequential trials was introduced to medical research many years ago,[15] but its use has not been reported often in the physical therapy literature.[16] The sequential method either groups patients in pairs in which each member is randomly assigned to one of two treatments, or permits comparisons of one patient on a series of trials. Comparisons made within a single patient on a series of trials are used when studying effects of chronic disease, while comparisons of paired patients are used when studying effects of acute diseases where time for study is limited.[15] In the situation where responses of paired patients are compared, patients are added and compared until a conclusion is drawn about which treatment is better. A "stopping rule" based on the results obtained in the investigation defines the way in which the decision to stop is made. The plan for stopping the investigation is made in advance of the trials and may be determined by formulas for binomial distributions.[6,15,20,21]

The sequential trials method offers economy of subjects and time by having a fixed upper limit to the number of subjects required in an investigation. The greatest reduction in sample size occurs when wide differences between the treatments are recorded. The method is useful when the researcher wishes to select the better of two treatments, when it is convenient to pair subjects on two different treatments, and/or when a study should be stopped for ethical reasons as soon as a decision can be reached about which treatment is better.[22] The design offers the researcher the ability to estimate a characteristic of a population with a desired level of accuracy.[15] A sequential trials design is not suitable when the above situations cannot be met and when considerable time is necessary to follow-up patients' responses to treatment. This situation would not permit economy of subjects because the study might include pairs of patients whose responses could not be determined until after substantial follow-up periods. Readers are advised to study details of analysis of sequential trials by reading the cited references.[6,15,20,21]

Quasi-Experimental Designs

Quasi-experimental designs lack random assignment of subjects to experimental and control groups; therefore, they do not meet all of the conditions of experimental design. Random assignment of subjects to experimental and control groups is not always possible. Although this group of design contains a good level of internal and external validity, they do not possess complete experimental control. Interpretation of results when using quasi-experimental designs must be done with some reservations.

Nonequivalent Control Group Design. This design is similar to the Pretest-Posttest Control Group Design discussed previously; however, it differs because subjects are not assigned randomly to the different groups.

$$O \quad X \quad O$$
$$O \qquad\quad O$$

By systematically assigning one intact patient group to the experimental groups and another intact group to a control group, a lack of randomization takes place. This condition of systematically assigning intact subject groups permits some biases to occur in the groups which will cause invalidity of the study. The groups may differ in some characteristics that may confuse the interpretation of the results. Using a pretest compensates somewhat for the lack of randomization.

Earlier such controls as randomization, either subjects to groups or groups to experimental treatments, and use of analysis of covariance were discussed as possibilities for reducing initial (pretest) differences between experimental and control groups. Again, use of these measures can compensate for the weakness of this design.[22]

The analysis of covariance is the statistical approach for handling data gathered with an experiment using this design. Occasionally the t test is also appropriate for analyzing data of this design.

Time-Series Design. A single group of subjects is measured at pretreatment and posttreatment. Between the measurement intervals treatment is administered to the group. The time-series design is a version of the pretest-posttest design and may be performed with or without a control group.[1]

The single-group time-series design involves the repeated measurement of a group of subjects prior to the administration of a treatment (independent variables) and following the treatment. The effect of the treatment, if any, is shown by a directional change in the line connecting the scores recorded before and after the administration of the treatment. The single-group time-series design does not include assigning subjects randomly to a group or the employment of a control group. The design contains history and instrumentation as threats to validity.[7]

A control group may be used with an experimental group in the time-series design and is called the multiple time-series design. Use of a control group corrects for the threats of internal invalidity by history and instrumentation effects. Although the control group does not receive treatment, data on the dependent variable are collected over the same periods for both groups so that comparisons can be made between the two groups of subjects.

The time-series designs are easily analyzed by conventional statistical methods. The t test can be used to compare mean scores of the last pretreatment and first posttreatment scores of the two groups. Caution must be exercised, however, in interpreting significant t ratios. The patterns of the lines connecting all measured mean scores must be considered in the interpretation so that a significant t ratio is in isolation from the direction of other lines. Lines that vary considerably may not change because of the experimental treatment. Figure 9.1 offers an example. Pattern A shows that performance was increasing prior to treatment so no effect is indicated. Pattern C is quite variable and performance was increasing prior to treatment. Pattern B shows a treatment effect because the line changed after the treatment was administered.

Single-Subject Designs

Single-subject designs involve measurements on one subject or patient receiving conventional or experimental treatment over a period of time. This design is similar to the time-series design but involves a single subject rather than a single group of subjects. It differs from the case report by using greater experimental control while the case report is limited to impressionistic description.[1]

Single-subject designs are used to explore effects of independent variables on the behavior of an individual.[23] They have been used to demonstrate treatment effects on a patient,[24,25] and behavior modification of students in a classroom.[1] Three characteristics are common among single-subject designs: (1) the dependent variable (the subject's performance) is continuously and repeatedly measured across time, (2) the subject serves as his or her own control when comparing performances pretreatment and posttreatment, and (3) the multiple measurements provide some evidence of the treatment effectiveness. The designs enable the observer to examine

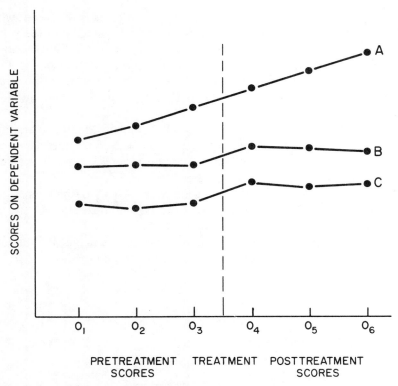

Figure 9.1. Possible patterns of a single group time-series design. O_1 to O_3 indicates mean pretreatment scores and measurement intervals, the broken vertical line indicates the administration of treatment, and O_4 to O_6 shows the mean posttreatment values and intervals.

changes in subject performance as they occur and with several data points, the observer may later predict subject performances.[23] I take the position that single-subject designs are useful in pilot work that may eventually lead to experiments using group designs and are good documentation sources of patient management and, therefore, of considerable value as a progress note. Single-subject designs require measurements of quantitative data which are good physical therapy documentations. As mentioned earlier a single subject may not be representative of a population or provide a firm basis for scientific prediction and inference. Caution must be exercised in generalizing about patterns of a single-subject design.

When data points are joined by lines, patterns in data are established which provide the essential information for interpretation. Patterns are interpreted visually, the primary method, or statistically. Visually, the observer or researcher notes the degree of variability, trend, and level of the pattern produced by multiple measurements across time. The variability effect consists of dissimilarity of scores recorded for a particular experimental condition. The direction that the pattern takes is the trend, while the level of the pattern is reflected in the amount of change in the values of the data.[23] Variability of scores is of great concern in single-subject designs. It can be examined within a specific measurement period (e.g., pretreatment) and across measurement periods (e.g., treatment-posttreatment). The plotted data points will help depict variability, trend, and level patterns (Fig. 9.2).

Patterns are not evaluated by conventional statistical methods and may be controversial. The *t* test can, however, be used to compare mean scores between pretreatment and posttreatment measurements. If many measurements are available, analysis of variance can be used.[23]

Single-subject designs may be considered as A-B-A designs where the nontreatment condition or period of time is symbolized as A, and the treatment condition or period of time is symbolized as B.

The A-B design. In this variation of single-subject designs, the therapist determines the dependent variable to be measured and measures it repeat-

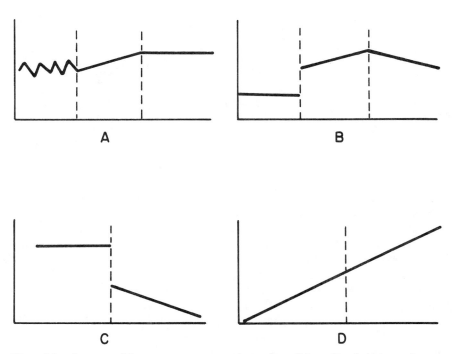

Figure 9.2.   Some possible patterns across experimental conditions: Graph A shows changes in variability and trend, Graph B shows change in level but no change in treatment, Graph C shows changes in level and trend, and Graph D shows no change. The dotted lines represent treatment period.

edly during the pretreatment or baseline period.

```
O   O   O   X   O   X   O   X   O
A           .               B
            .
```

This condition of pretreatment measurements may be a problem for clinicians who are obligated to immediately treat patients after an initial assessment. For patients having chronic problems (e.g., neurological), a delay of treatment until several measurements can be taken may not pose a problem. Measurements are continuously taken during the experimental treatment period. Approximately the same length of time and number of measurements should be observed for each phase (nontreatment and treatment) of a single-subject study.

The A-B-A design. This design is an extension of the simpler A-B design where a posttreatment phase is measured following the treatment, otherwise the same steps as the A-B design are followed.

```
O   O   O   X   O   X   O   X   O   O   O   O
A       .   B               .       A
        .                   .
```

Although this design has good internal validity, the observed treatment effect is dependent upon the particular baseline conditions imposed in this study. That is, the therapist can conclude only that the treatment effect occurs consistently for that particular baseline.[1]

The A-B-A-B design. The design introduces two within-subject replications of treatment to satisfy somewhat the ethical question of reduced treatment time to accommodate the pretreatment time.

```
O   O   O   X   O   X   O   X   O   O   O   O   O   X   O   X   O   X   O
A       .               B       .       A       .               B
        .                       .               .
```

Ending the study with a treatment phase strengthens the interpretation of treatment effects.[7]

Analysis of Covariance

The analysis of covariance is a statistical procedure used to control for initial differences between groups. If pretest scores indicate that the dependent variable is different between groups, then analysis of covariance can adjust scores on the dependent variable for the initial differences on some other variable (the covariate). Usually the posttest scores are adjusted for initial pretest differences.

The analysis of covariance is similar to matching groups for increased control on a variable. With this technique groups are placed on parity with respect to the control variable and then compared.[26] That is, the effect of an extraneous variable is controlled prior to the testing for group differences from the experimental treatment by removing it.

The analysis of covariance is a rather complex and lengthly statistical procedure that is difficult to compute by hand. It is recommended that a statistician and a computer program be used for analysis.

Designs for Analyses of Variance

In experimental research the investigator is often interested in comparing more than two treatments or variables in a single experiment. The randomized, randomized blocks, factorial, and repeated measures designs will be discussed briefly for the purpose of introducing terms and concepts that appear frequently in research literature. No attempt is made in this book to fit these particular designs to the proper statistical calculations. These mixed designs that are discussed are for analysis of variance. Summary tables that coincide with these designs are also presented.

The randomized design is the proper scheme to use with the one-way analysis of variance presented in Chapter 10. "One-way" implies that a single response measure is involved with the analysis of variance design. The remaining designs (factorial, randomized blocks, and repeated measures) are presented only for the purpose of acquainting the student with terms that will be used in the research literature, since the researcher studies more than one variable in most investigations. The appropriate procedures of analyses for these designs are covered in most books of intermediate level statistics.

Randomized Design. This design permits the means of two or more independent random groups of subjects receiving variations of a single response measure to be compared for difference. A single response measure is a variable that is common to all treatments, but treatments may be varied. In the example of Table 10.5 the intramuscular temperatures (dependent variable) of the gastrocnemius were measured before and after application of heat by hot packs, infrared, short wave diathermy, and ultrasound. The temperatures were measured by a thermistor and the fictitious data in the table represent the difference between before and after values. Twenty-eight subjects were assigned randomly to four different treatment groups so that seven subjects are treated in each of the treatment groups. The general design for the random samples used in the example of Table 10.5 was

$$
\begin{array}{cccc}
 & & 1 & \\
A & B & C & D \\
\hline
S_1 & S_2 & S_3 & S_4
\end{array}
$$

where 1 represents the one independent variable (heating agent); A, B, C, and D represent each (level) heating agent of hot packs, infrared, short wave diathermy, and ultrasound, respectively; and *S1, S2, S3, S4* are the samples, each containing seven randomly assigned subjects. Since subjects are assigned randomly to one of the groups and receive a particular treatment without being influenced by another form of treatment, the groups constitute independent random samples of subjects and a randomized design. This design may also be called a one-way analysis of variance because only one independent variable (heating agent) is used. An unlimited number of levels (heating agents) may be used as long as the same dependent variable (intramuscular temperature) is measured from subjects in the sample of each level. In the cited example four heating agents were used to cause elevation of heat; a fifth level could have been a control group or some other heating agent.

In reading the research literature, many tables representing the various methods of ANOVA will be encountered. In the randomized design (one-way ANOVA) used for collecting and analyzing data contained in Table 10.6 the investigator could report the analysis as shown in Table 9.2.

If the results from the study described above are to be meaningful, controlled variables must be sex, mass, and ages of patients; type, severity, and location of the injury; and duration of the injury. If these variables are not similar in characteristics, then the effects from the treatments will give ambiguous results with respect to any of the variables outlined. For example, if sexes and ages were not similar, the researcher cannot determine whether the most favorable effects are attributable to the type of heat, the healing power of the younger subjects, or the sex characteristics of the subjects. Uncontrolled variables in a simple randomized design can interact with treatment or other effects to influence or contaminate (confound) the outcome. Control of variables is critical in this design.[27] The one-way analysis of variance is the proper statistical method for this design. The analysis of variance enables the measured scores to be broken down into the proportion presumed to be due to the treatment or experimental effects (X_T) and into a proportion that can be attributed to error or chance variation (X_E). Thus, the randomized design for two or more groups

Table 9.2
Summary of One-Way Analysis of Variance with Equal Sized Samples (Example for Table 10.5)

Source of Variation	Sum of Squares	Degrees of Freedom	Mean Square	F
Between (heating methods)	0.370	3	0.123	1.051*
Within (error)	2.810	24	0.117	
Total	3.180	27		

* Not significant at .05 level.

compared on a single response measure can determine the components of the measured score, $X = X_T + X_E$.

Factorial Designs. The researcher would be limited in ability to test complex problems if only the randomized design was available for studying different treatment effects of a single independent variable. Factorial designs enable the researcher to compare concomitantly two or more treatment (independent) variables within the same experiment. These designs enable the researcher to use the same subjects for estimating the effects from the two or more variables, and this results in economy of subjects and time. Also, two or more variables are permitted to affect the outcome of the results and, therefore, each variable (main effects and independent) may influence another variable (main effects and independent) to cause interaction (crossing of levels of experimental effects to confound effects). That is, one or more independent (main) variables may affect the dependent variable but also two or more independent (main effects) variables may have a joint effect (interaction) on the dependent variable.

In biofeedback training of patients having tension headaches, acceptable practice includes the use of audio and visual modes of feedback. Some physical therapists prefer autogenic (self-suggestion) to progressive relaxation (muscular contraction and relaxation) techniques with electromyographic biofeedback. An experiment can be designed to contrast groups of patients using audio or visual modes with patients receiving autogenic and progressive relaxation techniques. If two independent variables (modes and techniques) are compared and each variable has two different levels (modes: audio and visual; techniques: autogenic and progressive relaxation) the design is a 2×2 factorial design. The patients are chosen and assigned randomly and independently for each level of the design. This 2×2 factorial design can be depicted as

$$1$$

		A	B
	A	S_{111}	S_{121}
2	B	S_{211}	S_{221}

where 1 is one independent variable (modes) with two levels A (audio) and B (visual), and 2 is the second independent variable (techniques) with levels A (autogenic) and B (progressive relaxation). A total of four samples (cells) must be obtained with an equal number of subjects in each sample or cell. If eight patients, in the above example, are assigned to each cell, then a total of 32 patients are required. The first subscript number of the cell (S) designates the row, the second subscript number designates the column, and the third subscript number designates the subject for the purpose of identifying a particular subject. For example, S_{215} is the fifth subject of the audio-progressive relaxation sample.

The summary of the analysis for the 2×2 factorial design is shown in Table 9.3.

In designs that are more complex than the randomized design, treatment variables that may influence each other in the variance are partitioned out into interaction. Sometimes the interaction of variables is the most valuable portion of an analysis. Each factor (main effect) is also partitioned out into individual components for examination of the influences. Many combinations of factors can be analyzed in a factorial design but the example here is basic to the design class.[28]

In addition, the error proportion can be determined. The factorial design offers flexibility to the researcher for studying as many variables and levels of variables as desired. The complexities and number of subjects groups of the design increase as the numbers of variables to be studied increase. A $3 \times 2 \times 4 \times 5$ factorial design which restricts the data from one subject to one data cell requires 120 groups and with 20 subjects assigned randomly to each one of the groups, a total of 2,400 subjects would be required in the experiment. This particular design is very complex and unlikely to be used often, but could technically be computed.

Randomized Blocks Design. A randomized blocks design may be conceptualized as a basic factorial design to which one or more block factors have been added.[27] A block is a classification variable in which subjects are placed into sub-groups or blocks. Subjects in each block may be assigned at random to any number of manipulated treatments with the restraint that each treatment occurs only once in each block.[29] Classifying subjects is similar to adding another variable to the design for study. Sex is often a significant factor when men and women are used in an experiment and the researcher wants to know what differences may occur between subjects of different sexes on the other variables being investigated. By blocking or sub-grouping subjects according to sex, the experiment becomes relatively homogeneous. The blocking technique reduces the error component. The equation to represent the concept is $X = X_T + X_E$ where X_T is broken into components of treatment factors, interaction between

Table 9.3
Analysis of Variance Summary for a 2×2 Factorial Design

Source	SS	DF	MS	F
Columns (main effect-modes)	SS_1	1	$SS_1/1$	MS_1/MS_w
Rows (main effect-techniques)	SS_2	1	$SS_2/1$	MS_2/MS_w
Interaction (modes-techniques)	$SS_{1\times2}$	1	$SS_{1\times2}/1$	$MS_{1\times2}/MS_w$
Within (error)	SS_w	$4\,(n-1)$	$SS_w/4\,(n-1)$	
Total	SS_T	$4\,(N-1)$		

treatment factors and blocks, and blocks. The 2 × 2 factorial design discussed previously is compared with the randomized blocks design where patients have been blocked into levels of severity, mild and severe (Table 9.4).

The summary table for randomized blocks design will differ from the 2 × 2 factorial design by blocks replacing rows and interaction replacing interaction and error, respectively. In the randomized blocks design, the interaction factor serves as the error factor, thus eliminating the component of interaction by main effects.

Repeated Measures Design. Repeated measures implies that each subject involved with the experiment is measured for each response measure (variable) being investigated. In four angles of knee extension with and without a wedge under the knee during maximum isometric contraction of the knee extensors, each subject will be measured for each of the six levels. In the randomized blocks and factorial designs, separate groups of subjects were used for each factor measured. Repeated measures design may be built into the randomized blocks and factorial designs.[27]

Since each subject is exposed and measured on each response measure, much of the variability that exists between different subjects is automatically limited. The sensitivity of the experiment is increased. The subject serves as his own control.[30] Pairing or matching of subjects improves the homogeneity of groups of subjects and was discussed in the two-group and randomized blocks designs. In the repeated measures design, the ideal pair for a given experimental subject is achieved by having each subject to be his own match.[27]

The design in Table 9.5 is very conservative for subjects. Each subject serves as his own control making this design useful for very sophisticated analyses. Also, all main effects or treatments can be given to each subject or measurements can be made on any designated factor.[27]

The notation of the numbering sequence (e.g., X_{321}) for this design is first subscript number = level of first factor ($X_{3..}$), second subscript number = level of second factor ($X_{.2.}$), and third subscript number = subject ($X_{..1}$).

Summary of data broken down by a 4 × 2 × 25 factorial design of

Table 9.4
Variation in a 2 × 2 Factorial Design and a Randomized Blocks Design

		2 × 2 Factorial Design				Randomized Blocks Design	
		1				1	
		A	B			A	B
	A	S_{11}	S_{12}		1	S_{11}	S_{12}
2					Blocks		
	B	S_{21}	S_{22}		2	S_{21}	S_{22}

Table 9.5
A 4 × 2 Factorial Design with Repeated Measure on Each Factor

		Subjects	A	1	B
A		1	111		121
		.	.		.
		.	.		.
		.	.		.
		n	$11n$		$12n$
	B	1	211		221
		.	.		.
2		.	.		.
		n	$21n$		$22n$
	C	1	311		321
		.	.		.
		.	.		.
		.	.		.
		n	$31n$		$32n$
	D	1	411		421
		.	.		.
		.	.		.
		.	.		.
		n	$41n$		$42n$

Table 9.6
Summary of Analysis of Variance of Maximal Isometric Force of Knee Extensors with and without a Wedge

Source	SS	DF	MS	F
A (wedge)	64.98	1	64.98	1.43*
AS (Error)	1,088.02	24	45.33	—
B (angles)	25,278.52	3	8,426.17	16.23†
BS (error)	37,372.98	72	519.06	—
AB (interaction)	696.18	3	232.06	1.01*
ABS (error)	16,441.14	72	228.34	—
S (subjects)	61,082.18	24	2,545.09	—
Total	106,965.68	199		

  * Not significant at .05 level.
  † Significant at .01 level.

analysis of variance with repeated measurements on each factor, knee angles and wedge-on-wedge[31] is shown in Table 9.6.

The reader may see tables similar to Table 9.6 in the research literature but should not be perplexed; since the abbreviations are known as sum of squares (SS), degrees of freedom (DF), mean square (MS), and the F ratio, respectively. The significance of the F ratio is given in the table or

Table 9.7
Cumulative Summary of the Research Processes Presented

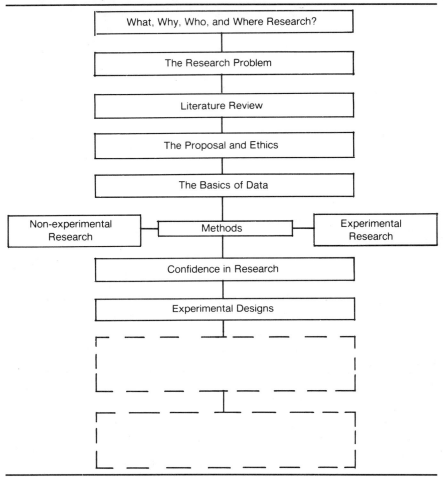

at the bottom of the table and indicates the outcome of the analysis for quick and easy interpretation of the findings.

These designs enable the researcher to make comparisons involving highly homogeneous material, thus increasing the power of the test; to conserve on the number of subjects required for any given investigation, because each subject is used more than once; and to reduce any history or maturation effects, because subjects are repeatedly measured over time.[27]

One problem with the use of repeated measures design is the carry-over effects caused by repeated physical performances which each subject must engage in to complete all measurements of the variables being studied. In strength measurements the researcher must avoid causing muscular fatigue because of the repeated performance over all measures for the purpose of collecting data through repeated measurements. Therefore, subjects tested on too many measures over a long period of time may yield data that are confounded by unwanted variables.[32]

The ANOVA is extremely versatile and can be adapted to most of the designs presented. There are methods available that can handle data for samples of unequal size.[27,30] The reader is advised that the "designs" presented in this chapter are not mutually exclusive (one variable cannot be used with another variable), but are used in various combinations. For example, a study might be prospective and longitudinal with subjects selected by a stratified sampling technique and the independent variable administered by means of a double-blind design.

SUMMARY

The established objectives and nature of the experiment will determine the appropriate design to be chosen. Several sources of internal and external validity are discussed briefly to acquaint the reader with the need for establishing suitable control in experimental research. Various designs are presented that can be selected by the researcher depending upon the variables to be controlled in his or her study. Selection of the appropriate experimental design is paramount so that any change in the posttest can be assigned only to the treatment that was manipulated by the researcher. For greater detail about the designs included in this chapter as well as additional designs the reader is advised to consult such authors as Borg,[1] Gay,[7] Campbell and Stanley,[8] Dayton,[27] Winer,[30] and Keppel.[33] Table 9.7 provides a summary of the research process presented thus far.

REFERENCES

1. Borg WR, Gall MD: Educational Research: An Introduction, ed 3. New York, Longman, 1979
2. Curwen MP: The clinical trial: An exercise in logic. Physiotherapy 56: 482–486, 1970
3. Slater SB: Let's reduce the understanding gap. 2. The design of clinical research. Phys Ther 46: 265–273, 1966
4. Gonnella C: Let's reduce the understanding gap. 2. The method: What and Why? Phys Ther 50: 382–385, 1970
5. Kelimbet ZA: Review of research methods as they apply to physiotherapy, with emphasis on the clinical trial. Physiother Canada 28: 35–37, 1976
6. Cox DR: Planning of Experiments. New York, John Wiley & Sons, Inc, 1958
7. Gay LR: Educational Research: Competencies for Analysis & Application, ed 2. Columbus, OH, Charles E. Merrill Pub Co, 1981
8. Campbell DT, Stanley JC: Experimental and Quasi Experimental Designs for Research. Chicago, Rand-McNally & Co, 1967
9. Lehmkuhl D: Let's reduce the understanding gap. Part III. The experimental design: What and Why? Phys Ther 50: 1716–1720, 1970

10. Ethridge DA, McSweeney M: Research in occupational therapy. Part III: research design. Am J Occup Ther 25: 24–28, 1971
11. Schenck, JM, Forward EM: Quantitative strength changes with test repetitions. Phys Ther 45: 562–569, 1970
12. Makrides L, Richman J: Research methodology and applied statistics, Part 5: experimental design. Physiother Canada 33: 6–14, 1981
13. Bracht GH, Glass GV: The external validity of experiments. Am Educ Res J 5: 437–474, 1968
14. Meyers LS, Grossen NE: Behavioral Research Theory, Procedure, and Design. San Francisco, WH Freeman and Co, 1974
15. Armitage P: Sequential Medical Trials. Springfield, IL, 1960
16. Gonnella C: Designs for clinical research. Phys Ther 53: 1276–1283, 1973
17. Cox KR: Planning Clinical Experiments. Springfield, IL, Charles C Thomas Publishers, 1968
18. Silverman FH: Research Design in Speech Pathology and Audiology: Asking and Answering Questions, Englewood Cliffs, NJ, Prentice-Hall, Inc, 1977
19. DeLateur B, Lehmann J, Stonebridge J, et al: Isotonic versus isometric exercise: A double-shift transfer-of-training study. Arch Phys Med Rehabil 53: 212–216, 1972
20. Rao CR: Linear Statistical Inference and Its Applications, ed 2. New York, John Wiley & Sons, Inc, 1973
21. Armitage P: Statistical Methods in Medical Research. New York, John Wiley & Sons, Inc, 1971
22. Burdette WJ, Gehan EA: Planning and Analysis of Clinical Studies. Springfield, IL, Charles C Thomas Publisher, 1970
23. Wolery M, Harris SR: Interpreting results of single-subject research designs. Phys Ther 62: 445–452, 1982
24. Ostendorf CG, Wolf SL: Effect of forced use of the upper extremity of a hemiplegic patient on changes in function. Phys Ther 61: 1022–1028, 1981
25. Martin JE, Epstein LH: Evaluating treatment effectiveness in cerebral palsy: single-subject designs. Phys Ther 56: 285–294, 1976
26. Currier DP, Mann R: Muscular strength development by electrical stimulation in normal individuals. Phys Ther 63: 915–921, 1983
27. Dayton CM: The Design of Educational Experiments. New York, McGraw-Hill Book Co, 1970
28. Cain RB: Elementary Statistical Concepts. Philadelphia, WB Saunders CO, 1972
29. Ferguson GA: Statistical Analyses in Psychology and Education, ed 5. New York, McGraw-Hill Book Co, 1981
30. Winer BJ: Statistical Principles in Experimental Design, ed 2. New York, McGraw-Hill Book Co, 1971
31. Currier DP: Evaluation of the use of a wedge in quadriceps strengthening. Phys Ther 55: 870–874, 1975
32. Singer RN: Experimental Research. In Hubbard AW (ed): Research methods in Health, Physical Education, and Recreation, ed 3. Washington, Am Assoc Health Phys Educ Rec, 1973
33. Keppel G: Design and Analysis: A Researcher's Handbook. Englewood Cliffs, NJ. Prentice-Hall, 1973

Part Three

HYPOTHESIS TESTING

10

Parametric Tests

Research is performed to answer specific questions relevant to physical therapy; i.e., to contribute to the body of knowledge. A researcher conducts studies only after having knowledge about the problem of interest; that is, the researcher operates within some frame of reference and the study is directly related to a problem within the reference. Raw data represent recorded observations which, upon examination, may imply certain conclusions or trends intuitively. Although this approach can sometimes yield information for making important inferences, failures in interpretations may often occur because the meaning of the data is not always obvious. Chance variations may mask information which suggests different conclusions than mere visual examination of the data would reveal. Chance variations can sometimes produce regularities as well as irregularities. If the researcher is deceived by what the data are showing, an erroneous conclusion can be disseminated and adopted. The science of statistics has been developed to help the researcher make fewer errors when inferring from collected data.

Research is performed to uncover information not obvious by other methods. The researcher performs experimental and non-experimental research in which results from two or more different groups or techniques are compared. The researcher performs research to test hypotheses. What are hypotheses? How are they tested? How does the researcher know whether a hypothesis is right or wrong? This chapter will attempt to answer these questions and offer some methods for analyzing experimental data. Expressions using the word "experiment" will pertain not only to experimental but to non-experimental research as well. Non-experimental research becomes experimental whenever two different methods are compared. For example, two different types of admission interviews may be compared or three forms of a written test administered to the same group of students.

HYPOTHESES AND HYPOTHESIS TESTING

Hypotheses

The term hypothesis has been defined in many different ways. A hypothesis is an idea based upon some plausible or factual knowledge about a problem. A hypothesis is a conjecture or an idea about the relation between two or more variables. Wilson[1] has defined a hypothesis as a trial, idea, or a tentative suggestion about the nature of things. Kerlinger[2] defined a hypothesis as a conjectural statement, a tentative proposition, about the relation between two or more observed phenomena or variables. A statistical hypothesis is an assumption about a parameter of a population.[3] Hypothesis testing is using data from a sample to support or refute a statement about the population.[4]

In Chapter 2 the concept of a problem was discussed and was defined as an answerable question, or an interrogative sentence. A problem asks, but a hypothesis states. Both a problem and a hypothesis express a relation between two variables. A hypothesis is always in declarative form and carries clear implications for testing the relation between the variables.[2] The problem asks, but cannot be tested in question form. To answer the research question, the researcher must make a declarative statement about what the specific relation is. For example, a hypothesis migh be: "Dynamic exercises are better than isometric exercises for increasing strength throughout the entire range of joint motion," "An ergometer causes less energy expenditure than a treadmill for a given load," or "Ice packs and hot packs are equally effective for treating patients having chronic low back strains." These statements are in declarative sentence form; they are statements that can be tested. They are hypotheses.

Examination of the above three hypotheses reveals that they differ in more ways than the content area to be tested. They also differ in the way that the statements are directed. The first hypothesis states that dynamic exercises are better than isometric exercises under a specific condition. The use of the word "better" implies that the mean of dynamic exercise data must be larger than the mean of isometric data if the hypothesis is true. The second hypothesis states that the ergometer should require less energy than the use of a treadmill in performing a particular amount of work. This hypothesis is opposite that of the first hypothesis because the mean value of the ergometric data is believed to be less than that calculated for treadmill data. If the calculated mean values were actually reversed in the first two examples, the hypotheses would be false. These two hypotheses indicate direction, each hypothesis indicates a specific but opposite direction that could be tested to determine whether they are true statements (hypotheses). The third example is somewhat different from the first and second hypothesis. Note that the third hypothesis represents a special case in hypothesis testing and is referred to as the "null" hypothesis. Null means without value, without significance, or amounting to nothing.[5] In hypothesis testing, the null hypothesis implies that the difference between the means of the different variables is equal to zero, that there is no difference between the means, or that the effect of each variable is the same. The null hypothesis is used commonly in experimental research because of its simplicity.

A researcher usually does not know the exact scores of a population; he does not know the mean or standard deviation of the population. In fact, the researcher seldom, if ever, knows details about the population, so hypotheses are formed about the population's parameters. The hypothesis is a convenient statement about the parameters and it can be tested. Hypothesis testing enables the researcher to compare theoretical results with those obtained by experimentation. The null form serves as a simple starting point by stating that no difference exists between two variables, i.e., the two variables are related. Since the null form states that no difference exists between variables, an alternate hypothesis must be developed which states that a difference does exist between the variables. Thus, two outcomes are possible for a research investigation. Gathering and analyzing data are ways of determining whether theoretical and experimental results are in agreement or whether the difference in results warrants rejection of the theory. The null form of hypothesis testing offers the researcher a simple, convenient, and versatile way of testing the probability of agreement between theory and observation. The null hypothesis is a clear and unambiguous statement.

Further examination of the three exemplary hypotheses should disclose the fact that none of these hypotheses offers the researcher an alternative decision. If the null hypothesis states that the means of the various variables are equal, what about the circumstance where the means are not equal? That is, if the mean differences are tested statistically and are indeed found to be different, all the researcher can say is that the hypothesis is false if two groups are involved. What about the situation where three of five means are equal (or nearly equal) but two means are different? In hypothesis testing the researcher must have two hypotheses, an original and an alternate hypothesis. The null hypothesis is used most commonly as the original hypothesis and can be written symbolically as H_0 (read as H sub zero). The null hypothesis, "Ice packs and hot packs are equally effective for treating patients having chronic low back strain," can be expressed as an equation. Suppose data collected from using ice packs are designated as sample A, and sample B represents data from using hot packs. Since testing hypotheses are really testing the difference between means of two variables and since statistics are unbiased estimates of parameters, then the equation expressing the null hypothesis can use symbols for parameters.

The exemplary null hypothesis can be written as $\mu_A = \mu_B$ or as $\mu_A - \mu_B = 0$ (μ represents the mean of the population). The alternative hypothesis can also be expressed as an equation, H_1: $\mu_A \neq \mu_B$ or $\mu_A - \mu_B \neq 0$. In narrative form, the alternate hypothesis can be stated as "Ice packs and hot packs do not have the same effect on patients having chronic low back strains." These two hypotheses now offer the researcher choices in decision making. If the statistical analysis indicates that the mean differences are the same, the researcher then concludes that the null hypothesis is true, and rejects the alternative hypothesis as being false. In practice, the researcher, because of background knowledge or frame of reference, usually hopes that the data will support the alternative hypothesis. If collected data support the null hypothesis then the different treatments (ice and hot packs) have the same effect, but if the data support the alternative hypothesis by indicating that a significant difference occurs between means, then the inference can be made that treatment A is better or worse than treatment B. In the situation where a significant difference between means occurs, the larger or largest mean then is inferred as being superior to the variable or variables having the smaller or smallest mean, respectively.

Hypotheses can be expressed as directional hypotheses, also. If a researcher has some evidence (personal observations or literature reports showed trend) to believe that one method should be better than another method, then a directional hypothesis can be stated. For example, a directional hypothesis is that dynamic exercises (A) are better than isometric exercises (B) for increasing muscular strength throughout the entire range of joint motion. The equation for this directional hypothesis (original) can be written: $\mu_A > \mu_B$. The alternate hypothesis then would be expressed symbolically as: $\mu_A \lesssim \mu_B$. Note that in statistics the symbol $>$ refers to greater than, $<$ refers to less than, and $-$ refers to as equal when used with a symbol of direction. The equation, $\mu_A \lesssim \mu_B$ can be read as the mean for ice pack effect (μ_A) is less than or equal to the mean effect for hot packs (μ_B). In this situation, the researcher would hope for support of the original hypothesis if hot packs are believed better than ice packs. The alternate hypothesis offers a choice of another outcome. If the researcher hoped that the data supported the ice packs, then the equation for the original hypothesis should have been written as $\mu_A > \mu_B$.

In experimental studies in which statistical analyses are made, the rule is that the researcher must devise two hypotheses. The hypotheses are formed (stated) before data are collected; the hypotheses can be stated in the protocol (Chapter 4). Data are collected for the purpose of confirming or refuting the hypotheses: hypothesis testing. The procedure in decision making is to choose one hypothesis as being true and reject the other hypothesis as being false. the decision of non-rejection or rejection of the null hypothesis is based on the outcome of the data analyses (difference between means).

Criteria for Rejection and Use of Hypotheses

Hypotheses are essential in the scientific approach; without them there is no way of explaining the collected data, dependent variables, or phenomena. Hypotheses must be written simply in terms of language for easy grasping by researcher and reviewers. Hypotheses should suggest investigations and arguments which, if they do not answer the specific question, will at least bring the researcher closer to the solution course. Hypotheses are used for contrasting, comparing, or verifying the relation of two or more variables at some more or less remote period of time.[6]

Hypotheses provide direction to the nature of the data to be gathered and the method in which the data should be gathered. The methods for organizing and analyzing the data are decided by hypotheses, and the decisions and the inferences to be made are suggested by hypotheses. Failure to pose the proper hypothesis relative to the research problem being investigated may cause decreased proficiency of the investigation. Thus, the basis of experimentation rests on the ability of the researcher to devise productive hypotheses and design proper experiments to test them.

At this point, the introduction of some new concepts and review of some concepts presented previously should help in synthesizing the idea of hypothesis testing, direction, and how to determine whether a hypothesis is right or wrong.

INFERENCES FROM DATA

Descriptive Statistics

Sampling is the procedure of collecting data from a few subjects, events, or characteristics so that the researcher can learn something about a population. Sampling procedures make the theory of probability practical in research by enabling the researcher to use inductive reasoning to say something about universal characteristics; for example, ice packs are superior to hot packs in the treatment of patients having chronic low back strains. A statistic calculated from a sample is the best estimate of a parameter of the population. The best estimate of central tendency is the mean which describes the central most characteristic of a sample or if inferred to the population, the mean of the population. The mean is used in testing hypotheses because it is the average score of the data and is the best estimate of the average score of a population.

Hypothesis testing asks the question of whether the means of two groups differ or do not differ. In theory, the question is whether the difference between means reflects sampling from two different populations.[7] The question may be whether the difference between the means of two or more samples will be small enough to be attributed to sampling variability; that is, due to chance and, therefore, the means were taken from the same population, or be large enough to be attributed to effects of the experiment (i.e., due to means drawn from different populations). If the difference between the means is small (no significant difference), the researcher concludes that no true difference exists between the means of the populations (ice packs and hot packs are equally effective). On the other hand, if the difference between the sample means is large enough to be attributed to the effects of the experimental manipulation (significant difference), the researcher concludes that a true difference exists between the two methods of treatment (effects of ice > or $\leq$ hot packs).

Because of chance variations, means of samples can vary within the population. Suppose a sample of patients having rheumatoid arthritis is selected and the mean wrist extensor strength is found to be 10 kg. Another sample of patients having rheumatoid arthritis is selected in which many variables are controlled (sex, age, severity of disease, similar motion, and measured with the same instrument under similar controlled conditions), and the mean wrist extensor strength is subsequently found to be 13.5 kg. Sampling and measuring can continue indefinitely by drawing subjects independently and randomly. Each mean strength value calculated is not exactly the same as that calculated for any other sample but yet when analyzed statistically, no significant difference is found. That is, all means may have ranged from 10 to 14 kg but the data support the null hypothesis that no difference exists between wrist extensor strength of patients having rheumatoid arthritis, given specific controlled conditions. Another way of interpreting the null hypothesis when the means range within certain values that are not statistically different is to say that the means do not differ from zero. The researcher can state that the mean differences were due to chance variations and that the samples were drawn from the same parent population. Now, if all possible samples are drawn from a parent population and the mean of each sample is calculated and then placed into a single sample, the single sample will be a distribution of sample means rather than a single sample of raw scores or values. The standard deviation of the sample of means (standard error of the mean, $s_{\bar{x}}$) can be calculated to represent the variability of the sample of means. If the standard error of the mean is squared, the variance of the sample is formed (Chapter 5). When dealing with experimental and control groups of subjects in a research study, which can be conceptualized from Figure 10.1, the variance can be visualized as occurring from two sources.

The method of determining the standard error of the mean in Figure 10.1 has no practicality; we had to determine its value by drawing all possible samples of a parent population. This situation would be similar

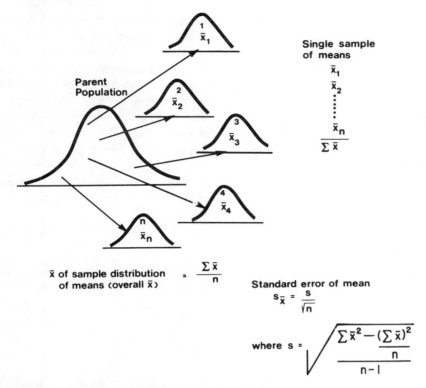

Figure 10.1. Samples are drawn from a parent population.

to taking measurements directly from the population, a feat that is physically and economically impossible for a researcher. Fortunately, an estimate of the standard error of the mean can be calculated from raw data collected from any one of the samples; for example, sample 1 of the figure. Since the variability of the means of all possible random samples depends upon the number of scores in a sample and the standard deviation of the data of that sample, the formula used for determining the standard error of the mean ($s_{\bar{x}} = s/\sqrt{n}$) can be used for a single random sample.

Within-groups variance is the variability that occurs within a particular sample: for example, variance occurring within sample 1 in Figure 10.1. Just as the means can be different for every sample so can the variances of each sample be different. Within-groups variance refers to the difference between scores of subjects within the same sample, and can be caused by the instruments, the researcher, individual strength differences of subjects measured, fatigue, or even amounts of enthusiasm.

The second source of variance is referred to as between-groups variance. If one group of patients is given ice packs and another group is given hot packs and the dependent variable is total number of treatments, the difference in the mean number of treatments between two groups is partially reflected by the between-groups variance. Returning to Figure 10.1, the between-groups variance can be represented as the variance occurring between group two and group four. Between-groups variance is the difference of group means from the overall mean and can be represented symbolically as: s^2 total $= s^2$ within-groups $+ s^2$ between-groups. Note: Use of variance here is not quite correct. In partitioning the variability which occurs in methods of hypothesis testing (viz, analysis of variance) the sum of squares is used correctly (Chapter 5). Sum of squares is in effect, only a proportion of the variance computation presented for determining variance. For reason of convenience in approaching the topic of significance, variance is used.

Degrees of Freedom

In calculating the variance and standard deviations (Chapter 5), the symbol, $n - 1$, appeared in the formula

$$s = \sqrt{\frac{\sum X^2 - \frac{(\sum X)^2}{n}}{n - 1}}$$

Degrees of freedom is a concept which enables the statistic, in this case, the standard deviation, to be an unbiased estimate of the population's standard deviation. Degrees of freedom (df) is the number of scores in an array that are free to vary when such constraints as the mean and the number of scores within the array must remain fixed. For example, in a sample with a mean of 50 and $n = 20$, 19 $(n - 1)$ scores are free to vary (19 df). In other words, if you have 20 scores which provide a mean of 50 where the mean and number of scores must remain the same (fixed), 19 of the scores can be altered to any other 19 scores chosen arbitrarily without changing the mean value of the data or the total number of data. In the equation $s^2_{total} = s^2_{within} + s^2_{between}$ the degrees of freedom for s^2_{total} is calculated by $n - 1$, the degrees of freedom for $s^2_{between}$ is calculated by subtracting 1 from the number of groups (K samples) or $K - 1$, and the degrees of freedom for s^2_{within} is found by subtracting the df for between-groups variance from the df for variance total, $df \, s^2_{within} = df \, s^2_{total} - df \, s^2_{between}$.

Significant Difference

Researchers can determine whether the difference between the means of two or more variables is consistently different by similar amounts. The researcher really wants to know whether the difference between two means is truly different and how reliable is the difference. Two methods are available to the researcher to solve the dilemma. A study can be repeated many times and if the differences between means remain similar, then the researcher can conclude that the differences are true and consistent. This approach is analogous to measuring the entire population to determine the true or real situation, and both approaches (repeated studies and measuring a population) are the best approaches in absolute terms. As discussed previously, in practice these approaches are costly and time consuming and are not used routinely. The alternate approach to this dilemma is to apply statistical methods to the data to determine whether differences between the means of samples are different statistically. Earlier, the standard deviation calculated from a sampling distribution of means was called the standard error of the mean and is expressed by the symbols $s_{\bar{x}}$ or SEM, and the equation $s_{\bar{x}} = s/\sqrt{n} \; or \; (s_{\bar{x}}^2 = s^2/n)$. The standard error of the mean (SEM) of a sample of means in practice has the same effect as repeating a study many times for determining the reliability of the differences between means. In effect, this statistic when used in computing the t ratio (t test) is somewhat similar to within-groups variance which is actually computed in the analysis of variance. In the concept of significant difference, a ratio is formed of the between-groups variance to the within-groups variance. The ratio is calculated and formed from the data collected from two (t test) or more variables (analysis of variance, ANOVA), and is referred to as the obtained value (t or F ratios). Once the statistic representing the obtained value between two or more variables is computed, the researcher must determine whether the value of the computed statistic (t or F ratio) could be attributed to chance or attributed to the effects of the experimental treatments. At this point, the theory of probability is applied to test the hypotheses. If the difference between means is more probably due to chance, then the conclusion is that the original hypothesis is true. On the other hand, if the difference between means is more probably due to the effects of the treatments than chance, the original hypothesis is rejected and the alternative hypothesis is accepted as being true.

Levels of Significance

In hypothesis testing the obtained ratio which is calculated by subjecting the collected data of the sample or samples to statistical procedures must be compared with a calculated probability of the statistic. That is, the obtained value (ratio) from the data is compared to a baseline value appropriate to the statistical test used in analyzing the data for the particular design chosen for the study (e.g., t test or ANOVA). The appropriate baseline (that which fits the design) is in effect, the level of significance. The level of significance is an arbitrarily designated level of confidence or probability which the researcher sets for accepting the null hypothesis. The level of significance is associated with the researcher's probability or risk of committing an error when accepting the null hypothesis. The concept provides a way of comparing a calculated statistic (ratio of differences between means and their standard error) with a norm for the purpose of committing fewer errors in the decision making process. Note that the researcher must specify the level of significance in advance of the collection of any data. The appropriate time and place to state the arbitrarily chosen level of significance is when writing the proposal (protocol). The hypotheses and level of significance should never be contrived after the data have been collected. Researchers must maintain a degree of ethics in the conduct of a study and the level of significance is stated in advance to indicate what risk the researcher is willing to take in making the conclusion or inference about the study. For most purposes in physical therapy the 5% (0.05) or 1% (0.01) level of significance is satisfactory. The nature of the study assists the researcher in the determination of the level of significance. In Chapter 7 the concept of error was discussed and because research deals with prediction, estimation, and probability, the true outcome or score is never really known (unless every member of the population is measured). That is to say, error is ever present and for this reason the researcher takes a risk when making a conclusion or inference from an experiment. How much risk is the researcher willing to take? The level of significance serves to answer the question. If the 5% level is selected, then the researcher in effect is stating that he is willing to be wrong five times out of a 100 chances. Another way of stating this is that if the study was repeated 100 times, the outcome would vary from the true course five times. Thinking positively the researcher may say that the outcome of his study will be correct 95 times out of 100 trials. This is a practical use of the probability theory. Suppose the researcher is unwilling to risk being incorrect five times out of 100 and, therefore, chooses the 1% level of significance (LOS). By doing this, the researcher has decreased the risk to being wrong only one time in 100, but in decreasing risk he has subjected the data to more rigorous scrutiny.

In Chapter 5 the concept of the normal curve was presented. The time is now appropriate to bring back some discussion of the normal curve. The unit normal curve has a mean of zero and a standard deviation of ± 1.0. Also, the normal curve can be sectioned into areas by means of the standard deviations and the areas can be used as probabilities.

Look at Figure 10.2. If you add the percentages of area on both sides of the mean, about 95% of the area is represented between ±2 standard deviations (SD) and about 99% of the area is represented between ±3 SD. When the researcher selects the 5% LOS, he is really setting the limits for rejecting the original hypothesis at ±2 SD from the mean.

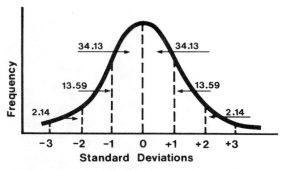

Figure 10.2.   Normal curve showing areas between ordinals at different standard deviations.

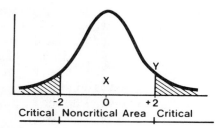

Figure 10.3.   Critical and non-critical areas under the normal curve; LOS = 0.05.

Suppose the researcher collects appropriate data for ice packs and hot packs in the treatment of patients having chronic low back strains and the unit of measurement is total number of treatments (TNT). The appropriate test is selected for testing the data (t test), the appropriate calculations are made, and the researcher arrives at an appropriate obtained value to the t ratio. The obtained value is now compared with the value appropriate to the selected LOS. The value appropriate to a particular LOS is found in a table of norms and is called the critical value. So in essence, the obtained value is compared with the critical value. If the calculated probability of the statistic is higher than the LOS established for the study, the original hypothesis will be true, no difference between means. That is, if the obtained value (t ratio) is smaller than the critical value of the table for the appropriate LOS, the original hypothesis is thought to be true. This situation is illustrated in Figure 10.3; when the 5% LOS has been selected, the null hypothesis will be accepted if the obtained value falls between the hatched areas.

If the obtained value (X) is less than the critical value (Y), the original hypothesis is accepted because the 5% LOS sets the limits at ±2 SD and

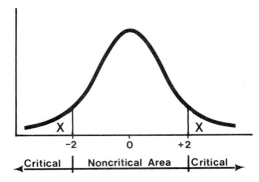

Figure 10.4. Critical and non-critical areas under the normal curve; LOS = 0.5.

any obtained value falling within the area X (non-critical) between ±2 SD is less than the critical value which established the limits at +2 SD and −2 SD. This situation also indicates that the calculated probability of the obtained value from the collected data (statistic) is higher than the LOS established for the study; therefore, the researcher accepts the original hypothesis. The use of ±2 SD is used as an example; in the normal curve, 2.5% of the area of the curve actually falls to the right of +1.96 SD above the mean and 2.5% falls to the left of −1.96 SD below the mean at the 0.05 LOS.

Conversely, the original hypothesis is false if the calculated probability of the statistic (obtained value) is equal to or less than the LOS established. The obtained value will be larger than the critical value (tabular value) established for the specific LOS when the original hypothesis is less tenable than the alternate hypothesis.

In the situation where the obtained value (calculated ratio) exceeds the critical value (tabular ratio), the original hypothesis is false because the obtained value X falls outside the limits of the non-critical area established by X at the 0.05 level (Figure 10.4). The researcher can conclude that the two samples were not drawn from the same population, that the obtained value was not due to chance variation, but that presumably, the obtained value was due to the effects of the treatment intervention (experimental method). If ice and hot packs were compared, ice packs having the smaller mean TNT, and if the obtained value exceeded the critical value at the 0.05 LOS, the researcher could designate the original hypothesis as false, choose the alternate hypothesis as true, and conclude that ice packs are superior to hot packs in the treatment of patients having chronic low back strains. The inductive reasoning (inferring from the specific or experimental results to the general or population) is based on the results of the samples and inferred to the population. Remember, if the 0.05 LOS was selected and only one experimental study was conducted, the researcher has no guarantee that the data and conclusion were not erroneous. The conclusion could have been based on data obtained among those five times out of 100 occurrences (this will be discussed later).

The probability level (LOS) that is established by the researcher is also referred to as alpha (α). If the calculated probability of the statistic is greater than (>) α, then the original hypothesis is accepted and is stated as being non-significant or true. If the calculated probability of the statistic is equal to or less than ($\leq$) α, the original hypothesis is false and the results of the calculated data are termed significant statistically or significantly different from zero.

Tails

Another new concept must be introduced at this point to clear up the muddy water. When the researcher specifies the level of significance (α), the limits of critical and non-critical areas under the normal curve are established. On the basis of the established limits (0.05 or 0.01 LOS), the collected data once calculated are compared to a baseline or norm in the form of a ratio. The baseline value varies according to the LOS selected. Earlier, the statement was made that the researcher decreases the risk of being incorrect when going from the 0.05 level to the 0.01 level of significance. In so doing, the areas under the curve change by increasing when going from 0.05 to the 0.01 level because instead of using ± 2 SD, the researcher now uses ± 3 SD at the 0.01 LOS. Note that as the levels change from 0.05 to 0.01, the area increases, the tail limits shift peripherally, and the probability increases. As the researcher decreases his risk of drawing wrong conclusions from the data, the restrictions for reaching significance are increased. That is, the critical values increase in size at the 0.01 LOS from those at the 0.05 LOS and, therefore, the obtained values must be larger for the 0.01 level than for the 0.05 level. One does not get anything free so the researcher must pay the price of decreasing risk by increasing the magnitude of the obtained ratio to exceed the critical value in order to accept the true hypothesis. In effect, this means that the effects of the experimental treatment or method must also be greater at the 0.01 level than at the 0.05 LOS in order to become significant.

Now, at the time the researcher selects the appropriate design, test, and level of significance for the experimental study, the number of tails must be selected. Returning to Figure 10.3, you will note the hatched areas at either end of the normal curve. These hatched areas are referred to as tails and in this particular illustration two tails are shown. Ordinarily, two tails are used in testing hypotheses when no direction is indicated. The null hypothesis is such a case where no direction is indicated by the wording or equation, $\mu_A = \mu_B$. The researcher really does care what direction the data

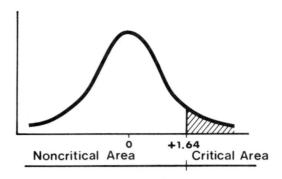

O   +1.64
Noncritical Area   Critical Area

Figure 10.5.   Non-critical and critical areas for one-tailed test; $\alpha = 0.05$.

take when forming the null hypothesis but cannot bias the data collected or outcome. In practice, the researcher hopes to accept the alternate hypothesis and conclude that a particular treatment is statistically significant or better than another. If one views hypothesis testing with this situation in mind, then the alternate hypothesis is really the more important hypothesis. Since the alternate hypothesis, when accompanied by the null hypothesis does not indicate direction either, $\mu_A \neq \mu_B$, but merely indicates that a difference does occur, the obtained value from the data can fall outside of the established limits (level of significance arbitrarily selected) either in a positive or negative direction. That is, if the obtained value exceeds the critical value, the researcher may designate the null hypothesis as false and choose the alternate hypothesis that a significant difference occurs, then that difference can occur outside the mean and limits to the right of the normal curve (positive tail) or to the left of the normal curve (negative tail). Two tails are working for hypothesis testing when no direction is indicated in the original hypothesis.

Going back to the hypothesis that ice packs are better than hot packs for the treatment of patients having chronic low back strains, you will note that direction is indicated by the word "better" which implies that the researcher possesses some prior knowledge (personal observations or review of literature) that one method of treatment might be better than another but the two methods have not been tested to determine which is better under specific conditions. Hypotheses of $\mu_A > \mu_B \gtrless \mu_B$ indicated direction and required one tail in testing because the researcher has indicated prior to data collection that one method is more (positive direction, above mean) or less effective (negative direction, below mean) than another (Figure 10.5).

The one-tailed test requires a smaller critical value (1.64 at the 0.05 LOS) for significance than does a two-tailed test; however, the restriction

Table 10.1
Conditions in Rejecting Hypotheses

	True Hypothesis	False Hypothesis
Do not reject the hypothesis	Decision is correct	Type II error
Reject the hypothesis	Type I error	Decision is correct

for a one-tailed test is rigid because it requires prior knowledge about the variables being compared. The two-tailed test is more commonly used in hypothesis testing than the one-tailed test. Tailed-testing applies to the t test but in the ANOVA the F ratio is mostly presented as a one-tailed test, so the researcher need be concerned about tails mostly when using the t test (procedures for t and ANOVA tests are discussed later in this chapter).

Errors

Errors are ever present in measurement and testing theory. The risks involved in selecting the level of significance were discussed briefly. Even though the researcher selects the LOS arbitrarily and in so doing indicates the risk he is willing to take in making conclusions and inferences, errors will be present regarding the decision in not rejecting or rejecting the original hypothesis. The errors associated with selecting hypotheses are called Type I and Type II errors. A Type I error is made when the original hypothesis is really correct but is ignored by the researcher in favor of the alternate hypothesis which is really incorrect. A Type II error is made when the original hypothesis is really incorrect and is considered true by the researcher rather than dropping it in favor of the alternate hypothesis which is really correct. The idea of Type I and II errors may be conceptualized if summarized in tabular form (Table 10.1).

The ability of a test to expose a false original hypothesis is related to its power. A statistical test has high power when a false original hypothesis is exposed at a high level of probability.[3] The level of significance relates to the power of the test but generally the 0.05 and 0.01 levels are sufficient for most studies in physical therapy. If the experimental treatment contains considerable risks or hazard to patients, then higher levels of significance are essential. For example, in pharmacological experiments where a particular drug may cause secondary complications or even death, a very high significance level must be used before accepting a potent drug for marketing; perhaps 0.0001 LOS may be selected. For situations like this, animals (rats) are used experimentally before the drugs are tested for human reactions. The theoretical idea is to avoid Type I errors whenever possible by selecting proper designs, tests, and levels of significance. Many researchers consult statisticians when planning a study and seek assistance for experimental designs and tests. This view has merit and is certainly recommended for the beginning researcher. Statistics and research design are a science and must be learned before their models can be applied to an investigation.

Type I and Type II errors and power of a test are discussed in many textbooks of statistics; the interested student is referred to the recommended books at the end of this chapter (Suggested Readings).

ANALYSIS OF DATA

The *t* Test

The *t* test, sometimes called Student's *t* test, is used appropriately only for experiments involving the two-groups design. The two-groups design refers to the variable that is measured on each of two independent groups. Designs are discussed in Chapter 9. The *t* test is not appropriate for comparing more than two groups because chance of error in interpreting significance is increased greatly when used for multiple comparisons. The *t* test is often misused in the literature, a good discussion is given by Michels.[8] Note that the "*t*" is always a lower case letter and should be written properly. The *t* test would be appropriate for studying the effect of a particular ultrasonic dosage (e.g., 1.5 watts/cm^2/unit time) on peripheral nerve conduction. The conduction is measured in advance of the ultrasound (pre), ultrasound is administered (treatment), and then the conduction is measured 3 minutes following ultrasound (post). Determination of any difference between mean values, before and after treatment, would be appropriate analysis for the experiment. Another example could be the comparison of the mean difference (difference between pretreatment and posttreatment means) of nerve conduction from ultrasound on peripheral nerve to the mean difference of conduction obtained from a sample that was not subjected to any treatment (control). The two groups of data could then be analyzed for determining statistical significance.

The *t* test is a rugged and flexible test. The test can be adapted to different situations. Three situations where the *t* test is appropriate will be presented with the appropriate calculations.

_t_ Test (Independent Samples, Equal Size). This variation of the *t* test examines the significance of a difference between the means of two samples or samples that have been drawn from the same or different populations.[3] Assumptions that are made when using this test are that two samples (*X* and *Y*) are independent and randomly distributed, are of equal size, and are drawn from normally distributed populations having equal variances.[3,4] The formula for determining the ratio of *t* is:

$$t = \frac{\bar{X} - \bar{Y}}{s_{\bar{x}-\bar{y}}}$$

where $s_{\bar{x}-\bar{y}}$ is the standard error $= \sqrt{s_{\bar{x}}^2 + s_{\bar{y}}^2}$ and $df = n_x + n_y - 2$.

Suppose we are interested in testing whether a hip angle of 70 degrees causes a difference in quadriceps force which is different from that of a hip angle of 80 degrees when subjects are performing knee strengthening exercises. The null hypothesis, H_0: $\mu_x = \mu_{y'}$ will be tested against the alternative hypothesis H_1: $\mu_x \neq \mu_y$, at the 0.05 level of significance. A sample of subjects (volunteers) will be collected and tested for maximum isometric muscular force (knee positioned 60 degrees from full extension) with hips angled at 70 degrees (X). Another sample of equal size will be measured under exactly the same controlled conditions but their hips will be angled at 80 degrees (Y) by a back support.[9] Since we do not know whether quadriceps force will be increased, maintained, or decreased by changing the hip angle from 70 to 80 degrees, no direction is indicated in the hypothesis (2-tailed). The samples contain eight measures only for illustrative purposes. Calculations are shown in Table 10.2.

The obtained data from the computation of the exemplary data yield a t ratio of 2.150. This obtained value is compared with a baseline value (critical value) found in Appendix, Table C. Table C gives the probabilities with which various values of t will be equaled or exceeded in random sampling from a normal curve. The appropriate degrees of freedom for the example ($n_x + n_y - 2$ or $8 + 8 - 2 = 14$ df) is determined, and then the

Table 10.2
Computation of the Independent t Test with Equal Sample Sizes: Effects of Hip Angles on Quadriceps during Knee Strengthening Exercise

X (kg 70°)	Y (kg 80°)
42	30
48	41
55	52
50	42
48	35
62	55
55	43
40	32

$$\sum X = 400 \qquad\qquad \sum Y = 330$$
$$(\sum X)^2 = 160{,}000 \qquad (\sum Y)^2 = 108{,}900$$
$$\sum X^2 = 20{,}366 \qquad\qquad \sum Y^2 = 14{,}172$$
$$\bar{X} = 50.00 \qquad\qquad \bar{Y} = 41.25$$
$$s_x^2 = 52.29 \qquad\qquad s_y^2 = 79.93$$
$$s_{\bar{x}}^2 = \frac{s_x^2}{n} = 6.54 \qquad s_{\bar{y}}^2 = \frac{s_y^2}{n} = 9.99$$

$$s_{\bar{x}-\bar{y}} = \sqrt{s_{\bar{x}}^2 + s_{\bar{y}}^2} = \sqrt{6.54 + 9.99} = \sqrt{16.53} = 4.07$$

$$t = \frac{50.00 - 41.25}{4.07} = 2.150 \qquad t_c = 2.145_{(0.05, 14df)}$$

row of the table (left-hand column) containing 14 degrees of freedom is entered. Because the test was two-tailed, read down from the top of the table for 0.05 LOS until the row for 14 df is met. The critical value "2.145" is located. Since the obtained value $t = 2.150$ exceeds the critical value $t_{c(0.05,14df)} = 2.145$, our decision is to accept the alternative hypothesis.

$$t_{\text{obtained}} > t_{\text{critical}} \therefore H_0{:}\mu_x = \mu_x \text{ is false}$$

The results of this example can be interpreted to mean that a hip angle of 70 degrees is superior to a hip angle of 80 degrees for enhancing quadriceps force of subjects performing knee strengthening exercises isometrically.

t **Test (Independent Samples, Unequal Sizes).** Occasionally during the process of conducting a two-groups experiment, subjects fail to report for testing, or for other reasons subjects cannot be obtained for two groups of equal size. In the previous example the standard error of the means common to both samples was found by the formula,

$$s_{\bar{x}-\bar{y}} = \sqrt{s_{\bar{x}}^2 + s_{\bar{y}}^2}.$$

When samples are unequal in size, the scores of the smaller sample will contribute more to the variance estimate than will scores of the larger sized sample. This situation creates an advantage for one sample which cannot be accepted if a comparison between two samples is to be made without bias. The mathematical procedure to prevent bias between samples having unequal sizes is to weight the variances rather than average the variances as was done in the previous example. The weighted procedure used to prevent bias between variances of two unequal sized samples is called pooling variances.[3] The pooling is performed during the computation of the sample variances, and therefore, the formula is somewhat different from that used previously for obtaining the variance.

$$s_{\text{pooled}}^2 = \frac{\left[\sum X^2 - \dfrac{(\sum X)^2}{n_x} \right] + \left[\sum Y^2 - \dfrac{(\sum Y)^2}{n_y} \right]}{df_x + df_y}$$

The degrees of freedom (e.g., df_x) are equal to $n - 1$ in each case.

The unequal sized samples, in addition to pooling variances, cause a change in the formula for determining the standard error of means ($s_{\bar{x}-\bar{y}}$) and is expressed by the formula

$$s_{\bar{x}-\bar{y}} = \sqrt{s_{\text{pooled}}^2 \frac{(n_x + n_y)}{n_x n_y}} \quad \text{or}$$

$$s_{\bar{x}-\bar{y}}^2 = s_{\text{pooled}}^2 \frac{(n_x + n_y)}{n_x n_y}$$

The computation of an exemplary problem will serve to illustrate the procedure of the t test for two unequal sized, independent samples. Suppose we are interested in testing whether the use of a biofeedback method (X) is effective in reducing spasm. A sample of patients having whiplash injuries to the cervical region accompanied by secondary spasm of the trapezius is measured for electrical activity of the trapezius, treated by biofeedback therapy for 1 week, and remeasured for electrical activity of the trapezius (X). Another sample of patients having similar injuries is not treated for 1 week, is measured and remeasured for electrical activity of the trapezius, and serves as a control (placebo) group (Y). Since we are interested in testing whether the use of biofeedback method (X) is effective in reducing spasm, a directional hypothesis is indicated because "reducing" implies direction (1-tailed t test). Hypotheses are formed as H_0: $\mu_x \geqslant \mu_y$ and H_1: $\mu_x < \mu_y$ at the 0.05 level. Hypotheses are formed as H_0: $\mu_x = \mu_y$ and H_1: $\mu_x \neq \mu_y$ at the 0.05 level. Table 10.3 shows the computation for the exemplary t test of independent samples of unequal sizes. The scores represent differences between premeasurements and postmeasurements of microvolts. The obtained value from the computation of the exemplary data yielded a t ratio of -2.603. This obtained value is compared with the critical value found in the Appendix, Table C, for a one-tailed t test (read down from the top of the table) for 0.05 LOS and 10 df to locate the number "1.812." Since the obtained value exceeded the critical value (left

Table 10.3
Computation of the Independent t test with Unequal Sample Sizes: Comparison of Biofeedback Method and Control Group (Artificial Data)

X (BF, μV)	Y (Control, μV)
30	44
25	45
15	33
5	16
12	32
10	
28	
$\sum X = 125$	$\sum Y = 170$
$(\sum X)^2 = 15{,}025$	$(\sum Y)^2 = 28{,}900$
$\sum X^2 = 2{,}803$	$\sum Y^2 = 6{,}330$
$\bar{X} = 17.86$	$\bar{Y} = 34.00$
$n_x = 7$	$n_y = 5$

$$s^2_{pooled} = \frac{\left[2{,}803 - \dfrac{15{,}625}{7}\right] + \left[6{,}330 - \dfrac{28{,}900}{5}\right]}{6 + 4} = 112.09$$

$$s_{\bar{x}-\bar{y}} = \sqrt{\frac{112.09\,(7 + 5)}{7 \times 5}} = \sqrt{38.43} = 6.2$$

$$t = \frac{17.86 - 34.00}{6.2} = -2.603 \qquad t_{c(.05,\,10df)} = 1.812$$

side of normal curve), the decision is to accept the alternative hypothesis that a difference between the means exists.

$$t_{\text{obtained}} > t_{\text{critical}} \therefore H_0: \mu_X = \mu_Y \text{ is false}$$

The object of biofeedback therapy is to get relaxation of the contracted muscle; in this case decreased microvoltage in sample X (biofeedback) indicated a reduction in spasm which was a favorable effect. No significant difference was found between sample means before the experiment was begun; therefore, the researcher can conclude that the significant difference obtained between means was attributed to the experimental treatment, biofeedback. Biofeedback therapy appeared to be effective among the sample of patients having spasm of the trapezius musculature. The independent distributions of this example were biofeedback therapy and control (placebo), while the dependent variable was the measured electrical activity (microvolts). The samples were independent of size n_1 and n_2 from two normally distributed populations with unequal variances.

Paired t Test. Matching or pairing members of one sample with members of another sample is a method of reducing variability and thus increasing the power of a test. The paired or dependent t test is a test that is appropriate

Table 10.4
Computation of the Paired t Test: Radial Nerve Latencies after Two Methods of Ultrasound

X (Ultrasound, msec)	Y (Ultrasound-electrical stimulation, msec)	$X - Y$ D	$D - \bar{D}$ d	$(D - \bar{D})^2$ d^2
2.3	2.5	−0.2	−0.12	0.0144
2.5	2.2	0.3	0.38	0.1444
2.4	2.6	−0.2	−0.12	0.0144
2.0	2.5	−0.5	−0.42	0.1764
2.6	2.5	0.1	0.18	0.0324
2.5	2.4	0.1	0.18	0.0324
2.6	2.5	0.1	0.18	0.0324
2.4	2.6	−0.2	−0.12	0.0144
2.5	2.5	0	0	0
2.4	2.7	−0.3	−0.22	0.0484
		−0.8		0.5096

$$\bar{D} = \frac{\sum D}{n} = \frac{-0.8}{10} = -0.08$$

$$S_D^2 = \frac{\sum d^2}{n - 1} = \frac{0.5096}{9} = 0.0566$$

$$S_{\bar{D}}^2 = \frac{S_D^2}{n} = \frac{0.0566}{10} = 0.0057$$

$$S_{\bar{D}} = \sqrt{S_{\bar{D}}^2} = \sqrt{0.0057} = 0.0755$$

$$t = \frac{-0.08}{0.0755} = -1.060 \qquad t_c(0.01, 9 \ df) = 3.25$$

to experimental designs which are contrived to reduce variability between groups. The paired t test is appropriate in the one-group design where pretest results are compared with the posttest results among the same members of a sample. The cross-matching design is appropriately used with the paired t test. Also, matching members according to similarity of scores obtained during pilot work is a suitable way of assigning subjects to the paired t test.[3] The assumptions for this test are that random samples of paired differences are from a normally distributed population of differences.[4]

Consider a sample of subjects whose right and left superficial radial nerve (sensory) latencies from the distal third of the forearm are measured after receiving an application of ultrasound and ultrasound-electrical stimulation over the location of the nerve branch, respectively. Measurements of the latencies from the right arm are designated X, while those recorded from the left arm are assigned Y. The null hypothesis is stated as H_0: $\mu_X = \mu_Y$ and the alternative hypothesis as H_1: $\mu_X \neq \mu_Y$ at the 0.01 level of significance, two-tailed. The test deals with the differences between each pair of scores rather than the difference between means of the samples. Formulas for each step in reaching the t ratio are somewhat different from those used in the independent t tests and will be presented in Table 10.4 with the computations. The t ratio is expressed by the formula:

$$t = \frac{\bar{D}}{s_{\bar{D}}}$$

where $\bar{D}$ is the mean, $\bar{D} = \sum D/n$, and $s_{\bar{D}}$ is the standard error of the mean, $s_{\bar{D}} = \sqrt{(d^2/n - 1)/n}$.

Note the change in degrees of freedom compared with that calculated for independent t tests. In independent t tests the degrees of freedom was calculated as $n_x + n_y - 2$ but in paired t tests the pairs are considered as one group and so the degrees of freedom is calculated as $n_{xy} - 1$. Pairing or matching scores in the two groups reduces variability, which in turn has the effect of decreasing the size of the standard error.[3] If the data were treated as independent samples, the df would have been 18 rather than 9. The critical value for the 0.01 level and 18 df is 2.878 whereas the critical value for this paired t test example with 9 df is 3.25 (2-tailed, Table C, page 332). Since the critical t values for the paired t test are greater than that required by the independent t test of similar sized groups, the former requires a greater obtained value for rejecting the null hypothesis. Thus, the researcher using the paired t test can place more confidence in his decision about the null hypothesis.

In the example, the obtained t value of -1.060 was less than the critical value t_c (0.01, 9 df) = 3.25 so the null hypothesis H_0: $\mu_x = \mu_y$ is true. The rate of nerve conduction is effected similarly by ultrasound and ultrasound-electrical stimulation.

Interpretation of the *t* Tests. One of the objectives in a course of research methods is to improve the student's ability to read the research literature. Reports of research studies in which *t* tests were used are not always informative about type of test (independent or paired), the number of tails (1 or 2), and levels of significance. Authors of research studies owe the readers this particular information. Also, the *t* tests are sometimes used improperly for multiple comparisons but the test is really only effective in comparing two distributions. Two unrelated variables should not be tested with the *t* test; for example, effects of isokinetic exercise (force) and effects of manual therapy (range of joint motion) on elbow extension. If isokinetic and manual therapy effects are treated as two methods effecting the variable motion (range of) of the elbow joint the *t* test for independent groups may be used.

The ability of a test to assist in accepting an original hypothesis when it is true and in dropping the hypothesis when it is false is very important to the researcher. Three conditions will improve the power of *t* tests. The first condition is to decrease the magnitude of the variance. The next is to increase the difference between means, and the third condition is to increase the size of the sample. Increasing the numbers of scores in samples will reduce the size of the standard error of the difference which has the effect of enlarging the *t* ratio.

Some assumptions about the *t* tests have been mentioned. Morehouse and Stull[3] have provided a clear discussion about the basic assumptions of the independent *t* tests. Conclusions drawn from the independent *t* tests will be suspect if the variables are not distributed normally. If for some reason scores are skewed (clustered into a certain region of the curve) or if the researcher has some doubt about the distribution of data, then perhaps non-parametric tests should be considered. For example, if strength (force) measurements are being converted into + or − symbols or into descriptive terms (fair or poor) as in the manual muscle test, the non-parametric tests (Chapter 11) should be used to analyze the data. One assumption is that the scores of one group do not influence in any fashion, the scores of the other group (independence). When scores are matched or paired, the use of the independent *t* test is violated, the paired or correlated *t* test would be appropriate.[3] Tests are available for verifying the homogeneity of variances of the different groups. If the variances are markedly different, such tests should be used to determine homogeneity. The student is referred to Cochran and Cox[10] for coverage of this topic. Wide divergence of sample sizes or extremely small samples are not recommended for use with the *t* tests. The *t* test tables go as low as 1 *df*, so values are available for very small samples; however, small amounts of information are not always representative of the population characteristic and therefore should be avoided. Actually, only drastic violations of the basic assumptions will have serious consequences.[11] The use of large sample sizes in experiments using hypothesis testing is the best preventive medicine for nonviolation of basic statistical assumptions.[12]

The t tests are parametric tests that estimate the parameter of the populations being tested.

ANALYSIS OF VARIANCE

In the discussion of the sum of squares earlier in this chapter, between- and within-groups variability was mentioned as being a component of the total sum of squares. The t tests are a special case in which the between-groups sum of squares cannot technically be partitioned out of the total sum of squares. In effect, the mean difference serves in the function of the between-groups variability but is a weak and limited version of the concept of partitioning total sum of squares into within- and between-groups variability. This is not taking anything away from t tests because they are excellent tests for the job for which they were mathematically designed. Remember that the t tests can only adequately handle the comparison between two groups, and between-groups sum of squares cannot be partitioned out but must be relegated to the means of the different groups. The t ratio can be conceptualized as:

$$t = \frac{\text{difference between two means}}{\text{within-groups sum of squares}}$$

Analysis of variance (ANOVA) is a statistical method that divides the sum of squares $\sum (X - \bar{X})^2$ into additive parts with each part assigned to a known source, cause, or factor.[12] The sum of squares of groups is a large proportion of the total sum of squares and is generally explained in terms of variance, the F ratio (F) can be expressed as

$$\frac{\text{Mean square}_{\text{between}}}{\text{Mean square}_{\text{within}}}$$

ANOVA is an extension of the t tests because in its simplest terms it can be used to test the significance of the difference between the means of two or more populations.[12]

The null hypothesis for ANOVA is used similarly to the way hypotheses were used in the t tests. In the t tests the ratio involved the difference between two means (H_0: $\mu_1 = \mu_2$), whereas in ANOVA the ratio may include differences between more than two means. The null hypothesis in ANOVA might be H_0: $\mu_A = \mu_B = \mu_C \ldots \mu_n$. An alternative hypothesis is also used and is usually given in the narrative form, H_1: at least two means differ. Methods of accepting the hypotheses are the same for t tests and ANOVA. If variations between means are due to sampling variabilities, the null hypothesis is accepted; but if the variations are not attributed to sampling fluctuations, the null hypothesis is believed false. Unlike the t tests a significant F ratio tells the researcher that a significant difference exists between the smallest and largest means only. Other differences of significance must be determined by special post hoc (after-the-fact or retrospective) analysis. Methods of post hoc analyses will be discussed subsequently.

Since the F ratio is formed by sums of squares in the numerator and denominator, two different degrees of freedom are necessary in comparing the obtained F value to the baseline, critical F value. This condition influences the shape of the F distribution by causing it to be skewed positively.

The ratio (Fig. 10.6) deals with squared values and, therefore, no negative values are formed for the F distribution which results in the zero point being at the extreme left and the median being 1.0. Most F tables present critical values for one-tailed tests because most computed F ratios fall to the right of 1.0 in the F distribution.

Theory of Analysis of Variance

ANOVA, like the t tests, is a test for determining whether the difference between means of different samples was drawn from the same population. Unlike the t tests, the ANOVA is appropriate for testing the difference between more than two means and offers many more design options to the researcher than did the t tests. The differences between more than two means can be tested simultaneously and the pooled within-groups variance can serve as an estimate of error variance which is important to the researcher.

ANOVA is an arithmetic scheme and is accomplished by partitioning the sum of squares $[\sum (X - \bar{X})^2$ or $\sum X^2 - (\sum X)^2/n]$ into additive parts so that each additive part can be assigned a known source, cause, or factor. These additive parts of known sources, causes, and factors are used to

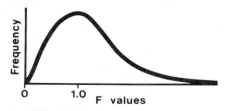

Figure 10.6.   Hypothetical F distribution.

estimate the variance of the population.[12] The simplest model on which ANOVA is based is the randomized model, the concept of randomness is the foundation of statistical probability. The partitioning of the total sum of squares (SS) can be expressed as $SS_{total} = SS_{between} + SS_{within}$. Different authors use different terminology for expressing the components of the total sum of squares; for example, between-groups SS are sometimes called treatment, and within-groups SS are sometimes called error SS. The total sum of squares is the sum of squares of the deviations from the overall mean for all scores, $\sum (X - \bar{X})^2$. Most books of statistics use a form of summation notation in ANOVA to differentiate sample and total values, and the student pursuing courses in statistics will become familiar with these. For illustrative purposes here a very simple method of using upper-case letters for total values and lower case letters for sample values is used. That is, x = sample values and X = total values.

The between sum of squares is the sum of the products for all samples of all scores in a given sample multiplied by the square of the deviations of a given sample mean from the overall mean.[3]

$$SS_{between} = \sum n_{all} (\bar{x} - \bar{X})^2$$

The sum of squares within is the sum of the squared deviations of all scores from their respective sample means.[3]

$$SS_{within} = \sum_{samples} \sum_{scores} (X - \bar{x})^2$$

The population variance can be estimated once the above calculations are completed by finding the mean squares (MS) of the partitioned parts.

$$MS_{between} = \frac{SS_{between}}{df_{between}}$$

where df is $K - 1$ (K = number of samples) being tested.

$$MS_{within} = \frac{SS_{within}}{df_{within}}$$

where df is $(N - 1) - (K - 1)$, N = total number of scores. The mean square for within is an extension of $(s_{\bar{x}}^2)$ and is a pooling of the sum of squared deviations from the means within all groups. Once the sum of squares and mean squares are calculated, the F ratio can be found by dividing $MS_{between}$ by MS_{within}.

$$F = \frac{MS_{between}}{MS_{within}}$$

Theoretically, if only sampling fluctuations have occurred between samples, the $MS_{between}$ will equal the MS_{within} and a ratio of 1.0 is formed. On most occasions with using ANOVA, the $MS_{between}$ will be larger than MS_{within} to provide an F ratio larger than 1.0. If experimental effects are at work in the study, the results will be evident in the F ratio when the $MS_{between}$ is many times larger than the MS_{within} value. Special F tables are available for comparing the obtained value from the computations to the critical value of the table (Appendix, Table D). If one thinks of df for MS_{within} being at the top of the F table, then little difficulty will be encountered when obtaining the critical value. Tables often have rows of values associated with the df_{within} rows and these represent different levels of significance. The appropriate row and level of significance must be found when locating the critical F value.

Example of One-Way Analysis of Variance

Computation of a hypothetical situation involving four methods of applying heat to the body is illustrated in Table 10.5. Because the one-way ANOVA is a randomized model, each sample contains different subjects who were assigned randomly to the different methods (samples). One-way refers to the one independent variable common to all samples. The

Table 10.5
Computation for One-Way Analysis of Variance with Equal Sample Sizes: Temperature Differences of Various Forms of Heat (Fictitious Data in Degrees)

Hot Packs	Infrared	SW Diathermy	Ultrasound	
2.0	1.6	2.3	2.3	
1.5	2.6	2.1	2.3	
1.8	2.5	2.3	2.1	
3.1	1.9	2.2	2.3	
2.2	2.2	2.1	2.5	
2.3	2.0	2.3	2.4	
2.4	1.8	2.4	2.9	TOTALS
$\sum x = 15.30$	14.60	15.70	16.80	62.40
$\sum x^2 = 34.99$	31.26	35.29	40.70	142.24
$\bar{x} = 2.19$	2.09	2.24	2.40	

$$SS_{total} = \sum X^2 - \frac{(\sum X)^2}{N} = 142.24 - \frac{62.4^2}{28} = 3.18$$

$$SS_{between} = \sum samples \frac{(\sum x)^2}{n} - \frac{(\sum X)^2}{N}$$

$$= \frac{15.3^2 + 14.6^2 + 15.7^2 + 16.8^2}{7} - \frac{62.4^2}{28} = 0.37$$

$$SS_{within} = SS_{total} - SS_{between} = 3.18 - 0.37 = 2.81$$

$$MS_{between} = \frac{0.37}{3} = 0.123 \qquad F = \frac{0.123}{0.117} = 1.05$$

$$MS_{within} = \frac{2.81}{24} = 0.117 \qquad F_{c(.05, \, 3 \, \& \, 24 \, df)} = 3.01$$

independent variable in the present example is methods of heating. The null hypothesis is H_0: $\mu_A = \mu_B = \mu_C = \mu_D$ and the alternative hypothesis (H_1) is that at least two means will differ. The 0.05 level of significance is used, the methods of applying heat are hot packs, infrared, short wave diathermy, and ultrasound. The intramuscular temperatures (dependent variable) of the gastrocnemius are measured for each application of heat by a thermistor.

In Table 10.6, the degrees of freedom for $MS_{between}$ is found by $K - 1$ samples ($4 - 1 = 3$), and for MS_{within} by $(N - 1) - (K - 1)$ or $[(28 - 1) - (4 - 1) = 27 - 3 = 24]$. F obtained $< F_{critical} \therefore$ accept H_0: $\mu_A = \mu_B = \mu_C = \mu_D$.

The obtained F ratio is less than the critical value of Table D in the Appendix; the conclusion can be made that the null hypothesis is true, the difference between the means is not significantly different from zero. If the hypothesis was true, then no difference in heating muscle is obtained by the different methods. The obtained F ratio would have to have exceeded 3.01 to be significant (i.e., accept the alternate hypothesis).

The ANOVA is extremely versatile and can be adapted to most of the designs presented in Chapter 9 (random, factorial, and repeated measures). Certain methods can be used to handle samples of unequal size, but these are not discussed in this book.

Post Hoc Analysis of Means

When the F ratio is tested for significance by comparing the obtained F value to a tabular value (critical value) and is found to exceed the critical value, the decision is to accept the alternative hypothesis. The alternative hypothesis is that at least two means are different. This acceptance of an alternate hypothesis that at least two means are different significantly is all that can be interpreted from a significant F value at this point. The interpretation is only that the mean having the smallest value is significantly different from the mean having the largest value when all means of the samples are rank ordered. What about the other means involved? If the F value is significant, the question is answered only by performing further analyses. Analysis of the significant means is called post hoc, postmortem, or a posteriori analysis. Several tests are available and are named after the men who developed them. These tests perform pairwise contrasts and are based on the avoidance of committing a Type I error. Because of their bases each bears varying degrees of conservatism and special tables are available for each procedure, although some procedures use similar tables. The procedures are presented according to their conservatism of the risk of the Type I error.

If the calculated F ratio in the above example was not significant (less than the critical value), no further analyses (post hoc) for the ANOVA is necessary. The null hypothesis would not be rejected.

Duncan Procedure. The Duncan procedure was designed for use with samples of equal size but sample means of unequal sizes can be compared by using the harmonic mean ($\overline{X}_h = n/(1/\sum X)$).[4] The standard error of a mean, $S_m = \sqrt{MS_{within}/n}$, is multiplied with an appropriate "multiple-range" value to provide an estimate of the standard error of the difference between ranked pairs of means. The level of significance is greater for pairwise contrasts for means separated by large numbers than for the small numbers of ranked positions.[13]

Newman-Keuls Procedure. Newman-Keuls procedure, sometimes referred to as Student-Newman-Keuls procedure, tests all pairwise contrasts at the same level of alpha so that the "studentized range" (special table) accounts for the magnitude or rank separation of the pair of means entering into a contrast. The studentized range protects the alpha levels (LOS) which vary according to the rank separation of pairs or means. The procedure is similar to Duncan's except for the protected levels of alpha. The two procedures are considered as middle-of-the-road post hoc analyses.[13]

Tukey Procedure. This procedure uses a fixed-range test that computes one critical value for all comparisons of means regardless of the number of steps that may separate the means. Tukey's procedure of "honestly significant difference" yields fewer significant differences than the previous two procedures. The procedure is easy to use, can be used for equal and unequal sized samples, and uses the "studentized range" table of Newman-Keuls.[3]

Scheffé Procedure. Scheffé's test involves the calculation of t ratios for each comparison followed by comparisons with a special critical t'. This procedure is the most conservative and will yield the fewest significant differences of the post hoc tests presented. The probability of committing a Type I error is never higher than the established alpha level in this test.[3]

Researchers must decide the risk they are willing to take when selecting post hoc tests (0.05 or 0.01 LOS). Review of the literature seems to favor the middle-of-the-road tests. Authors should report the type of post hoc analyses used in determining significance of the means in analysis of variance. The reporting of post hoc tests is usually found in the results section of the narrative report.

CORRELATION

Correlation is a method of determining the degree of association (correspondence, agreement, relationship) between two variables. The method of computing a correlation coefficient is appropriate for those research projects in which an attempt is made to determine relationships. Correlation is concerned then with a bivariate distribution where scores have been recorded for two variables or two sets of scores from a single variable. An example of the latter use is when you are interested in having patients perform some motor skill with the left and right hands and then determining the degree of association existing between the two performances (dexterity determinations). Karl Pearson, a behavioral scientist, devised a method known now as the Pearson product moment correlation method;[14] the coefficient is designated by the symbol "r". This symbol r when standing alone denotes Pearson product moment correlation and can be found in tables or narratives of reported research studies. Pearson product moment correlation should not be confused with other types of correlation such as rank order correlation to be presented in Chapter 11. The Pearson product moment correlation method is the most frequently used method of determining the agreement between two variables.

When two variables are correlated, the variables tend to vary together: (1) one variable systematically becomes larger, while the other variable systematically becomes larger; and (2) one variable systematically becomes larger, while the other variable systematically becomes smaller. In the first situation the variables are said to be correlated positively if both variables tend to vary in the same direction, larger or smaller. A person's height is usually correlated positively with body weight, both variables have a tendency to vary together in an upward (positive) direction. Coins could be said to vary in size with their values, the smaller the coin the less the value (the one- and ten-cent pieces are exceptions but the general trend holds true, although imperfectly). The second situation may occur where one variable tends to become larger and is paired with a variable which tends to become smaller; the variables in this situation are said to be correlated negatively. When a person becomes older (positive trend in age), muscular strength tends to become less (negative trend). In mathematics the negative sign masks the positive sign so that the correlation is a negative relationship (trends in different directions). Another example of negative correlation might be the correlation of items on a semantic differential scale where the descriptive terms are polar or opposites. For example, in the assessment of PAIN:

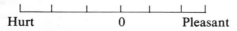

Hurt   0   Pleasant

The researcher would hope, however, that the results obtained from the instrument would correlate positively with some specific attitude.

The correlation coefficient not only detects the degree of variation between two variables but also detects the direction of variation. The coefficient is an index of relationship (correspondence, agreement, association) between two variables and is expressed as a single numerical value. The value can range from a perfect positive correlation of +1.00 to a perfect negative correlation of −1.00. The midpoint bisects the range and is designated by zero. A zero correlation indicates that no relationship exists between the two variables. The relationship between two variables can then take on any value (decimal number) ranging between +1.00 and −1.00; the coefficient is a continuous variable with set limits.

Scatter Diagrams

The examples of correlation cited can be graphed in a vivid fashion. A scattergram is a graphic illustration that shows the manner in which scores of two variables vary concomitantly. As a rule, the scores of the X variable are graphed on the horizontal axis of the graph, and scores of the Y variable are graphed on the vertical axis of the graph (in graphing correlation both variables are given equal standing, so either variable can be plotted on the X and Y axes). For purposes of illustrating different relationships between two variables, fictitious data will be used for the figures.

The scattergrams depicted are different because the points of the X and Y variables either follow a straight line (Figs. 10.7 and 10.11) or else depart from a straight line by varying amounts. A basic assumption of the Pearson product moment correlation method is that the association between the variables is linear, that the relationship between the variables follows a straight line. The magnitude of the correlation coefficient is reflected by the departure of the measures from the straight line. In Figures 10.7 and 10.11 all the points fall on a straight line (if the points are joined) and the relationships are perfect. In Figure 10.7 the scores of the X variable tend to increase, while scores on the Y variable tend to increase by equal amounts—a perfect positive correlation. The direction of the perfect correlation depicted in Figure 10.11 is negative because as scores of the X variable increase, the scores of the Y variable decrease by equal amounts. The relationships shown in Figures 10.8 to 10.10 vary in direction and magnitude.

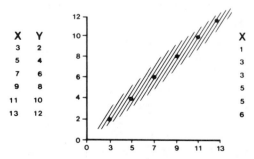

Figure 10.7. Perfect positive correlation. Note: In Figures 2 to 6, the shading around the points of the graphs is used to emphasize the relationships.

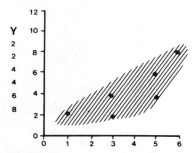

Figure 10.8. High positive correlation.

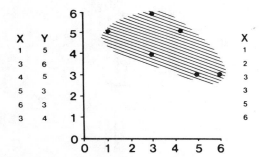

Figure 10.9. Low negative correlation.

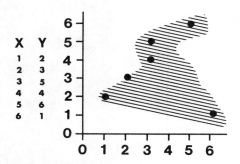

Figure 10.10. Low positive correlation.

Computation of Correlation

Several forms of the formula are available for computing the correlation coefficient but in keeping the theme of variance in statistical calculations, most formulas used in this book will have commonalities, variance. The

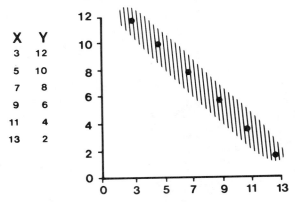

Figure 10.11   Perfect negative correlation.

basic formula for r is:

$$r = \frac{\Sigma XY - \dfrac{(\Sigma X)\,(\Sigma Y)}{n}}{\sqrt{\left[\dfrac{\Sigma X^2 - \dfrac{(\Sigma X)^2}{n}}{n}\right]\left[\dfrac{\Sigma Y^2 - \dfrac{(\Sigma Y)^2}{n}}{n}\right]}}$$

The n's in the denominators of the terms under the square root sign can be collected (n^2) by multiplying them, their square root taken $(n/1)$ and moved outside of the square root sign to form n/n which then cancels to give the formula:

$$r = \frac{\Sigma XY - \dfrac{(\Sigma X)(\Sigma Y)}{n}}{\sqrt{\left[\Sigma X^2 - \dfrac{(\Sigma X)^2}{n}\right]\left[\Sigma Y^2 - \dfrac{(\Sigma Y)^2}{n}\right]}}$$

where

$$\begin{aligned}
r &= \text{correlation coefficient} \\
\Sigma XY &= \text{sum of the cross-product of } X \text{ multiplied by } Y \\
\Sigma X^2 &= \text{sum of squared scores (also for } Y) \\
\Sigma Y^2 &= \text{sum of scores squared (also for } Y) \\
n &= \text{number of paired scores}
\end{aligned}$$

The formula caused three operations of division by the positions of n; therefore, a more convenient form of the formula which represents a savings in efficiency is:[3]

$$r = \frac{n\Sigma XY - (\Sigma X)(\Sigma Y)}{\sqrt{[n\Sigma X^2 - (\Sigma X)^2][n\Sigma Y^2 - (\Sigma Y)^2]}}$$

Table 10.6
Results and Computation of Test-Retest Reliability of Measurements Recorded from a Volume Cylinder Using Hands of Various Sizes

Test (mm of water displaced)	Retest (mm of water displaced)
36.0	36.0
18.0	17.0
22.0	22.0
17.0	16.0
24.0	24.0
20.0	23.0
20.0	18.0
8.0	10.4
12.0	16.6
14.0	15.6
13.0	12.8
22.0	24.0
16.5	15.0
17.2	16.4
10.4	10.0
22.8	19.6
15.0	16.0
10.4	10.4
9.8	10.0

$\Sigma X = 328.10$ $\Sigma Y = 332.80$
$\Sigma X^2 = 6{,}451.29$ $\Sigma XY = 6{,}475.82$ $\Sigma Y^2 = 6{,}563.20$
$(\Sigma X)^2 = 107{,}649.61$ $(\Sigma Y)^2 = 110{,}755.84$

$$r = \frac{n\Sigma XY - (\Sigma X)(\Sigma Y)}{\sqrt{[n\Sigma X^2 - (\Sigma X)^2][n\Sigma Y^2 - (\Sigma Y)^2]}}$$

$$= \frac{19 \times 6{,}475.82 - 328.10 \times 332.80}{\sqrt{[19 \times 6{,}451.29 - 328.10^2]\ [19 \times 6{,}563.20 - 332.80^2]}}$$

$$= \frac{13848.90}{\sqrt{14924.90 \times 13944.96}} = \frac{13848.90}{14426.61} = 0.95995 = 0.96$$

An example of testing for reliability of an instrument using some data should help with the use and understanding of the formula (Table 10.6). The reliability determined by the test-retest method in Table 10.6 is $r = 0.96$ which is highly correlated. The repeated measurements are dependent on the instrument (volume cylinder).

Interpretation of the Correlation Coefficient

The coefficient is an index of convenience which was developed in theory and modeled by the mathematical formulas for practical use. Because limits of $+1.0$ to -1.0 were chosen arbitrarily, the reader can only interpret the obtained index values in relative terms.[14] The coefficient is not a proportion or a percent. An r of 0.96 has the same value as an r of -0.96 but the concomitant variation of the two variables tends to vary in different directions. The numerical size of the coefficient does not permit an interpretation about the magnitude of the variables.

The coefficient value does not imply a cause and effect relationship between the two variables. The reader cannot determine the cause of relationship other than the way the scores actually vary with each other. Suppose separate groups of young adult women and men were tested for strength by measuring maximum isometric muscular contractions of the quadriceps. The bivariate distribution of scores yielded a value of $r = 0.98$; the researcher should not conclude that the quadriceps strength of women and men are equal or the same. In all probability, the women were athletic and endomorphic, while the men were sedentary and ectomorphic. Previous studies have indicated that women have about 70% of the strength of men.[9,15]

To avoid some problems of interpretation, the coefficient is squared. The coefficient of determination is the name given to the squared correlation coefficient, r^2, and was discussed earlier in this section. The r^2 value is the ratio of the explained sum of squares of variable Y divided by the total sum of squares of variable Y. If the coefficient of determination is used, then the value is a proportion of the retest variance which is associated with the preexisting variance. The coefficient of determination ranges between zero and $+1.00$ (squaring converts a negative score into a positive score). The r^2 value may be a better indicator or predictor of the relative importance of the different magnitudes of r than the correlation coefficient alone.[16]

Correlation can be used in experimental research as well as non-experimental research for determining relationships between two variables and hypothesis testing.

REGRESSION ANALYSIS

We have seen how the relationship of two variables can be projected through an index. Sometimes a single score of one variable can be predicted when the corresponding score of the other variable is known.[17] Regression analysis is the method used to determine the linear relationship between two variables when predicted values of one variable are desired. When a relationship exists between two variables, one can attempt to predict a score of one variable within the limits of the scores on which the correlation coefficient was based.[3] Correlation and prediction form close relationships and so one method can be projected to the other. Unlike correlation where each variable is given equal standing, regression analysis accords the X variable from which prediction is based as the independent variable and the dependent variable as the variable score which is being predicted, Y. This rule holds true when displaying the results of regression analyses in graphic form.

With the scattergram we were able to form a vivid image of the relationship of the two variables, and with the correlation coefficient a numerical value was assigned to provide a relative index of that idea. Now an equation will be introduced and it will express the relationship between two variables.

Computation of Regression Analysis

Like the method of Pearson product moment correlation, regression analysis also uses the assumption that the two variables are related in a linear fashion. If a scattergram is plotted and the geometric form does not resemble a straight line, but, for example, a curve line (curvilinear), the regression analysis discussed herein is not appropriate. The technique provided for regression analysis is only for the situation where the two variables resemble a straight line (linear relationship). The linear regression line is sometimes referred to as the line of best fit.[18] The equation for a straight line is:

$$Y' = a + bX$$

where

$Y' =$ the predicted Y value
$a =$ intercept of Y
$b =$ slope of the line
$X = X$ variable on which prediction is based

This equation of a straight line represents the relationship of a series of points formed by their coordinates. According to the above equation, the dependent variable, Y, will equal a when the independent variable equals zero. The point where the line of best fit and Y meet is the Y intercept or the distance on Y between zero and the point of intersection; b is the tangent of the angle formed by X and Y.[16] In Figure 10.12, the mean electrical activity in microvolts root mean square of the left anterior deltoid will be 5.2 when X (time in seconds) is zero, or the noise level of the electromyographic unit when the muscle is not contracting.

The regression line is computed by a method using the scores of a bivariate distribution and locating coordinate points for the average of the scores containing a minimum of error.[18] The symbols a and b in the equation are statistics computed from gathered data. The equation, $Y' = a + bX$, can be found by first solving for b and then for a.

$$b = \frac{\sum XY - \dfrac{(\sum X)(\sum Y)}{n}}{\sum X^2 - \dfrac{(\sum X)^2}{n}}$$

$$a = (\bar{Y} - b\bar{X})$$

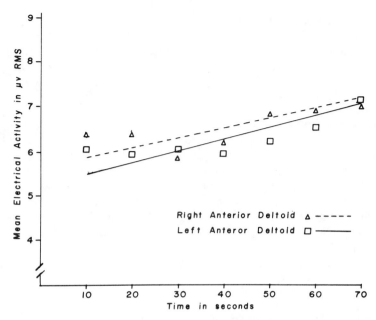

Figure 10.12   Voltage of contracting muscle as a function of time. (Reprinted with permission from Currier DP: Measurement of muscle fatigue. Phys Ther 49: 724–730, 1969).

Using data supplied in Table 10.7, a regression line can be formed from the scores for predicting future outcomes of the dependent variable. If the value of 45 seconds was recorded for X, the predicted Y' value would become, $Y' = 5.380 + 0.023 \times 45 = 6.420$ RMS (root mean square). If for some reason you were interested in predicting the electrical activity of the contracting muscle, established a particular amount of time (X), and solved for Y' in the equation, the Y' would be an estimate of the corresponding score on the other variable (electrical activity). Suppose we chose an X value recorded in the time column of Table 10.7 and solved for Y', let us say 40 seconds, the predicted Y' value would be 6.30 RMS. The predicted value of 6.30 is not the same as that of 6.06 which was obtained (Table 10.7) by actually measuring the electrical activity. The difference of 0.24 RMS between the two scores and expressed by our equation is not exact. The predicted score can, however, be considered as our best estimate of muscular activity without actually measuring the electrical activity of muscle contracting for 40 seconds. The larger the number of data examined and used in the computation of the equation, the better our estimate will become. One thousand data are better than 10 or 100 data. According to error theory, the predictor equation will never be perfect.

Determination of the correlation coefficient before the regression anal-

Table 10.7
Prediction of Electrical Activity of Muscle from Contraction Time

X Time (seconds)	Y Electrical Activity (RMS)
10	5.96
20	5.98
30	6.02
40	6.06
50	6.27
60	6.58
70	6.91
80	7.20
90	7.52
100	8.03

$\Sigma X = 550$ $\Sigma Y = 66.53$

$(\Sigma X)^2 = 302{,}500$ $(\Sigma Y)^2 = 4{,}426.24$

$\Sigma X^2 = 38{,}500$ $\Sigma Y^2 = 447.47$

$$\Sigma XY = 3{,}850$$

$$\bar{X} = 55.0 \qquad\qquad \bar{Y} = 6.65 \qquad r = .95$$

$$b = \cfrac{\Sigma XY - \cfrac{(\Sigma X)(\Sigma Y)}{n}}{\Sigma X^2 - \cfrac{(\Sigma X)^2}{n}} = \cfrac{3{,}850 - \cfrac{(550)(66.53)}{10}}{38{,}500 - \cfrac{302{,}500}{10}}$$

$$= \frac{3{,}850 - 3{,}659.15}{38{,}500 - 30{,}250} = \frac{190.85}{8{,}250} = 0.023$$

$$a = (\bar{Y} - b\bar{X}) = 6.65 - (0.023)55 = 6.65 - 1.27$$

$$= 5.38$$

$$Y' = 5.380 + .023X$$

ysis will assist the researcher in decision making, whether or not to compute a line of best fit. Unless the correlation coefficient is very high, the equation will not be a good predictor. Caution must be exercised in using linear regression for predicting. The relationship must be appropriate for what is being predicted. A high correlation can be demonstrated for quantitative electromyographic activity of muscle and muscular force during contraction. The association between the two variables is linear so that as force increases so does the electrical activity of muscle. Upon cursory observation one may be inclined to simulate this association into clinical practice for measuring the strength of a patient's involved muscle group. The difficulty arises when making intercomparisons with different individuals, different muscles of different individuals, and different muscles of the same individual because of several factors (age, sex, strength, fitness, impedance, and mass differences); the comparisons are very erratic. Sampling the electrical activity of one muscle cannot predict the outcome of another. The idea is appealing, however, but one must be cautioned about the appropriateness of predictor equations if the variables are not related from a physiological or conceptual view. The correlation coefficients may be very high between the two variables, but the coefficients are not indicative of cause and effect relationships.

TEST OF SIGNIFICANCE OF CORRELATION

Often one reads in the research report that the calculated correlation coefficient r was significant. This reporting of a significant r is often enough to warrant attention in improving the student's ability to read and interpret the literature. The use of the word "significance" or "significant" in testing correlation coefficients does not carry weight of importance as it did with the t tests or analyses of variance. The interpretation of a significant r only means that that particular coefficient value is not to be expected if the hypothesis that states that no relation between variables is true.[3] The distribution of r does not satisfy any distributions (normal, t or F) so far presented. The correlation coefficient, however, can be transformed into a t distribution where t is represented by the equation

$$t = \frac{r \sqrt{n - 2}}{\sqrt{1 - r^2}}$$

Hypotheses can be formed as a null hypothesis, $H_0: \rho = 0$, and as an alternative, $H_1: \rho \neq 0$. The letter "ρ" (rho) is the parameter for the statistic "r". When the null hypothesis is false, the interpretation is that the calculated r is statistically significant from zero. Another interpretation is that the value of the correlation coefficient obtained is unlikely to have resulted by chance variations if ρ was indeed equal to zero.[3] One must realize that the r value required to reach significance is dependent upon the sample sizes, and if a very large number of scores is included in the samples (e.g., $\geq 1,000$) the significant r value will be close to zero. Table C of the Appendix used for the critical values of the t distribution is used also for the transformed r values for determining significance. The levels of significance, again, are determined arbitrarily by the researcher. Hypothesis testing is similar to that used for the t tests and the F ratio. Ferguson has suggested that little importance should be given to the use of this formula when small samples sizes ($n = <20$) are used unless the coefficients are large.[12]

Upon observation, the difference between the obtained r value and zero is obvious and, therefore, using the above test would be fruitless. If some value other than zero is to be used to compare significance of the obtained r value, then a method of transforming the r value to a "Z_r," value is possible with use of a special transformation table. This method results in the comparison between Z and r having some importance. Ironically, authors seldom report the method of transformation used in determining significance of r in their studies. A conservative view would assume that the t transformation is used commonly in the literature, since the method

Table 10.8
Cumulative Summary of the Research Processes Presented

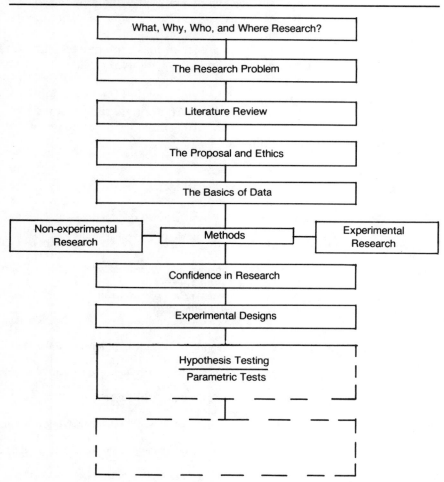

is frequently presented in many textbooks of statistics. The Z_r transformation uses natural logarithms in the conversion for improving parity with r and Z values. The significance of the difference between correlation coefficients can be performed through the Z_r-transformation methods for hypotheses testing. Again, a special table is available in many books of statistics for the convenience of the researcher who does not need to make the log transformations.[3]

SUMMARY

An hypothesis is a conjectural statement about the relation between two or more variables. If the hypothesis is clearly and specifically stated, it can be tested. The null hypothesis is a special form in hypothesis testing and implies that the difference between the means of the different variables is equal to zero. The null hypothesis is used commonly in experimental research because of its simplicity.

Hypothesis testing enables the researcher to make inferences, based on the collected data, with a relative degree of reliability. Hypothesis testing is based on the theory of probability.

This chapter answers what hypotheses are, how they are tested, and how risks in hypothesis testing are determined. Appropriate statistical tests are presented for testing hypotheses. Table 10.8 provides a summary of the research processes presented thus far.

REFERENCES

1. Wilson BE: An Introduction to Scientific Research. New York, McGraw-Hill Book Co, Inc, 1952
2. Kerlinger FN: Foundations of Behavioral Research, ed 2. New York, Holt, Rinehart & Winston, Inc, 1973
3. Morehouse CA, Stull GA: Statistical Principles and Procedures with Applications for Physical Education. Philadelphia, Lea & Febiger, 1975
4. Remington RD, Schork MA: Statistics with Applications to the Biological and Health Sciences. Englewood Cliffs, NJ, Prentice-Hall, Inc, 1970
5. Random House Dictionary of the English Language, Unabridged ed. New York, Random House, 1967
6. Cajal SR: Precepts and Counsels on Scientific Investigation: Stimulants of the Spirit. Mountain View, CA, Pacific Press Publishing Assoc, 1951
7. Meyers LS, Grossen NE: Behavioral Research Theory, Procedure, and Design, ed 2. San Francisco, WH Freeman and Co, 1978
8. Michels E: Letters to the editor: Use of the t-test. Phys Ther 50: 102–104, 1970
9. Currier DP: Positioning for knee strengthening exercise. Phys Ther 57: 148–152, 1977
10. Cochran WC, Cox GM: Experimental Designs, ed 2. New York, John Wiley & Sons, Inc, 1957
11. Boneau CA: The effects of violations of assumptions underlying the t-test. Psych Bull 57: 49–64, 1960
12. Ferguson GA: Statistical Analyses in Psychology & Education, ed 5. New York, McGraw-Hill Book Co, 1981
13. Dayton CM: The Design of Educational Experiments. New York, McGraw-Hill Book Co, 1970
14. Roscoe JT: Fundamental Research Statistics for the Behavioral Sciences, ed 2. New York, Holt, Rinehart and Winston, Inc, 1975
15. Williams M, Stutzman L: Strength variation through the range of joint motion. Phys Ther Rev 39: 145–152, 1959
16. Sokal RR, Rohlf FJ: Introduction to Biostatistics. San Francisco, WH Freeman and Co, 1973
17. Daniel WW, Coogler CE: Statistical applications in physical medicine: Part II. Am J Phys Med 54: 25–47, 1975
18. Alder HL, Roessler EB: Introduction to Probability and Statistics, ed 6. San Francisco, WH Freeman and Co, 1977

SUGGESTED READINGS

Daniel WW, Coogler CE: Beyond analysis of variance: A comparison of some multiple comparison procedures. Phys Ther 55: 144–150, 1975

Edwards AL: Statistical Analysis, ed 4. New York, Holt, Rinehart & Winston, Inc, 1974

Huntsberger DV, Leaverton PE: Statistical Inference in the Biomedical Sciences. Boston, Allyn and Bacon, Inc, 1970

Schor SS: Fundamentals of Biostatistics. New York, GP Putnam's Sons, 1968

Steel RGD, Torrie JH: Principles and Procedures of Statistics. New York, McGraw-Hill Book Co, 1960

11

Non-Parametric Tests

It is better to be satisfied with probabilities
than to demand impossibilities and starve.
F. C. S. Schiller

Statistical procedures are divided into parametric and non-parametric statistics. Chapter 10 included tests of significance (t, analysis of variance, correlation) upon which inferences could be made about the parent population. This group of statistics is called parametric. "Metric" refers to measurement procedures, while "para" refers to the assumptions about the population from which data were obtained.[1] Assumptions for parametric statistics are that the samples are random, that scores are independent of each other, that experiments are repeatable types with constancy of measurements from experiment to experiment, that data are about normally distributed, and that samples have similar variances.[2] The parametric group of statistics then requires certain methods having desirable characteristics which yield unbiased, consistent, efficient, and sufficient estimates of the population.[3] Calculations are sometimes demanding by requiring long mathematical procedures, and results are sometimes difficult to interpret or understand by those not well versed in mathematics.

All statistical tests have assumptions but non-parametric statistics refers to a class of statistics that does not require assumptions as rigid as those of the parametric class. "Non-para" implies this. Because this group of statistics does not require assumptions signifying a certain form of distribution or make statements about parameters or equality of variances, non-parametric statistics are sometimes referred to as distribution-free methods.[4] In statistics, robustness is the degree to which a test can stray from the assumptions before changing the probability too much. The non-parametric class trades the power (large sample sizes) of the parametric tests for robustness, (generality).[2,5] The assumptions are that the samples are randomly and independently chosen, and that the experiments are of repeatable nature. No assumptions about the shape of the distribution have to be met as in the parametric class; non-parametric tests can test the null hypothesis but the hypothesis is not stated in terms of parameters of parent populations. Non-parametric statistics do not estimate parameters either but test the null hypothesis in a general form that samples come from populations having the same distribution. The alternative hypothesis then tests that samples come from populations with different distributions. Attention must be drawn to the fact that methods which require few and weak assumptions about the populations which are being sampled are less efficient than the corresponding parametric methods. Chances of committing Type II errors are increased with the use of non-parametric statistics.[6] Table 11.1 groups statistics and statistical tests according to their classification, and appropriate use by design.

USES

Non-parametric tests are used in the behavioral sciences where there is no basis for assuming certain types of distributions. Siegel[5] advocates that non-parametric tests are to be used for nominal and ordinal levels of measurements, while parametric tests are appropriate for analyzing interval and ratio data. In practice, levels of measurement are sometimes "down graded" from ratio and interval to ordinal or nominal scales for convenience of a measuring instrument or interpretation. For example, muscular strength or force (force = mass × acceleration) is a variable which yields ratio data because a true zero point exists in the level of measurement.[5,7] Muscular strength is absent with paralysis (true zero point). The manual muscle tests converts the ratio characteristics of force (mass and acceleration) into an ordinal scale by assigning grades of relative position (N, G, F, P, T, O or 5, 4, 3, 2, 1, 0 scale). Williamsen[8] has countered that statistical tests are selected to meet certain aims or goals or to answer specific questions rather than to match levels of measurements with parametric or non-parametric procedures. Gaito[9] has also offered a good argument

Table 11.1
Summary of Statistics and Statistical Tests Presented in Book

Classification	One-group	Design Two-group	Multi-group

Non-parametric	mode
	median
	chi-square
	percentile
		chi-square
		median test
		Turkey quick test
		Rank correlation
		Wilcoxon matched-
		  paired signed-ranks
		  test
		Mann-Whitney U test
			Kruskal-Wallis one-
			way ANOVA

Parametric	mean
	coefficient of variation
	standard deviation
	correlation (r, R)
		t tests (independent
		  and paired)
		regression analysis
		  (linear)
			Analysis of variance
			(ANOVA)

against contaminating measurement theory with statistical theory. Levels of measurement are not used in the application of non-parametric statistical procedures in this chapter.

Calculations of non-parametric tests are generally very easy to perform[10,11] and to apply,[10] and have considerable intuitive appeal as shortcut techniques.[6] Caution must be exercised because of their ease and convenience to calculate. Non-parametric tests are to be used when the assumptions of parametric tests cannot be met, when very small numbers of data are to be used, and when there is no basis for assuming certain types or shapes of distributions.[8] Non-parametric tests are never to be substituted for parametric tests when the parametric tests are more appropriate. Parametric tests are more powerful than non-parametric statistics and deal with continuous variables, while non-parametric tests deal with discrete variables. Caution must also be exercised in using results from analysis of a non-parametric test for making inferences because small numbers of data are used and no assumptions about parent populations are made.

Non-parametric tests are used if data can only be classified, counted, or ordered; for example, rating staff on performance or comparing results from manual muscle tests. These tests should not be used in determining precision or accuracy of instruments because the tests are somewhat lacking in both areas.

ADVANTAGES

The techniques of non-parametric tests are generally simpler to calculate mathematically than are parametric tests which they replace.[6,11] These tests may be performed quickly and easily without the need for automated instruments (computers and calculators).[11] Non-parametric tests are easier to understand and explain. The tests have ease of calculation and reduced concern for assumptions and have been designed for small numbers of data including counts, classifications, and renumerations such as diagnosis, sexes, and professions. These tests are robust and can be used effectively in behavioral research.

DISADVANTAGES

Non-parametric tests are not as powerful as the parametric class and, therefore, are somewhat limited in their use in experimental research. The ease of calculation and reduced concern for assumptions have been referred to as quick and dirty statistical procedures.[12]

Non-parametric tests are available for determining relations and significance. Tests for conditions in which parametric tests were presented in Chapter 10 will be discussed for non-parametric tests.

RANK CORRELATION

Earlier, The Pearson product moment correlation (r) was presented for computing the association or relation between two variables. The uses of this method were for testing validity and reliability of instruments and correlational investigations. The rank correlation (ρ) of Spearman is a non-parametric method of computing correlation from ranks. The method is similar to Pearson's with the computed value ρ providing an index of the relationship between two groups of ranks. If the original scores are ranks, the computed index will be similar in value to that computed by the product moment method. The difference between the two methods is that the product moment method assigns weight to the magnitude of each score, while the rank method is concerned with the ordinal position of each score.[8]

The coefficient of rank correlation (ρ, rho) ranges from $+1$ when paired ranks are changing in the same order, to -1 when ranks are changing in reverse order. Zero is an indication that paired ranks are occurring at random to each other. The formula for rank correlation is

$$\rho = 1 - \frac{6 \sum d^2}{n(n^2 - 1)}$$

where $\sum d^2$ is the sum of squared differences between ranks, 6 is a constant, and n is the number of paired scores.

Suppose 10 student physical therapists were drawn at random from a large class; each student has been rated on a 10-point scale for a recent clinical experience and each student has a grade-point average. The coefficient of ranks will be computed to determine the extent of agreement between the two sets of scores (clinical experience rating and grade-point average). In the rank correlation method, the procedure is to replace the raw scores by assigning an appropriate rank to each score of each set. Ranks for each set correspond to the total number of scores in that set.

If the relationship was true (real data), it would be interpreted as a fair relationship between clinical experience ratings and grade-point averages of students. The example illustrates what happens when obtained scores are similar (tied ranks). When tied ranks occur (e.g., column Y of Table 11.2), each score is then assigned the average rank which the tied scores occupy. The GPA of 3.2, for example, had two scores occupying ranks 3 and 4, since ranks of 1 and 2 were occupied by scores of 3.6 and 3.5, respectively. The average rank for the scores of 3.2 was obtained by adding ranks (3 + 4) and dividing by the number of ranks being occupied (e.g., 3 + 4 ÷ 2 = 3.5 ranking).

Table 11.2
Computation of Coefficient of Rank Correlation: Clinical Rating and Grade-Point Average
(GPA) of 10 Student Physical Therapists (Artificial Data)

X (Clinical Rating)	Rank	Y (GPA)	Rank	(X − Y)	d^2
9.0	4	3.0	6.5	−2.5	6.25
8.0	6	2.9	8.0	−2.0	4.00
10.0	1	3.5	2.0	−1.0	1.00
6.0	9	3.0	6.5	2.5	6.25
8.3	5	3.1	5.0	0	0
7.0	8	2.7	9.0	−1.0	1.00
9.2	3	3.6	1.0	2.0	4.00
5.0	10	2.5	10.0	0	0
7.2	7	3.2	3.5	3.5	12.25
9.3	2	3.2	3.5	−1.5	2.25
					37.00

$$\rho = 1 - \frac{6\,(37.00)}{10\,(100-1)} = 1 - \frac{220.00}{990.00} = 1 - .22 = .78$$

Since ρ is equivalent to r of the product moment method, the assumption is made that ranks are the first integers or raw scores as in the product moment procedure. When a lot of tied ranks appear in the computation, in the above example, the sum of squares of ranks departs from the sum of squares of the first integers as in r^3. This departure affects the ρ value. When substantial tied ranks occur, the researcher is advised to use Pearson's product moment correlation method.

TESTS FOR SIGNIFICANCE

Non-parametric tests are available and these replace the three parametric tests presented in Chapter 10 (correlation, t, and analysis of variance). Representative non-parametric tests are provided in this section.

Rank Correlation

Rank correlation can be used for hypothesis testing. The hypothesis H_0: $\rho = 0$ and H_1: $\rho \neq 0$ can be tested for significance. For 20 paired scores or more, the formula $t = \rho \sqrt{(n-2)/(1-\rho^2)}$ approximates a t distribution with $n - 2$ degrees of freedom.[3,7,13] The $n - 2$ degrees of freedom is peculiar to testing the significance of r from zero and the slope of a line from zero.[3] The table for the parametric t distribution can be used as a baseline (critical values) for comparing obtained t for rank correlation and the critical t value (Appendix, Table C).

If the ρ value from 22 pairs of data was 0.78, the values can be substituted in the formula for t, the t value of 5.58 is then obtained

$$t = 0.78 \sqrt{\frac{22 - 2}{1 - 0.78^2}} = 0.78 \sqrt{\frac{20}{0.39}} = 0.78 \times \sqrt{51.28} = 5.58$$

and locating the critical value for the 0.05 level of significance for 20 df, we find a t value of 2.21 for a two-tailed test.

$$t_{\text{obtained}} > t_{\text{critical}} \therefore \text{ accept } H_1\text{: } \rho \neq 0$$

The results can be interpreted that the coefficient of $\rho = 0.78$ is significantly different from zero. The hypotheses having direction (one-tailed) can also be tested for significance by using the one-tailed levels of significance in the table for t distribution.

One-Group Test

Chi-Square. Occasionally one sample chi-square is used when the apportionment of subcategories (K) of a sample into mutually exclusive and exhaustive sets is to be compared with expected theoretical frequencies. The chi-square (χ^2) test is based on the difference between an observed frequency for some category (K) and that expected from a known probability. The assumptions are that the subcategories $(K_z\text{'s})$ are standard scores, have normal distributions, and are independent.[8] The null hypothesis can be written to show the probability of observed frequencies differing from expected frequencies, H_0: $D = O - E$ and an alternative hypothesis as H_1: $D \neq O - E$ where D is the difference, O is the observed frequency, and E is the expected or theoretical frequency. The formula for chi-square is

$$\chi^2 = \Sigma \left[\frac{(O - E)^2}{E} \right]$$

The categories (K) may be classes of a quantitative variable or components of a discrete or continuous variable. The χ^2 distribution is used to test significance in a fashion similar to that in which the t or F distributions were used. The null hypothesis states that no difference exists between the observed and expected frequencies; if the obtained chi-square value is less than the critical chi-square value, then the indication is good that observation agrees with expectation. On the other hand, an accepted alternate hypothesis means that a significant difference exists and cannot be explained by sampling variations. Tables are available for indicating the values required to select hypotheses. The degrees of freedom are $K - 1$ in the single sample chi-square, and the 0.05 and 0.01 levels of significance are generally used to determine significance.[3]

An example of the chi-square using fictitious data is illustrated in Table 11.3. Suppose the directors of a physical therapy department desired to

Table 11.3
Computation of Chi Square for Single Group: Preferred Use of Transcutaneous Electric
Nerve Stimulators (Fictitious Data)

TENS	O	E	$O - E$	$(O - E)^2$	$(O - E)^2/E$
A	10	22.5	−12.5	156.25	6.94
B	15	22.5	− 7.5	56.25	2.50
C	30	22.5	7.5	56.25	2.50
D	35	22.5	12.5	156.25	6.94
					$\Sigma = 18.88$

know which of four brands of transcutaneous electric nerve stimulators (TENS) was preferred by patients.

As shown in Table 11.3, χ^2 obtained = 18.88; χ^2 critical = 7.82 (0.05, 3 df) ∴ select H_1: $D \neq 0 - E$.

The hypothesis tested was whether the observed frequencies were equal to the expected frequencies (22.5). The value of 22.5 is derived from the probability of preferring any one TENS based on the opinions of 90 patients who were selected to use all four TENS units at various times. Since four TENS units were being observed and 90 patients used them, 90 divided by 4 is 22.5 or the theoretical expected frequency of preference. The values entered in the observed frequency column (O) are the frequencies of preference indicated by the 90 patients who underwent a trial period with each instrument. The obtained χ^2 value exceeded the critical value of χ^2. The hypothesis selected was in favor of the alternative hypothesis that the observed frequencies were not equal to the expected frequencies. The director might wish to eliminate one or two units of TENS based on the probability of their ever being preferred by patients as frequently as expected.

Appendix, Table E, can be consulted for the appropriate critical values at the desired levels of significance.

Two-Group Tests

Chi-Square. The 2×2, or four-fold, contingency table of the chi-square test is used to determine the significance of differences between two independent samples for nominal level measures. The hypothesis to be tested is whether the two samples differ on some variable with respect to the frequency with which sample observations can be classified.[5] In this use of chi-square, the number of degrees of freedom is $(2 - 1)(2 - 1) = 1$.[3] An example will serve to describe the test. Suppose a physical therapist studied the relation of skill acquisition of a novel activity among subjects having left and right arm dominance. The null hypothesis, H_0, stated that there is no difference between skill acquisition of left-handed and right-handed individuals. The alternate hypothesis, H_1, stated that right-handed individuals should do better than left-handed individuals in skill acquisition. The task for the seated-subjects was to obtain success in four successive trials of putting a ball into a distant basket.[14] Each subject (10 left-handed and 10 right-handed) was given 50 trials; the number of successes and failures were counted. The hypotheses were tested at the 0.05 level. The 2 × 2 contingency table shows the results of the experimental procedure (data are fictitious).

	Left	Right	
Success	A_{20}	B_{18}	38 $(A + B)$
Failure	C_{30}	D_{32}	62 $(C + D)$
	50	50	
	$(A + C)$	$(B + D)$	

The formula for calculating chi-square is

$$\chi^2 = \frac{N(AD - BC)^2}{(A + B)(C + D)(A + C)(B + D)}$$

where N = the total number of trials, and the letters correspond to specific blocks of the 2 × 2 contingency table.[3] The calculation of χ^2 from the above data may then be:

$$\chi^2 = \frac{100(20 \times 32 - 18 \times 30)^2}{(38)(62)(50)(50)} = \frac{1,000,000}{5,890,000} = 0.17$$

Appendix E is consulted for χ^2, $df = 1$, 0.05 level and the critical value, 3.84, is found. For $df = 1$, a $\chi^2 = 0.17$ indicates that no difference occurs between left-handed and right-handed individuals in skill acquisition of a novel task. The null hypothesis, H_0, is accepted.

The Median Test. Discrete and continuous variables are used with the median test. Note, however, that continuous variables are treated as discrete in this statistical design. The median is determined for the two samples combined; scores above the median and scores equal to and below the median are counted. This information is placed into a table showing categories of scores and their totals. A chi-square statistic with 1 degree of freedom (2 samples) is calculated to test the hypothesis. The null hypothesis, H_0: $Md_A = Md_B$ is tested against an alternative hypothesis that the two populations do not have the same medians, H_1: $Md_A \neq Md_B$.[5] The median test is used to determine whether two independent samples of nominal level measures came from populations that have the same median.[15]

The table for showing categories of scores and their totals can be displayed as

A	B	$A + B$
C	D	$C + B$
$A + C$	$B + D$	N

and the chi-square formula for the 2×2 tabular information can be calculated by the formula

$$\chi^2 = \frac{N(AD - BC)^2}{(A + B)(C + D)(A + C)(B + D)}$$

where N = total number of scores involved in all samples; A and C are values above the median of each sample, and B and D are scores equal to or below the median of each sample.

Consider a situation where the physical therapist wishes to know the number of hours in which the patient is free from pain following two different methods of treating "tennis elbow." The hypotheses would be H_0: $Md_a = Md_b$ and H_1: $Md_a \neq Md_b$ and tested for the 0.05 level of significance. χ^2 obtained = 0.20 $\lessgtr$ χ^2 critical (0.05, 1 df) = 3.84; $\therefore$ the null hypothesis H_0: $Md_a = Md_b$ is true.

In the example (Table 11.4), two groups of equal numbers (10) of patients having "tennis elbow" are each treated by a different method (a and b). All scores are placed in a single distribution and are rank ordered. The median (7) is determined. Scores in each column (A and C) larger than the median (7) are counted ($A = 4$, $C = 5$) and placed in the appropriate blocks of the table. Next, scores in each column (B and D) equal to or smaller than the median are counted ($B = 6$, $D = 5$) and placed in the proper squares of the table. The values entered in the labeled squares of the table are placed into the formula and solved for χ^2 (Table 11.4).

Since the obtained χ^2 value was less than the critical χ^2 value, the researcher would have no reason not to accept the null hypothesis and must conclude that no difference exists between the relief time provided by the two methods.

Table 11.4
Computation of the Median Test: Two Methods of Treating "Tennis Elbow"

Method a (hours of relief)	Method b (hours of relief)					
1	2					
4	1					
6	8		$>$	$\geqq$		
10	6					
8	12	a	4^A	6^B	10	
7	5					
6	9	b	5^C	5^D	10	
7	10					
17	15		9	11	20	
13	5					

median for combined groups = 7

$$\chi^2 = \frac{20 \ (20{-}30)^2}{(10) \ (10) \ (9) \ (11)} = \frac{2000}{9900} = .202$$

Tukey's Quick Test. Suppose a group of patients ($N = 10$) having had recent strokes are given a form of facilitatory training in an attempt to re-educate a certain group of muscles assessed to be non-functional. Each non-functional muscle group is tested for tone before therapy is begun and again at the termination of their biofeedback program. A group of normal subjects are also measured before and after the experimental period but do not receive any therapy (control group). The myotonometer is an instrument that measures the resting tone of muscle by determining the amount of tissue depression possible under controlled conditions. The unit measured is a "MTM" and is an arbitrary unit.[16] Table 11.5 shows the amount of change in muscular tone of each subject during the experimental period.

The results are analyzed by Tukey's quick test. The MTM is a numerical unit, but one that lacks great precision, and therefore, the data are better suited to non-parametric testing, as with Tukey's test, than to a t test. From Table 11.5 the largest value in each group is located. The experimental group (facilitatory training) has the largest value (21 MTM'S) and the control group's largest value is 6 MTM'S. The number of values in the experimental group larger than the largest value recorded for the control group (6 MTM's) is counted. Eight values in the experimental group are larger than the largest value in the control group. Next, the number of values in the control group that are smaller than the smallest value in the experimental group (3 MTM's) is counted. Five values in the control group are smaller than the smallest value (3 MTM's) of the experimental group. The two counts are added ($8 + 5 = 13$) and if the sum of the two counts is equal to or greater than seven the conclusion is that the effects of the two treatments (facilitatory training and placebo in example) are different. The number seven is fixed and is the criterion value to be used in the comparative phase of Tukey's quick test. If the sum of the two counts is less than seven, the conclusion is that the effects of the two treatments are

Table 11.5
Increase in Muscular Tone Following Biofeedback and Placebo Program (Fictitious Data)

Experimental Group (MTM units)*	Control Group (MTM units)*
4	2
15	6
3	1
15	3
9	1
11	2
16	4
21	3
8	2
10	4

* Difference between before and after treatment measurements; MTM = myotonometer units.

not different. In the example cited, the sum of the counts was 13; therefore, the conclusion was that the effects of facilitatory training are different from placebo effects.

In the event that both the largest value and the smallest value occur in the same group, the conclusion is that the two treatments do not have different effects.[11]

Wilcoxon Matched-Pairs-Ranks Test. This rank test is appropriate for two paired or related samples, and it considers the size and direction of the differences within pairs.[5] The difference (d) between each is found; if the paired numbers are equal, d is assigned zero. The difference (d) values may be negative or positive but are ranked by ignoring the sign. The smallest difference value is assigned the rank of 1 and so on. When tied ranks occur, each score is then assigned the average rank which the tied scores occupy (similar to that used for rank correlation). After determining the ranks the sign of the difference (ignored earlier) is now assigned to the particular rank. The original hypothesis can be formed that the sum of positive ranks will equal the sum of negative ranks. A large difference between the sums provides support for rejecting the original hypothesis that the paired measurements are from the same population. The sum of the negative and positive ranks are compared. The smaller of the two sums is assigned T. The researcher then compares T with the number of paired scores having signs (ignore zeros) and the level of significance selected. Appropriate tables for this test are found in Ferguson[3] and Siegel[5].

Suppose two groups containing eight subjects each are matched for sex, weight, and age and then rated by a perceived exertion rating scale (Chapter 6). One group rode a bicycle ergometer (X) and the other ran on a treadmill (Y) at a similarly fixed load and duration. The following are paired observations for X and Y:

X	15	19	16	14	17	18	16	17
Y	18	17	19	20	17	17	20	15
d	−3	2	−3	−6	0	1	−4	2
rank	−4.5	2.5	−4.5	−7	0	1	−6	2.5

The sum of the negative ranks is 22 and that of the positive ranks is 6. A Wilcoxon table indicates that for $n = 7$ (zero rank is ignored) at the point 0.05 LOS for a two-tailed test (H_0: $\mu_x = \mu_y$) the lower sum must be two or smaller to reject the null hypothesis. These data indicate that exertion from ergometer and treadmill activity of equal load and duration are perceived similarly by matched subjects.

When the number of ranks exceed 25 the Wilcoxon table cannot be used but a table containing values of z in the normal distribution must be consulted. This latter table can be found in standard statistical tests.[2-7] The negative and positive sums of ranks are found using the same approach for N of less than 25. The letter T is assigned to the smaller number, placed in a formula where z (the normal deviate)[3] is calculated,

$$z = \frac{T - \dfrac{N(N + 1)}{4}}{\sqrt{\dfrac{N(N + 1)(2N + 1)}{24}}}$$

where N is the number of ranks, and 4 and 24 are constants. Once z is found its value is located in a table of the normal distribution and the probability for a two-tailed or one-tailed test is determined for a particular level of significance.

Mann-Whitney U Test. This is a rank test for two independent samples and may be the best non-parametric alternative to the t test.[5] An example will explain this particular test.

Suppose an experimental group of five rabbits receive laser treatment to their contrived wounds (X), while a control group of seven rabbits do not receive treatment to their contrived wounds (Y). The Mann-Whitney test is chosen because two independent samples containing small numbers of subjects and days to complete healing are selected criteria. The null hypothesis is H_0: $\mu_x = \mu_y$, and the 0.5 significance level is selected. Consider the following scores and their ranks:

X	27	51	33	37	43		
rank	2	11	4	6	9		
Y	30	35	25	53	50	38	40
rank	3	5	1	12	10	7	8

Each score is given a rank in ascending order of size; that is, a rank of 1 is assigned to the smallest value. Next, the ranks are ordered according to their identity.

rank	1	2	3	4	5	6	7	8	9	10	11	12
group	Y	X	Y	X	Y	X	Y	Y	X	Y	X	Y

The U is found by determining the number of X scores preceding each Y score. The U is: $1 + 2 + 3 + 3 + 4 + 5 = 18$ (rank $2X$ precedes $3Y = +1$, ranks $2X$ and $4X$ precede $5Y = +2$, ranks 2, 4 and $6X$ precede $7Y = +3$, and so on). Consulting a Mann-Whitney U test table for $n_y = 7$ (larger sample size), locate U value (18) on left-hand margin, and $n_x = 5$ at top of the table. The probability of occurrence under the stated null hypothesis is 0.562. The null hypothesis is true and the decision is that the data are not supportive of rejecting H_0.

The above procedure is appropriate only when the larger sample size is eight or smaller. Different procedures and tables are used for samples ranging between 9 and 20, and larger than 20, respectively. Procedures and tables for the Mann-Whitney test can be found in Siegel.[5]

Test for More Than Two Groups

Kruskal-Wallis One-Way Analysis of Variance by Ranks. The Kruskal-Wallis one-way analysis of variance by ranks functions similarly to the conventional one-way analysis of variance. The null hypothesis to be tested is whether the differences among samples show true population differences or whether they represent chance variations that are to be expected among several samples from the same population.[5] Another view of hypothesis testing of the Kruskal-Wallis technique is that the ranks within each sample constitute a random sample from the set of numbers 1 through N.[13] The assumption, in using this test, is made that the variable being tested has a continuous distribution.[5]

Scores in all samples are combined and arranged in order of magnitude for the purpose of assigning ranks to each score. The lowest score is assigned the rank of 1. The scores are then replaced in their respective samples with their appropriate ranks. The ranks for each sample are summed ($\sum R$). An assumption is that mean rank sums ($\bar{R}$) should be equal for the samples and equal to the mean of the N ranks, $(N+1)/2$, if the samples (K) are from the same population.[3]

Equal and unequal sized samples may be used in the Kruskal-Wallis test because the sums of sample ranks ($\sum R$) are pooled in the formula. This pooling is similar to that of independent t tests of unequal sample sizes (Chapter 10).

The statistic "H" used in this test can be defined by the formula

$$H = \frac{12}{N(N+1)} \left[\sum \frac{R^2}{n} \right] - 3(N+1)$$

where N is the number of scores in all samples combined; $\sum R^2/n$ is the sum of scores in a particular sample squared, and divided by the number of scores in that particular sample; and n is the number of scores in a particular sample. The sum of scores, $\sum R^2/n$, is obtained by adding all of the groups' dividends together. The example shown in Table 11.6 is

$$\frac{68.5^2}{6} + \frac{46.0^2}{6} + \frac{56.5^2}{6} \text{ for}$$

$$\sum \frac{R_1{}^2}{n_1} + \sum \frac{R_2{}^2}{n_2} + \sum \frac{R_3{}^2}{n_3} \; .$$

The random sample distribution of H is approximated by a chi-square distribution of $K - 1$ degrees of freedom where K is the number of samples. The chi-square probability of Appendix, Table E, can be used to determine the significance of H when each sample contains more than five scores. Special tables (not included in this book) have been prepared for use in cases when there are only three samples with five or fewer scores in each.[5]

Tied ranks may occur and are averaged in a way that is similar to that used in rank order correlation. However, a special denominator is used with the formula for computing H. The H value is usually smaller if computed without the special denominator. The special denominator corrects the deficiency caused by tied scores. H is computed by the above formula and divided by

$$1 - \frac{\Sigma T}{N^3 - N}$$

where $T = t^3 - t$. In this situation, t is the number of scores tied at a particular level of tied ranks. When no tied ranks are involved, the special denominator is not used. The formula for H when ranks are tied is

$$H = \frac{\frac{12}{N(N+1)}\left[\Sigma \frac{R^2}{n}\right] - 3(N+1)}{1 - \frac{\Sigma T}{N^3 - N}}$$

Table 11.6 provides an example of the computation for the Kruskal-

Table 11.6
Computation of the Kruskal-Wallis One-Way Analysis of Variance by Tied Ranks: Methods of Teaching Pathokinesiology (Artificial Data)

Text and Lab (%)	Rank	Text (%)	Rank	Lab (%)	Rank
95	17	94	16	88	6.5
92	13.5	88	6.5	92	13.5
86	3.5	90	9.5	97	18
91	11.5	84	1	97	5
93	15	86	3.5	91	11.5
89	8	90	9.5	85	2
	$\Sigma = 68.5$		$\Sigma = 46.0$		$\Sigma = 56.5$

$T = t^3 - t$ ties	3.5	6.5	9.5	11.5	13.5
t (no. of ties)	2	2	2	2	2
$T(t^3 - t)$	6	6	6	6	6

$$H = \frac{\frac{12}{18(18+1)}\left[\frac{68.5^2}{6} + \frac{46.0^2}{6} + \frac{56.5^2}{6}\right] - 3(18+1)}{1 - \frac{30}{18^3 - 18}}$$

$$H = \frac{\frac{12}{342}[1666.75] - 57}{.995} = 1.34$$

Table 11.7
Cumulative Summary of the Research Processes Presented

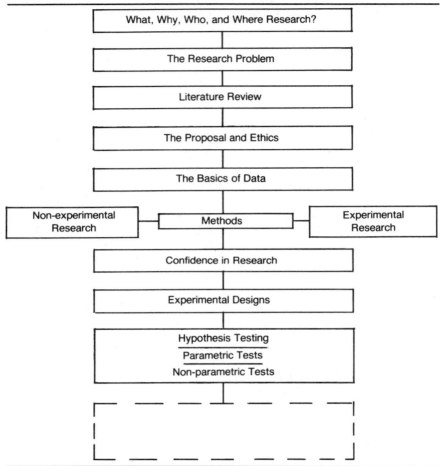

Wallis one-way analysis of variance by ranks when ranks are tied. Suppose three sections of a class of physical therapy students are taught pathokinesiology by three different methods (using a text and laboratory exercises, using a text, or using laboratory exercises). The students are given a test at the end of the instruction. All recorded scores are rank-ordered into a single (univariate) group. χ^2 obtained = 1.34 < χ^2_{critical} (0.05 LOS, 2 df) = 5.99; $\therefore$ accept H_0: $R_1 = R_2 = R_3$.

The Kruskal-Wallis one-way analysis of variance by ranks is indicated when assumptions for the parametric ANOVA are not suitable for the data, or when the level of data is less than interval measures.[5]

The obtained χ^2 value was less than the critical χ^2 value so the conclusion is that the three methods of teaching pathokinesiology were equally effective.

A few non-parametric tests that appear occasionally in the research literature have been presented. This introduction should enable the reader to understand some non-parametric statistics used in comparative research. Statistics presented in Chapters 10 and 11 are used with certain designs in controlled experiments. Some considerations for experimental design and control are presented in Chapter 9.

SUMMARY

Non-parametric tests refer to a class of statistics that does not require assumptions signifying a certain form of distribution or make statements about parameters or equality of variances. These tests are used for analyzing small sized samples. Non-parametric tests are performed quickly and easily, and are interpreted without difficulty. They are less powerful than parametric tests.

Tests of rank correlation and significance have been presented. Tests of significance included one-group, two-group, and multi-group designs. Table 11.7 provides a summary of the research processes presented thus far.

REFERENCES

1. Meyers LS, Grossen NE: Behavioral Research Theory, Procedure, and Design. ed 2. San Francisco, WH Freeman and Co, 1978
2. Schor S: Fundamentals of Biostatistics. New York, GP Putnam's Sons, 1968
3. Ferguson GA: Statistical Analyses in Psychology and Education, ed 5 New York, McGraw-Hill Book Co, 1981
4. Remington RD, Schork MA: Statistics with Applications to the Biological and Health Sciences. Englewood Cliffs, NJ, Prentice-Hall, Inc, 1970
5. Siegel S: Nonparametric Statistics for the Behavioral Sciences. New York, McGraw-Hill Book Co, 1956
6. Freund JE: Modern Elementary Statistics, ed 5. Englewood Cliffs, NJ, Prentice-Hall, Inc, 1979
7. Morehouse CA, Stull GA: Statistical Principles and Procedures with Applications for Physical Education. Philadelphia, Lea & Febiger, 1975
8. Williamsen EW: Statistical Reasoning. San Francisco, WH Freeman and Co, 1974
9. Gaito J: Measurement scale and statistics: resurgence of an old misconception. Psych Bull 87: 564–567, 1980
10. Weinberg GH, Schumaker JA: Statistics: An Intuitive Approach, ed 4. Belmont, CA, Brooks/Cole Pub Co, 1980
11. Daniel WW, Coogler CE: Some quick and easy statistical tests for physical therapists. Phys Ther 54: 135–140, 1974
12. Tukey JW: Quick and dirty methods in statistics. 2. Simple analyses for standard designs. In Quality Control Conference Papers. New York, Am Social Quality Control, 1951
13. McCollough C: Introduction to Statistical Analyses: A Semi-programmed Approach. New York, McGraw-Hill Book Co, 1974

14. Payton OD, Kelley DL: Electromyographic evidence of the acquisition of a motor skill. Phys Ther 52: 261–266, 1972
15. Cain RB: Elementary Statistical Concepts. Philadelphia, WB Saunders Co, 1972
16. Gordon AH: A method to measure muscle firmness or tone. Res Q J Am Assoc Health Phys Educ Rec 35: 482–490, 1964

Part Four

REVEALING
RESEARCH

12

Reporting Research

The culmination of investigative efforts is the report. Research is never complete until the results have been reported. The report is the opportunity for the researcher to communicate with the scientific community by disseminating his findings orally at professional meetings or by publishing in a professional journal. The scientific community receives the report and responds. This response is formed through questions or correspondence, or any replication or extension of the reported research. Thus, communication is established between the researcher and the scientific community. Through the reporting process the researcher and his findings are scrutinized by his colleagues. Unless they are reported, the findings are lost forever and few can benefit from the researcher's time and efforts.

This section will discuss reporting the research findings through written and oral presentations with the major emphasis on publication.

PUBLICATION

The final step of the process of research is the publication of the results.[1] However, publication in a reputable scientific journal is not the ultimate outcome; the ultimate outcome of research is to improve health.[2] Some therapists may question the need to publish a study, particularly when the results did not support the investigator's original hypothesis.

Why Publish?

Publication is essential if physical therapy is to continue to grow.[1] In 1960, Worthingham[3] stated that the realm of empiricism can be removed from physical therapy only through research presented and reported in the literature. She faulted physical therapists for their lack of contributions to the literature. Of 1,800 National Foundation physical therapy scholarships, 14% of the recipients had undertaken graduate study, but only 6% of these had contributed to the professional literature.[3] An informal survey of the authorship of articles appearing in PHYSICAL THERAPY during the period between 1970 and 1974 has provided evidence to indicate that some weaknesses of 1956 have been corrected. The percentage of authors, having obtained graduate degrees, who contributed to the Journal during the 5-year period ranged from a low of 55% (1974) to a high of 71% (1971).[4] In spite of the increased contributions of physical therapists with graduate degrees, a proportionate increase of publishable papers has not kept pace with the increased Association membership.[5]

Michels[6] has repeated the words of A. C. Ivy[7] that the most easily committed error in physical therapy is to believe that the treatment has worked if the patient improves following the therapy. The same amount of improvement may have occurred without treatment.[6] We must produce evidence that what we do to patients is effective and without it patients cannot enjoy their full recovery potential. Documentation of scientific evidence supporting the efficacy of techniques and procedures must be made through publication.[8] The results of research must be communicated to others so that the information can be integrated into the world of science which can only expand through the accumulation and interpretation of such communication.[9] The researcher has the obligation of informing others who might wish to replicate the study.[10] The published report provides a vehicle for igniting sparks (ideas) among other interested investigators and serves to inform them of completed study in order to avoid duplicating an invalid approach. Others can read the report, alter their design or method, and perhaps improve upon the reported approach to an answerable question. A published study may also be valuable to the reader if a new twist has been given to an old idea, if literature has been reviewed critically, if an author's experiences are shared, and if illuminating situations are cited.[11]

The researcher is derelict in responsibilities to colleagues and peers if results of a study are not published. After all, why was a study undertaken and deserving of one's time and energies if the outcome is not shared? This question may be answered by offering several reasons. Writing for everyone is difficult and time consuming. Perhaps the investigator does not submit a manuscript for publication because of fear of rejection. Writing requires additional time and energies beyond those required to conduct the study and perhaps an individual feels overwhelmed by the process and trauma associated with manuscript preparation. Or was the outcome of the study unexpected or undesired? The purpose of formulating a hypothesis is to test the specific declarative statements regardless of the outcome. The report makes a valuable contribution to the professional literature regardless of whether the data supported the original or the alternative hypothesis. Either way, someone will be satisfied by the outcome and, therefore, the report possesses value. Perhaps a reader will make some minor revision of the design methods used and will subsequently resolve the problem by repeating the study.[1] Researchers must publish their results to contribute to the body of knowledge of physical therapy.

Format for Publishing Research

Published studies are expected to meet the same literary standards of organization and precision that apply to all forms of scientific or technical writing.[12] No exceptions can be made for physical therapists. I have heard many physical therapists claim that many Journal articles are too technical or do not have clinical application. Rejection of the misunderstood is a trait of human nature. Perhaps the therapist who makes such a statement that Journal articles are too technical or inapplicable to his practice is admitting that he does not understand research reports.

More than ever we must write clearly and concisely. We must convey our thoughts in as few words as possible using words that everyone understands. Writing, to be effective, must be understood. The reader should be able to understand the author's message without difficulty and the interpretation should be obvious.

The potential author should select the journal to which he will submit his manuscript and familiarize himself with that journal's style. Each professional journal will have a certain style and format to be followed when writing for that particular journal. Most journals devote space in each or a few issues for "Instructions to Authors" which may differ according to the particular journal. Researchers who plan to submit their work for publication are strongly advised to consult the instructions of each particular journal to which they hope to publish. The information is intended to assist potential authors by stating the style and format in which submitted manuscripts are to be received. Specific formats are given for tables, illustrations, and references. Much of the information contained in this chapter will assist the researcher in submitting research manuscripts to PHYSICAL THERAPY. I believe that physical therapists should submit most of their research reports to their own professional journal because: (1) Good research articles upgrade or maintain high quality levels of a journal. (2) More physical therapists read their own journal than those of other disciplines. Thus, the research results can be shared directly with those who will benefit the most from the information. (3) Publishing in the researcher's own professional journal is good for the profession by contributing to its growth and body of knowledge. Because physical therapists frequently pursue graduate study outside of their own profession (e.g., anatomy or physiology), they often publish in other journals in order to maintain an alliance with a particular discipline. Although this situation results in a loss of many good research reports to PHYSICAL THERAPY, it does broaden the exposure of physical therapy.

Components of Journal Research Reports

These components of a research report should serve as a guideline when writing a report. Research is generally reported as a journal manuscript, a thesis, or a formal document to a funding agency. The essential components are the same.

1. Title. The title of a manuscript is an important part of the paper because the reader often decides whether or not to read a paper on the basis of the description of the paper's contents.[13] The brief title conveys the major aspects of the paper and should contain key words which represent the major aspects.[13-15] Because titles of reported studies are used for indexing purposes, the author should avoid the use of "A," "An," "Use of," or "Study of" in the beginning of the title.[14]

2. Abstract. The abstract, a brief summary presenting the major sections of the research report, can take the place of a summary section in the paper. Abstracts should include the rationale for conducting the research, describe the design and methods, and summarize the results and conclusions. Most journals restrict the length of abstracts to 150 words, so a suggested strategy in writing the abstract is to conceive of a narrative containing a key statement or thought from major sections of the paper.[13] The abstract should be written last, since it is a brief condensation of the entire study.

3. Introduction. This section is the beginning of the main report which sets the stage for the paper by presenting the framework on which the study was conceived. The word "introduction" is not used as a heading of the paper but is understood without labeling. Specifically, the introduction contains the purpose, the background for the study, and review of literature relevant to the theme or topic of the paper. Information included in this section should be a synthesis of reports logically arranged in sequential and chronological order.

4. Review of Literature. If the literature review is extensive, this area may be removed optionally from the introduction and placed into a separate section using the above heading. The literature review provides the background for work done by others, discrepancies in previous attempts at resolving the identified problem, and support to the rationale presented later in the discussion section. The literature review provides a valuable service to readers by giving them the opportunity to read about the topic in greater detail and saves the interested reader considerable time and effort in locating relevant information.

5. Method. This section describes, in sufficient detail to allow interested investigators to replicate the study if desired, the subjects (number, type, height and weight, ages), the sampling method, materials, instrumentation, procedures, design, and statistical methods used in the study.[13] The method section should include what the author did and the technical detail.[15] For clarity, the section may be divided into sub-sections according to subjects, apparatus, procedure, and design, but wording should be succinct.

6. Results. The researcher must decide how best to describe the results just as he did in deciding what tests were appropriate in analyzing them so that all pertinent information is "squeezed" from the data. Findings of the study and statistical analyses (e.g., level of significance, significance, and post hoc tests if appropriate) are presented in this section. No discussion takes place; only the reporting of the results. Descriptive statistics commonly presented include the mean, standard deviation, and correlational values if appropriate to the study. Tables, or figures, or both, are suggested to reduce the length of the narrative report and to provide visual information for quick and easy interpretation. The same data should not be presented in both the narrative and table; only the highlights of tabular statistics are included in the narrative. Excessive statistical detail should not be reported because many readers do not understand statistics. Raw data are usually not presented because descriptive statistics provide representation of a group of numbers with a single value, a statistic, which enhances reader interpretation. Statistical findings in the narrative should be limited to the most pertinent; other details may be presented in tables, footnoted, or made available upon request.[16] Organization of statistical reporting in the results section is important. A few sentences should identify the dependent variable and how scores were obtained. Results should be reported from the general to the specific. Values of central tendency and variability are reported first to provide the background for the inferential statistics which usually are presented last.[16]

7. Discussion. The results are explained and interpreted in this section. Deductions are made from the data analyses. The literature review may be brought in to support the data of the study or the author may contradict reports cited in the literature. Inconsistencies borne out by the data of the study or extensions of present theory suggested by data are discussed. Rationale for the outcome of the study is given. The interpretation and discussion of the results must be consistent with the findings. If analyses indicated that the difference between means was not significant, then this should be stated, but the author should not go beyond the limits of the research findings. That is, if the null hypothesis is accepted, the author should not state that one mean was still higher than another or that the data still showed a trend in spite of the accepted hypothesis. This approach misleads the reader and is erroneous. Statistical findings are usually reported in the results section and interpreted in the discussion section. If the statistics precede the interpretation in an organized fashion, interpretation and writing are simplified for the author and reading is easier for his audience than if the sections were combined. Occasionally, the results and discussion sections are combined but this requires more writing skill than if presented separately.[16]

8. Summary and Conclusion. The summary of the study was given in the abstract and need not be repeated at the end of the study. Research reports published a few years ago included a summary, but more and more journals are using the abstract instead. Since the abstract replaces the summary and precedes the main body of the manuscript, readers may take delight in this shortcut to reading the literature. Conclusions, based on the results, are stated briefly and are a separate section of the paper. If no abstract is given as a section of the report, then the conclusions are given as part of the summary and conclusions section.

9. References. Journals usually specify the style in which references must be cited in the text. Generally, the reference list follows at the end of the paper, and references are cited chronologically in the order of their citation in text or alphabetically depending upon journal requirements. The potential author must consult the "Instructions to Authors" section of each journal when citing references. The recommended style is that used by PHYSICAL THERAPY.[14]

Each reference cited in the paper is indicated by a superscript of an Arabic numeral at the end of the sentence or series of sentences pertaining to the work of the author being cited. The same superscript is used whenever the reference is cited. If the reference is a Journal article, the format is: author's last name followed by initials without internal punctuation; only three authors are listed, then "et al" is indicated and followed by a colon; title of the article with only the first letter of the first word capitalized; a period follows the title; name of the journal is abbreviated according to the form used by INDEX MEDICUS, no punctuation is used; volume number of the journal followed by a colon; inclusive page numbers for the first and last page of the article followed by a comma; the year is the last item; no punctuation follows the year. An example of a journal reference is:

Nelson RM: Facial nerve excitability: Its reliability, objectivity and descriptive validity. Phys Ther 51: 387–390, 1971

A reference cited for a book is slightly different from that of a journal article to enable the reader to easily differentiate between them. Superscripts are used for citing both references and may be listed in chronological order. The sequence of a book reference is: author's last name followed by initials without internal punctuation and after three authors the words "et al" are used preceding a colon; the title of the book is given with the first letter of each word capitalized with the exception of articles, conjunctions, and prepositions, and this is followed by a period; if more than one edition of the book has been printed then a comma replaces the period following the title, followed by "ed", the edition number and a period; the place of publication is given by the name of the city and state or country with internal punctuation, followed by a comma; publisher's name is given with internal punctuation and followed by a comma; and the year is placed at the end without any punctuation following. Page numbers also should follow the date of publication when cited. An example is:

Hawker M: Geriatrics for Physiotherapists and the Allied Professions. Philadelphia, PA, N.B. Lippincott Co, 1976, p 61

If the book is one of a volume, the volume number follows the date of publication. Miscellaneous examples of references are:

No Author
Style Manual, ed 4. Washington, Am Phys Ther Assoc, 1976

Editor of Book[14]
Le Veau B (ed): Biomechanics of Human Motion, ed 2. Philadelphia, PA, W.B. Saunders Co, 1977

Annual Reviews (yearbook)[17]
Am Physiol Assoc, Annual Review of Physiology, city, pub, 1977

Encyclopedias[18]
Encyclopedia Britannica, 1973 ed, s.v. "Physical Therapy"

Theses and Dissertations
Nelson RM: Effects of Elbow Flexion on Motor Nerve Characteristics Theses. Boston, MA, Boston University, 1972

Paper Read at a Meeting[14]
Name: Title. Read at the Annual Conference of the American Physical Therapy Association, St. Louis, 1977

Authority for additional citations should be consulted in the style manual of the respective journal[14] or in books for writers.[17,18]

Before beginning to write the research report, an outline of the report's contents is beneficial to the writer. The easiest approach is to follow the sequence of components of the research report just presented. Using the section headings and filling in the outlined requirements of each section will provide an "instant" guide to be followed. Each outline is modified and adapted to the purpose and nature of the report but generally the outline will follow the suggested outline shown in Table 12.1. More detail about writing the report is presented later in this chapter.

Some components of the written research report, the title, introduction, method and references are also parts of the proposal (Chapter 4). Thus, 50% of the final written report is already prepared. After writing the

Table 12.1
Suggested Outline for the Written Report

Component	Suggested Contents
Title:	1. Concise description of study
	2. Place important words of the research in title (dependent variable, method, key words for indexing)
Introduction:	1. Nature of the problem, background, what led to study
	2. Purpose and scope, significance of outcome
	3. Literature review, synthesis of past studies
Method:	1. Describe subjects, instrumentation, procedures, design
	2. Provide sufficient detail for replication by readers
	3. Emphasize new or unique approaches
Results:	1. Describe general results, descriptive statistics
	2. Identify tables and figures
	3. Report analyses, LOS, specifics
Discussion:	1. Discuss major cause and effects relation, present major conclusions that data supported
	2. Discuss the evidence provided by the data, refer to tables and illustrations
	3. Discuss and compare data with work of others from literature review, point out differences, recommendations
Conclusions	1. Briefly emphasize conclusions discussed
Abstract:	1. Purpose
	2. Methods
	3. Results
	4. Conclusions

proposal, collecting and analyzing data, only the results, discussion, conclusion, and abstract sections remain to be written.

Abstracts of Current Literature

Students may write abstracts of current research literature as partial fulfillment of course work or these abstracts may be written to be submitted for publication. The abstract is a summary of a recent article having appeared in some health-related journal. PHYSICAL THERAPY requires this format:

Heading. The heading includes this information in sequential order: title of article with the first letters of words capitalized excepting articles, prepositions, and conjunctions, and this is followed by a period; last names and initials of the first three authors (additional names are cited as "et al"); enclosed in parentheses is the affiliation of the author(s) including city and state or country; abbreviation of the journal as listed in LIST OF JOURNALS INDEXED IN INDEX MEDICUS;[19] volume number followed by a colon; inclusive pages; and year of publication. An example is:

Influence of Isometric Exercise and Passive Stretch on Hip Joint Motion.

Mederros JM, Smidt GR, Brumeister LF, et al (University of Iowa, Iowa City, IA) Phys Ther 57: 518–523, 1977

Text. The body of the abstract includes the purpose of the research, the procedures, the results, and conclusions. The abstract, no longer than 250 words is written in the past tense. No comments or judgments about the article are to be given because the abstract is a factual report describing the article.

Form. The abstract must be typed, double-spaced on standard size paper; two copies should be submitted, an original and one duplicate copy. The first paragraph is not indented, but all other paragraphs have the first line indented. The abstractor's name, typed in uppercase letters, is flush with the right margin at the end of the review.[1,14]

Figures and Tables*

Readers of scientific publications frequently do not read each article in its entirety, but readers often look at the figures and tables which, if presented well, may entice the reader to read the article. Figures and tables are appealing and informative visual presentations of research results or text material. Because authors wish to reach as many readers as possible, authors must be familiar with the general principles of constructing figures and tables. This section provides authors, or potential authors, with information which may be of assistance in the visual presentation of their results.

Figures

Figures are used to provide an overview of the results of the study or presentation and should observe simplicity. Detailed information or results are not to be placed in figures. Figures may be drawings or photographs to illustrate text material or graphs which show comparisons or trends.

Drawings and Photographs

A drawing or photograph serves to clarify text material so that the reader sees clearly the subject which the author is presenting. For instance, readers might have difficulty understanding what the author is trying to present unless a picture accompanies the text. The picture should be clear and as uncluttered as possible. The item should be photographed against a plain background and should be in the forefront of the picture. In submitting photographs to a journal, authors must remember that photographs will usually be reduced to fit in one column or part of one column. If the

---

* This section on figures and tables has been reprinted from PHYSICAL THERAPY 55: 768–772, 1975 by permission of the American Physical Therapy Association.

photograph is cluttered with excessive material, the important point which the author wishes to illustrate will be lost completely in the reduction. Photographs accompanying articles should be black and white glossy prints. Instantly produced pictures usually do not have as good a contrast as black and white prints.

Often, line drawings are more effective than a photograph. A line drawing effectively omits everything which is not essential to the understanding of the points which the author is trying to make.

Graphs

Graphs, like photographs, provide instant communication to the reader. By looking at a graph the reader can readily observe the trends or comparisons which, if presented in the text, might be obscure. Graphs should be fully self-explanatory and should not require numbers within the body of the graph. A key, however, which identifies the different effects or methods may be placed within the body of the graph (Fig. 12.1).

The author is responsible for the impression which a graph conveys; therefore, he must present the graph in a manner which will not deceive the reader. The spacing of units or divisions along the horizontal scale (abscissa) and vertical scale (ordinate) must be proportioned similarly. Disproportioned spacing of units along one scale will overemphasize one variable or characteristic and thus deceive the reader.

Bar graph. One of the simplest types of graphs for presenting discontinuous data is the bar graph which appears in Figures 12.1 and 12.2. The

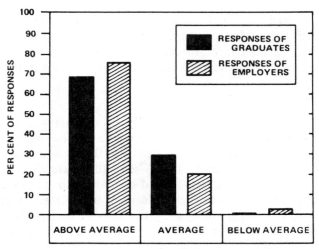

Figure 12.1. A simple bar graph. Note spacing between bars and key in the graph. (From Conine TA: A survey of the graduates of a professional physical therapy. Phys Ther 52: 855, 1972.)

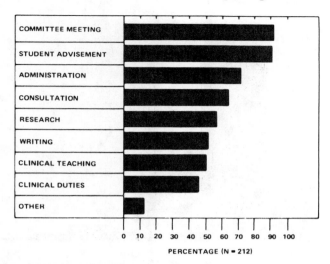

Figure 12.2. A bar graph with horizontal rather than vertical bars. (From Conine TA: Teacher preparation based on functions and opinions of educators. Phys Ther 53: 876, 1973.)

bar graph presents frequencies of things or events by a series of bars or rectangles placed horizontally or vertically with the length or height of the bars proportional to the amount or frequency of the things being measured. Usually each bar is separated by uniform spaces which are generally one-half the width of a bar and which enable the reader to make comparisons among data quickly and conveniently.

Histogram. A histogram is similar in form to a bar graph; however, it presents continuous or grouped data and shows the frequency of things occurring within each group. The histogram is constructed by representing scores or observations which have been grouped on the abscissa, while representing the frequency of the scores or observations on the ordinate. The bars of histograms are adjacent to each other so that the reader can readily discern the frequencies which the author is trying to show (Fig. 12.3).

Broken-line graph. A broken-line graph is useful for comparing changes occurring in one characteristic with changes occurring simultaneously in another characteristic. The graph is constructed by plotting pairs of points of corresponding values of the two characteristics and joining the consecutive points by a series of straight lines. The independent variable is plotted on the abscissa and the dependent variable is plotted on the ordinate. The graph is adapted conveniently to show different effects and methods which affect the two variables (Fig. 12.4).

Pie graph. The pie or circle graph is used most frequently to represent apportionment of a whole into its component parts. The component parts can be expressed as percentages, probabilities, or fractions of a whole

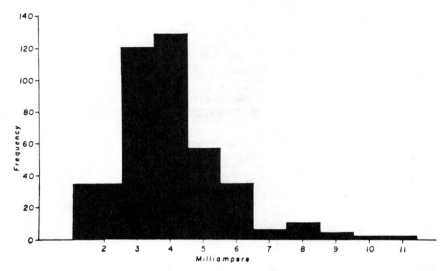

Figure 12.3. A histogram. Note that bars are adjacent to each other for ease in discerning the frequency of grouped data. (From Nelson R: Facial nerve excitation ability: its reliability, objectivity, and descriptive validity. Phys Ther 51: 387, 1971.)

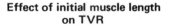

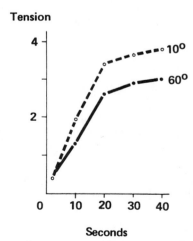

Figure 12.4. A broken-line graph showing how the changes in one variable influence changes in a second variable. (From Bishop B: Vibratory stimulation: Part 1. Neurophysiology of motor response evoked by vibratory stimulation. Phys Ther 54: 1273, 1974.)

quantity. Labeling within the apportioned areas is permissible in the pie graph in order to prevent cluttering (Fig. 12.5).

Tables

Tables provide for the orderly and detailed arrangement of data. Tables provide clarity and increased meaning to data which the narrative form of presentation often fails to accomplish. When data are presented in the tabular form of columns and rows according to logical and pertinent classifications of the subject matter, the reader can interpret the results of the article readily and conveniently.

Tables should clarify or emphasize certain aspects of the text but should not repeat the text. Often tables can present detailed material easily in less space than would otherwise be required in the text (Fig. 12.6).

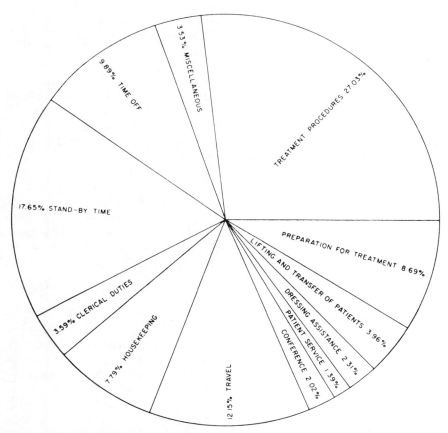

Figure 12.5. A pie graph is used to show values of parts in relation to a whole. (From Gray JM: Function of nonprofessional physical therapy personnel. Phys Ther 44: 103, 1964.)

TABLE 1. *Summary of Analysis of Variance for Muscle Tension During Test and Retest*

Source	SS	df	MS	F
Subjects		40		
Test	14653.51		366.34	
Retest	17820.20		445.51	
A (Elbow angles)		2		
Test	3629.89		1814.94	34.02[a]
Retest	5539.19		2769.59	60.90[a]
AS (interaction)		80		
Test	3023.51		37.79	
Retest	3638.34		45.48	
Total		122		
Test	21306.91			
Retest	26997.73			

[a] Significant at 0.01 level.

Figure 12.6.   A table can be used to present statistical data with greater clarity than can be done in the text. (Modified from Currier DP: Maximal isometric tension of the elbow extensors at varied positions. Part 1. Assessment by cable tensiometer. Phys Ther 52: 1043, 1972).

In constructing tables, authors should limit the table to as few points as possible. Complex tables will be passed over because they make tedious reading. In developing a table, authors should think of the size of a Journal page. A table is limited usually to one column in the article and must be limited to no more than two columns unless it is presented sideways in the text which, of course, makes it difficult to read. Only common abbreviations should be used in a table. The title of the table should indicate precisely what the table is about. Each column and row of numerical data or variables must be labeled clearly with an identifiable unit. The same number of decimal places should be used when reporting data of the same characteristic. Zeros should be used in a table to indicate "none" if the rest of the data is numerical. If data are not available, a series of dots (. . .) should appear in the appropriate column.

Summary and Conclusions

Good figures and tables can enhance a written presentation by offering variety and convenience to the reader. Remember, figures present an overview and are kept simple and uncluttered; tables are reserved for presenting detail. Although the most commonly used figures and table have been presented, the variations of ways in which data can be displayed are really dependent upon the imagination of the author. The author presenting pictorial information, however, must follow the general rules and guidelines.

Common Faults in Writing

No infallible guide exists for good writing nor any assurance that an individual who thinks clearly will be able to write clearly.[20] Although scientific journals have a certain form to be followed in manuscript writing, this section provides some of the aspects to be considered when writing the research report.

Punctuation. Clarity is achieved by good punctuation. The punctuation used in the research report should follow the rules of current usage. The writer should seek authoritative sources for proper punctuation.[14,20,21]

Brevity. When writing, the author must have something to say and be able to end it.[22] Effective scientific writing conveys the thought or idea of the author to the reader directly, clearly, and succinctly.

Sanger[23] has offered some rules for writing: be simple, be specific, and be short. The best writing contains no unnecessary words and is presented in simple language. The vocabulary should be simple but appropriate. Good writing is interesting and alive, and can be expressed with brevity.[23] Any time a five-word sentence can be stated just as effectively as a 10-word sentence, then the latter sentence contains too many words. Sentences can often be reduced in length if the writer puts the manuscript away for a few days and then returns to it; freshness of ideas may prevail when approached after a rest from the labors of writing. The author must review sentences critically to avoid misinterpretations.

Verb Tenses. Past tense is usually suggested, since the research has taken place prior to the writing of the report.[13] The present tense is used in the presentation of the results, tables and illustrations;[21] for example, "Table 2. Summary of Analyses of Variance on Effect of Varied Back Positioning on Force of Knee Extensor Muscles,"[24] Both the past and present tenses are used in the discussion of results.[21]

Diction and Accuracy. The reader has difficulty in interpreting what the author is saying or is confused when words and phrases necessary to complete a thought are omitted, ambiguous statements are made, poor organization is present, points are raised but not discussed, or when erroneous tables or figures are labeled inaccurately.

Phrases must relate to a specific word when used or else the phrases are dangling words without meaning. Sometimes modifying words are misplaced in the sentence, and this destroys the emphasis desired. The normal order of the subject and verb should not be reversed.[25]

Jargon is language peculiar to particular groups; jargon is unintelligible discourse for individuals outside of the particular group or profession. De Bakey[25] has called this imprecise language "gobbledygook." The writer must avoid the use of words which may be understood by some but cannot be understood by most people. Abbreviations such as PRE or ROM or the word "plinth" may qualify as jargon. Flowery wording may also be labeled as jargon. Use of jargon or long unfamiliar words is often an attempt to confuse readers or to appear "learned," but the fact is the learned writer uses simple short words for effective writing.[22]

Other Concerns. The use of "It is," "There are," "This," and other indefinites causes the reader to look for the proper subject rather than providing the reader with the subject which "it" acts to substitute; complicated sentences result in misinterpretation and lack of smoothness in sentence transitions.[22]

The writer must be careful in compound construction or use of modifiers in a sentence. If a phrase, clause, or word is put into a sentence for additional information or explanation, and is not an essential part of the sentence, it is set off by commas. Without the use of commas the reader cannot tell a verb or noun from all the modifiers.

The word "parameter" is frequently used to mean the characteristics of a trait or event. The word pertains to measures of a population in the science of statistics and is a mathematical term. If used in writing to express something other than a mathematical measure of the population, parameter is misused.

Numbers less than 10 are expressed in words and numbers greater than 10 are expressed by Arabic numerals. An example might be, the active motion of the elbow was only five degrees but the passive motion was 15 degrees. Decimal and fractional amounts are usually written in Arabic numerals, 3.8 kilograms. In scientific writing the metric system is used to express weights and measures. Temperatures are expressed in Celsius (centigrade). Abbreviations of the metric system are usually acceptable in the body; for example, 15 cm.

Footnotes are used in the body of the paper to provide product information such as manufacturer's name and address, or explanation of tables. Specific symbols are used in sequential use of superscripts (*, †, ‡, **).[14]

Writing the Report

The research report is a statement of facts and an interpretation of those facts,[21] and requires greater attention and higher standards than other kinds of writing.[25] Poor writing blocks efficiency, wastes the reader's time, and fails to communicate effectively.[25] Just as a plan is important for the composition and conduct of the research study, the written report must also be planned for effective communication. This section will attempt to provide guidelines for writing the report.

Guidelines for Writing the Report

Keep the outline present (in view) when writing. Organize resource materials (reprints, notes, data sheets, tables, books) for ease of reference. Arrange the resource materials so that similar information is grouped together for logical order of reporting. Writing a topic sentence for each group helps to fill in the outline; no more than five main topic sentences should be used for effectiveness in any section. The last point to be presented will usually be the point the reader remembers so the most important point(s) should be placed last.[25] Write a rough draft of the complete paper without stopping or regard to detail or sentence structure. Write for flow of ideas in the organized plan.[21,26] Put the rough draft aside for 1 or 2 weeks and then return to the paper with a hypercritical approach for detail, correct word usage, and further development of ideas. Several rewrites will be necessary. "Good writing does not exist; only good rewriting." Consider the reader of the report. One of the most difficult tasks of writing is wording the paper so as to anticipate the reader's questions, and to present the paper in a manner that enables the reader to grasp the meaning and interpretation quickly and easily. Writing for the reader and revision of the paper are essential and cannot be overemphasized.[5]

Statements should be documented if they provide specific information or may be open to question. Credit is given for the original work and ideas.[26]

When you think the report is in good form, give it to knowledgeable critics and to those with little or superficial knowledge of the topic. Your best critic will be frank and will offer the most constructive suggestions. If the reviewer with little or superficial knowledge of the topic understands the report then the "average" journal reader will also understand. This "behind the scenes" review helps to produce a finished product of worth. The most competent and prolific scientific writers of any profession go through the process of revision, revision, and preliminary critical reviews.

Once a young potential writer (neophyte) was called to the office of the chairman of the faculty's editorial committee where a caustic critique of the poorly written paper was begun. Upon termination of a thorough critique by the chairman, the neophyte was ready to end a writing career in disgust; the chairman, who was renown in his field, then produced a handful of letters and postal cards representing rejection notices for manuscripts over which he had spent countless hours and effort in preparation. The conversation ended; the neophyte left the room without saying more than "Thank you." The moral of the story is that if you are going to engage in research and fulfill your obligation to communicate the results, be prepared to accept criticism of your writings from friendly and unfriendly reviewers, journal reviewers, and peer reviewers. Even with thorough planning and following suggested writing procedures, difficulties in the process of publishing research reports will occasionally be encountered. Professionals must accept the challenge and not be deterred by minor setbacks caused by the publication process. Persistence, perseverance, and some callus will enable the therapist to survive in the research arena. You may even find research and publication challenges, which may make your professional life more stimulating and satisfying.

Copy right release statements are required by journals published in the United States of America. Instructions to Authors of a particular journal usually provide a sample of the statement that must accompany the manuscript on a separate sheet of paper. The statement must be signed by each author.

Submission of the Research Report for Publication

Once the final draft is complete and submitted for consideration for publication, a period of time elapses before a decision is reached about the manuscript. Time varies according to the workload of the volunteer reviewers, but ranges from about 2 to 6 months. The course which your paper follows after leaving your hands has been described for PHYSICAL THERAPY in "Whatever Happened to My Paper" by Davies.[27] Upon receipt of your manuscript by the Journal office, an acknowledgment of receipt is sent to you and the manuscript is sent to be reviewed by two or three reviewers. One of the consulting editors may be asked to review the manuscript, also. The reviewers determine whether the paper should be accepted, rejected, or revised along with suggestions for improvement. You are notified of their decision. Few manuscripts are accepted outright; about 60% to 65% are rejected because of poor writing. A few of the papers are rejected because the topic has been overexposed, or because the topic is not appropriate for the Journal. A rejection does not imply that the manuscript will not be reconsidered; a rejection means reconsideration if a major revision is performed as suggested. If the decision of the reviewers was revision, follow the suggestions and resubmit the revised paper.

The revised paper is treated as a new manuscript. To control bias, the manuscript may be sent to other reviewers. The time for this review is usually less than that of the original submission because the manuscript should be more readable. Once accepted, the paper is scheduled for future publication; the scheduling may vary according to the topic and length of the paper. About 3 months before publication, the paper is subjected to necessary editing by the Journal editors and readied for submission to the managing editor.[27]

The managing editor is responsible for preparing your paper for the printer. The type size for the different parts of the paper is selected, and the manuscript is marked. Next, the paper goes to the printer where it is rearranged and marked for magnetic tape before the actual printing. The tape is used to make galley proofs; the galley is a proof printed from the type made from the tapes. Major revision cannot occur at the galley level. A copy of the galley proofs is mailed to the principal author for checking for typographical errors and for correction. The returned galley copy is rechecked by Journal staff for accuracy. The managing editor lays out the format of the article as it will appear in the Journal and returns the master galleys to the printer. A series of correctional readings and transfer of copies takes place between the Journal editorial staff, the printer, and printing plant personnel until the final form is authorized for placement on photosensitive aluminum plates. The image from the plates is printed on paper which is folded, collated, trimmed, and encased in a cover to assume the appearance of a Journal issue. The process of printing requires 2½ months after all the other preparation of the Journal staff which requires about 3 months.[27] A year or longer can transpire between submission of your original manuscript until the printed product is delivered to your peers.

Review by Editors

What do journal reviewers look at when reviewing a manuscript? The reviewers may have different reviewing styles but similar criteria are used for judging the merits of the manuscript. The ultimate decision of their review is based on whether the manuscript is worthy of publication and whether the principles for good writing were followed by the author(s). Reviews by manuscript reviewers are made independently, but each reviews the manuscript for: appropriateness of the title for indicating the contents of the paper; organizational structure to determine if logical sequence is followed; contents and their details; writing style; and quality and quantity of illustrations and references.[28,29] Failure to state how and why results of the study are important to physical therapy is cause for manuscript rejection.

Since the objective of publishing research reports is the dissemination of truth, the reviewers check each section of the manuscript for accuracy and technical details. An overview of the paper is judged for imagination, creativity, interest, and its contribution to physical therapy.[28]

Several factors are considered by reviewers when checking contents of a manuscript. Logical sequence and development of the topic must be apparent. The supportive rationale must be relevant and sufficient. The assumptions presented must be valid and consistent with the purpose of the study. The detail of the study must follow the sequence and proper information of components of the report; method, results, discussion, and conclusion. The conclusion must be based on the experimental design of study and method of analysis, and it must be supported by the findings.[29]

Revisions, Responsibility?

"The editor of a scientific journal may be likened to a combined producer and director of a television series. Like a producer, he is responsible for selecting material that is interesting and important to his audience; like a director, he is also responsible for presenting it in an appealing and compelling way. Like both, he is subject to certain constraints that are imposed by his budget, his authors, his audience and his sponsors."[30]

The editor's task is to inform the author of the dilemma of major revision of what may have been considered a masterpiece by the author and to educate the author through guidance to bring about improvement and revision without discouragement. If the editor prepares the revision, then the question of authorship is raised. The editor should give the author the chance to improve the manuscript according to suggestions without insisting too much on specific methods of expression. When accepted for publication, the editor has the additional task of facilitating the reader's comprehension by means of clarity, simplicity, and shortness without lowering standards of scientific writing.[30]

The author's task is to submit a paper written with clarity, simplicity, brevity, and accuracy. I believe that the manuscript is the author's responsibility and that the editors only guide and advise. After all, the principal author receives the credit for the article and also benefits from the assistance of the reviewers. The author should not be discouraged and disgruntled with the decision of revision or rejection. All is not lost! If the time and effort were worth performing the research and submitting the report in the first place, the additional time and effort required for rewriting are certainly worthwhile. Poor writing is not the fault of the editors. They are protecting the readers of the Journal from poorly written, poor quality communication when they reject manuscripts.

The reader benefits from the revisions which occur before publication and is assured of some protection against the atrocities of poor writing. The reader does not have guarantees that the study is accurate or that the information is factual when he reads a scientific article because the outcome of a single, "one-shot,"[7] study is based on probability and a Type I error may be committed without anyone's knowledge. The reader does, however, have some guarantee that the style, purpose, organization, and contents are consistent with good writing principles because of the numerous reviews. Errors can go undetected in the writing-publication process. Reviewers and editors do their best but occasionally slip up and miss an error in the data computations, a misprint, or an incorrect reference. Although publication of scientific reports is the joint responsibility of the author and the editors, readers must learn to discriminate among speculation, hypothesis, inference, and fact.[7]

What the Reader Must Ask

Crocker[12] has given eight questions asked by journal referees in an attempt to increase the reader's ability to interpret and evaluate the research report. These questions and brief discussion follow.

1. Is the research problem or purpose clearly defined? Although the problem and purpose of research are different, the author should provide information about the research problem, operationally define the variables, and give the purpose of the study. This information is usually found in the introduction section of the article.

2. How does this research question relate to the current body of knowledge in the profession? The significance of the study is indicated in the literature review and conclusions.

3. How were data gathered? The author should have stated how data were gathered in the method section and provided the unit of measurement (found in method or results sections, or in the tables). The data gathering method is usually indicated by a description of the instrumentation such as a questionnaire, interview, strain gauge, or graphic recorders. The author should convince the reader that the method was appropriate for the design and solving the identified problem.

4. Is the size of the sample sufficient to answer the question? Journal referees (reviewers) are often impressed with large-sized samples but a large-sized sample is not always essential. Experimental "overkill". is possible.[31] Crocker suggested that authors should report the percentage of the population in the sample and the raw number in the sample so that readers may judge the appropriateness of sample size.

5. What is the sampling procedure? The author should state how subjects were obtained for the study. Sampling procedures are usually found in the method section. Subject attrition should also be discussed in the paper in the discussion section.

6. Are the design procedures of the study described? Procedures are supposed to be described in sufficient detail so that any interested reader could replicate the study (necessary for determining reliability of the study) and are discussed in the method section. The design is sometimes described in the method or results section, depending on how worded.

7. Are appropriate statistical procedures used? If correlational or comparative studies are presented, then the correct statistics must be used to describe and analyze the data. The level of statistical significance should be reported and post hoc analyses if appropriate.

8. Is the article well organized? The suggested format of components of a research report must be followed unless the author of the report is justified in deviating from the standard reporting procedure. The style of reporting must be looked at in a critical fashion to judge the research and the facts presented. If ambiguous sentences are encountered, the reader must read and interpret with suspicion.[12]

If these eight questions are followed by the author of a report, then publication is assured. Answering the questions is good exercise for the student to learn the principles of good writing, the essentials of a research report, and the methodical evaluation of the written report.

THE ORAL REPORT

The oral report, like the written report, is used to communicate the results of research. The speaker must organize the presentation for audience appeal. The report must be prepared with the audience in mind, keeping the report at the knowledge level of the audience. A report can be given to several groups, each group having a different level of knowledge about the subject, but the essential features of the message can be given to each group. The speaker must consider the composition of the audience, what they expect from the presentation, and what is the most important information to give them. The speed of delivery of an oral presentation is slower than reading a written report; therefore, less information can be given in an oral report. Reading aloud at a slow pace takes between 2 and 3 minutes per typed page. Voice aspects must also be considered along with audio and visual aids.

The oral report cannot be used for the written report and vice versa. Each report is used to communicate the results of research but the mode of each is different and, therefore, each requires different styles, format, and emphasis of content. Readers are strongly urged not to submit for publication a report prepared for oral presentation without alteration and re-amplification.

Format of the Oral Report

The oral presentation contains an introduction, a description of the procedure, and a discussion of the results. The introduction must catch the attention of the audience and provide the background for the study. Since the attention of the audiences rises and falls during most presentations, the beginning and ending of the report are perhaps the most important parts.[32] Keeping this in mind, the presenter must make his most important points conspicuous during introductory and closing remarks. The introduction of the oral report is similar to that of the written report. The speaker can present the events that led up to the study, the problem that was derived from the events or review of the literature, and the purpose for conducting the study. Meeting or conference formats place limitations on the time allotted for the presentation of scientific papers. The time may vary between 10 and 60 minutes, but the usual time is 10 to 15 minutes per report. The introduction should be kept short; a suggested time for introducing the study orally is eight to 10% of the total time allotted.[33]

The study method is important. Because of time limitations, sampling and measuring procedures must be described clearly and concisely. Visual aids are valuable to emphasize a point or to reduce time for describing instrumentation. A picture can save many words, particularly if the procedure was complex and innovative. The speaker must decide before the presentation which aspects of the method are important and set priorities or orders of presentation. Elaborate descriptions of subjects and designs can be reduced or eliminated. The time devoted to this portion of the oral report should be 17% to 25% of the total time allotted.

The results are reported, not discussed, at this point. Slides are valuable in presenting statistical data and results, and will increase the audience's understanding or appreciation of the explanations. Slides may include tables and graphs. Slides may be repeated for emphasis. The pertinent features of the findings are presented as simply as possible. The research findings are one of the most important features of the presentation. The pace of talking should be slower for presenting the findings than the pace for the introduction and method portions. Seventeen to 21 percent of the total presentation time should be allotted to permit audience understanding of pertinent points.

The discussion of the results follows and is the featured portion of the report. The speaker interprets the results and develops the theory for or against the findings. Pertinent literature is cited to support or contradict the data. Practical applications of the new knowledge can be discussed. Twenty-nine to 50 percent of the total time should be given to the discussion.[33]

The remaining 8% of the time is devoted to a brief summary and conclusions. Conclusions presented separately can serve to emphasize the discussion by repetition of important features. Usually, the rules governing oral reports allot additional time for a question and answer period.

To hold the attention of a difficult audience, Small and Kause[32] have suggested a provocative and unconventional pattern for oral presenters: Begin with conclusions, then justify the conclusions with the findings, and finish with a review of the literature. Table 12.2 provides guidelines for presenters of research studies to National Conference, American Physical Therapy Association.

Common Errors in Oral Reports

Some common errors have been noted by Johnson[33] as too extensive a review of literature, failure to identify the purpose of the study, too much material for the time allotted, failure to integrate literature with results, failure to rehearse the talk prior to the presentation, and poor slides.

Mistakes made when preparing slides can be disturbing to audiences. The amount of detail included on the slide should be clear and simple, like a figure in the written report. The audience is given limited time to view and obtain the information, so each slide should contain one thought; for example, no more than six lines of copy per slide. Tables should contain more data than figures, but care must be taken to avoid clutter on a slide. Generally, graphs have better audience appeal than tables. Closely printed slides are to be avoided because of difficulty of reading them at some distance away from the screen. Color slides are more attractive than black

Table 12.2
Guidelines for Presenters and Discussants of Original Investigative Studies[a]

The session for Original Investigator Studies is to provide a mechanism of communication through which physical therapists may present the results of their investigations. These sessions follow the pattern of similar meetings of other organizations. A format of these sessions has been developed and considerations for presenters are offered.

Distribution of Time (25 minutes per paper)
1. The presenter is allocated 15 minutes.
2. Five minutes are reserved for audience questions and comment. (The discussant has five minutes, if used.)

Suggestions for the Author
1. Assume that the audience is composed of interested physical therapists.
2. Do not spend time on the elementary aspects of the subject, and do not "speak down" to your colleagues.
3. Convey ideas in short, clear statements, using understandable terms.
4. Relate only the main points by restricting the amount of material presented. Leave the details for answers to questions the discussant or the audience may ask.
5. Speak at relaxed pace so that the audience comprehends what you say.
6. Rehearse your talk before one or more experienced speakers and invite constructive criticism. Remember that the chairman of the session will allow you to speak for *only* 15 minutes.
7. Do not burden the listener with numerical data he cannot assimilate.
8. Allow sufficient time to summarize the main points established in your paper and explain how the findings may be applied to physical therapy.
9. Do not end your talk with a comment, such as, "That's all I have" (which is awkward and weak), or by saying "Are there any questions?" (which precludes applause and amounts to assuming the duties of the chairman of the sessions). Instead, make your final statement in a firm voice, and as a courtesy you may wish to thank the audience for their attention. The chairman will introduce the discussant.

[a] Adapted from Guidelines for Presenters and Discussants of Original Investigator Studies and Special Interest Papers. National Conference, APTA. Reprinted by permission of the American Physical Therapy Association.

and white, but the amount of information contained in one slide is the most important concern. Black and white slides are effective if prepared properly. Color slides are more expensive, but have great audience appeal, especially when colors are mixed and arranged differently in each slide. The change in color, design, and style can break the monotony and hold an audience's attention.

Slides should be 5×5 cm (2×2 inches), clean, and marked for order of presentation and position of entry into the projector. Arrangements for the presentation of slides should be made in advance of the presentation so that proper equipment is available. When remote projection is not possible (from speaker's platform), a copy of the presentation marked to show location of slides can be of great help to the speaker and the projectionist. Use duplicate slides for ease and efficiency when referring back. Unless experienced and skilled in the preparation of slides, the presenter should seek the skill of an expert.

Table 12.3
Cumulative Summary of the Research Processes Presented

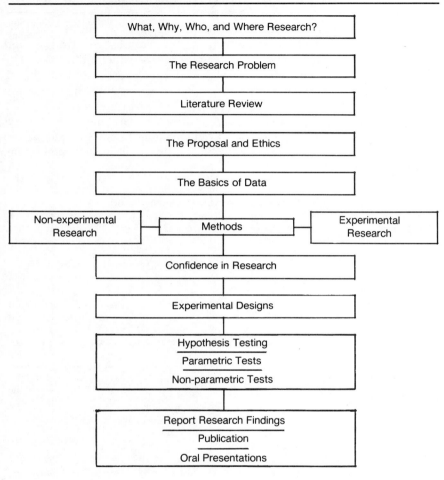

SUMMARY

The culmination of investigative efforts is the report. Research is never complete until the results have been reported. The oral and published reports provide the researcher an outlet for sharing the results of the investigation with colleagues.

Writing is not an easy task. It requires considerable effort and practice on the part of the researcher. The researcher is required to follow a certain format when preparing a manuscript for publication in a particular journal. The research report usually contains a title, abstract, and introduction, review of literature, method, results, discussion, and conclusion sections.

Editors prefer manuscripts that are informative, thought provoking, or interesting. All submitted manuscripts are reviewed thoroughly and evaluated for content, organization, contribution, grammar, and style.

The oral report, like the published report, is used to communicate the results of research. Although the oral report requires organization and similarities of the written report, it cannot be used for publication. The mode of the oral report differs from the published report and, therefore, requires different styles, format, and emphasis of content. The discussion of the research results is the featured portion of the oral report.

The reader should now have an appreciation of the research process and be able to understand and to interpret research literature better than before reading the contents of this book. Table 12.3 provides a summary of the research process as presented in this book.

> The investigation of nature is an infinite pasture-ground, where all may graze, and where the more bite, the longer the grass grows, the sweeter is its flavor, and the more it nourishes.
>
> T. H. Huxley
> Administrative Nihilism

REFERENCES

1. McLaren HM: So you want to conduct a clinical study. Physiother Canada 25: 219–244, 1973
2. Mapwell C: Clinical Trials Protocol. Surrey, Eng, Stuart Phillips Publications, 1969
3. Worthingham C: The development of physical therapy as a profession through research and publication. Phys Ther Rev 40: 573–577, 1960
4. Boone D: A survey of the authorship of articles appearing in PHYSICAL THERAPY during a five year period. Presented at a meeting of the Journal Committee of PHYS THER, 1975
5. Nelson C: Editorial readers and writers—help! Phys Ther 56: 807, 1976
6. Michels E: The 1970 presidential address. Phys Ther 50: 1579–1590, 1970
7. Ivy AC: The essentials for success in therapy. Phys Ther Rev 20: 259–260, 1940
8. Magistro CM: The 1976 presidential address. Phys Ther 56: 1227–1239, 1976
9. Lathrop RG: Introduction to Psychological Research. New York, Harper & Row, 1969
10. Ethridge DA, McSweeney M: Research in occupational therapy. Part VI. Research writing. Am J Occup Ther 25: 210–214, 1971
11. Fishbein M: Medical Writing: The Technic and the Art, ed 4. Springfield, IL, Charles C Thomas, 1978
12. Crocker LM: Let's reduce the communication gap: Guidelines for preparing a research article. Phys Ther 54: 971–976, 1974
13. Meyers LS, Grossen NE: Behavioral Research Theory, Procedure and Design. ed 2. San Francisco, WH Freeman and Co, 1978
14. Style Manual, ed 4. Washington, Am Phys Ther Assoc, 1976
15. Hislop HJ: The rudiments of the scientific paper. J Am Phys Ther Assoc 44: 58–59, 1964
16. Gonnella C: Let's reduce the understanding gap. 4. Data presentation: guidelines for authors (and readers). Phys Ther 53: 871–875, 1973

17. Turabian KR: A Manual for Writers of Term Papers, Theses and Dissertations, ed 4. Chicago, The University of Chicago Press, 1973
18. Campbell WG: Form and Style, Theses, Reports, Term Papers, ed 6. Boston, Houghton Mifflin Co, 1982
19. List of Journals Indexed: Index Medicus, 1983, Bethesda, MD, Nat Lib Med, 1983, pp 11–75
20. Strunk W Jr, White EB: The Elements of Style, ed 3. New York, The Macmillan Co, 1978
21. Trelease SF: How to Write Scientific and Technical Papers. Cambridge, MA, The MIT Press, 1969
22. Davies EJ: Let's reduce the communication gap: That's not what I meant! Phys Ther 54: 750–753, 1974
23. Sanger J: "Fog" in your pen? J Am Phys Ther Assoc 46: 512–515, 1966
24. Currier DP: Positioning for knee strengthening exercise. Phys Ther 57: 148–152, 1977
25. De Bakey L: Competent medical exposition: The need and the attainment. Bull Am Coll Surg 52: 85–92, 1967
26. De Bakey S: Basic principles of good writing. Am Op Room Nurse J 15: 69–72, 1972
27. Davies EJ: Let's reduce the communication gap: Whatever happened to my paper? Phys Ther 54: 509–510, 1974
28. Strohm BR: Let's reduce the communication gap: What associate editors look at. Phys Ther 55: 266–267, 1975
29. Lister MJ: Manuscripts: What you always wanted to know. Phys Ther 57: 1007–1012, 1977
30. De Bakey L, Woodford FP: Extensive revision of scientific articles—whose job? Scholarly Publishing 4: 147–151, 1973
31. Michels E: Opinions and comments of readers: Use of the t test. Phys Ther 50: 581–585, 1970
32. Small WP, Krause U: An Introduction to Clinical Research. Edinburgh, Churchill Livingston, 1972
33. Johnson PB: Oral Research Reports. In Hubbard AW (ed): Research Methods in Health, Physical Education, and Recreation, ed 3. Washington, Am Assoc Health Phys Educ Rec, 1973

SUGGESTED READINGS

George SA: Photographs that speak. Phys Ther 57: 1381–1382, 1977
Pal AC: Writing good abstracts: It's a tough job. Phys Ther 58: 175–177, 1978
Lister M (ed): Advise to authors: An Anthology. Washington (DC), APTA, 1982
Witt P: Research Writing Tips. Washington (DC), APTA, 1981

APPENDIX

Appendix

Table A

EXAMPLE OF A RESEARCH PROPOSAL

A. Title of Study
Electrical stimulation effect on localized blood flow

B. Name of Investigator(s)
Dean P. Currier, Ph.D.
Professor, Physical Therapy
University of Kentucky

Cynthia Reed, M.S.
Graduate Student in
Physical Therapy, UK

C. Specific Aim(s) of Study
To determine whether sinusoidal current of 2,500 Hz frequency, modulated at 50 Hz, increases blood flow to muscle stimulated at intensities of 10% and 30% maximum voluntary contraction (MVC).

D. Significance of Study
Electrical stimulation (sine; 2,500 Hz modulated at 50 Hz, 15 sec on/50 sec off timing cycle) is currently being used by physical therapists and athletic trainers in their treatment of patients having various musculoskeletal problems. No study has been published to show that electrical stimulation with the specific above current characteristics increases blood flow to the stimulated muscles. Most of the information from the manufacturer appears to have come from the Russian literature, anecdotes, and research done using electrical stimulators that are no longer marketed. Often new electrical stimulators are marketed with approval of safety standards but their efficacy is not substantiated by research. This study will test the validity of claims that electrical stimulation with the specific current characteristics outlined increased blood flow to muscle.

E. Related Research
Calf muscle blood flow has been studied while using voluntary contractions graded according to force and frequency.[1-4] Recent studies by

Richardson and Shewchuk[3] showed that postexercise blood flow to the calf muscles increased by increasing the frequency of contractions and by increasing muscular force at a given frequency. In another study blood flow was found to increase over that of rest during contractions of 7.5 and 15% MVC but not when 30% MVC force was sustained.[4]

The rhythmic muscular contractions produced by electrical stimulation, which controls recruitment and frequency of motor unit activity, have been reported to increase peripheral circulation. Wakim[5] found that significant increases in blood flow to dog muscle resulted when the muscle was directly stimulated at rates of 8 to 32 Hz by use of surface electrodes placed on the skin over a particular muscle. Randall and co-workers[6] reported a greater hyperemia following electrical stimulation (oxygen debt) than that occurring during contraction of the stimulated muscle. Folkow and Halicka,[7] using stimulus rates between 1 and 60 Hz on the cat gastrocnemius muscle, found that blood flow decreased progressively as the stimulus frequency was increased. Using various stimulus frequencies and levels of muscular contractile forces, Petrofsky et al[8] found that blood flow increases during most levels of contractions but to a greater extent immediately following contraction regardless of the level of contraction force.

Review of the literature indicates that blood flow to muscle has not been reported when using contractions graded according to force produced by electrical stimulation having current characteristics outlined (sine; 2,500 Hz modulated at 50 Hz, and 15/50 sec timing cycle).

F. Plan of Study

Subjects

Healthy men and women volunteer subjects, 18 to 30 years of age, will participate in the study. Each volunteer will be instructed about the procedure of the study and risks involved prior to their consenting to participate. A proper consent will be obtained from each subject in writing and prior to their participation in the study. No risk should be encountered by the subjects. Ten or more subjects will be used.

Procedure

1. Each subject will lie prone with the right leg in a comfortable resting position of extension, abduction, and external rotation.
2. A Doppler unit will be used to locate the popliteal artery and once located the greatest blood flow measurement will be taken. Pretreatment, 1, 5, and 10 min and postmeasurements (1, 3, and 5 min) will be taken.
3. Electrodes from the selected electrical stimulator will be secured on the skin over the gastrocnemius muscle. Electrical stimulation will be administered for 10 min with a 15-sec "on" and 50-sec "off" timing

sequence during the 10-min treatment phase. Two phases of electrical stimulation intensities will be given, 10% and 30% MVC.

G. Time, Space, Equipment
1. Time.
   The study will require 6 months to complete from the approval date. During this period of time, volunteers will be obtained, data collected and analyzed, and the results prepared for oral and written presentations.
2. Space.
   Laboratory space is available.
3. Equipment.
   All necessary equipment and supplies are available. Instrumentation will consist of Electrostim 180-2 unit for 2,500 Hz sinusoidal current to elicit muscular contractions. Measurement of blood flow will use a 5.4 kHz Doppler blood flow unit that will be interfaced with a Beckman R612 graphic recorder.

H. Cost Analysis
1. MEDLINE search of literature $_____
2. Art work (graphs, illustrations, slides) for
   oral and written presentation $_____
3. Computer use, personnel $_____
4. Travel to and from _____ to present findings $_____

Signature of Principal Investigator   Date

REFERENCES

1. Barcroft H, Millen JLE: The blood flow through muscle during sustained contractions. J. Physiol 97: 17–31, 1939
2. Barcroft H, Dornhorst AC: The blood flow through the human calf during rhythmic exercise. J Physiol 109: 402–411, 1949
3. Richardson D, Shewchuk R: Effects of contraction force and frequency on postexercise hyperemia in human calf muscles. J Appl Physiol: Respir Environ Exercise Physiol 49: 649–654, 1980
4. Richardson D: Blood flow response of human calf muscles to static contractions at various percentages of MVC. J Appl Physiol 51: 929–933, 1981
5. Wakim KG: Influence of frequency of muscle stimulation on circulation in the stimulated extremity. Arch Phys Med Rehabil 34: 291–295, 1953
6. Randall BF, Imig CJ, Hines HM: Effect of electrical stimulation upon blood flow and temperature of skeletal muscle. Am J Phys Med 32: 22–26, 1953

Table B _____

SAMPLE CONSENT FORM

Electrical Stimulation Effect on Localized Blood Flow

I, _____, freely and voluntarily consent to participate in a research project under the direction of Dr. Dean Currier to be conducted in the physical therapy research laboratory.

I understand that knowledge of physiological effects of electrical stimulation is necessary in physical therapy of various musculoskeletal problems. This knowledge may lead to more effective treatment that may speed up the recovery process. The purpose of this study is to determine whether stimulus intensities of 10% and 30% maximum voluntary contraction (MVC) will increase blood flow to the muscle being stimulated.

A thorough description of the procedures has been explained, and I understand that the only risk is soreness of the contracting muscles. The electrical stimulation may be somewhat uncomfortable while the current is "on."

I understand if I have any questions regarding my participation in this project, I can call Dr. Dean Currier at 233-5941.

I understand it will be necessary for me to participate in two testing sessions. Each session will last up to 60 minutes. Procedure: (1) The strength of plantar flexion will be measured pretest by a Cybex dynamometer and tolerance to electrical stimulation will be obtained. (2) Lying prone in a comfortable relaxed position, the popliteal or posterior tibial arteries will be assessed by a small probe placed on the skin. (3) Electrical stimulation will be given for 10 minutes at any intensity that is 10% and 30% MVC (treatment). (4) The arterial blood flow will be assessed following the electrical stimulation (posttest).

I understand that I may withdraw my consent and discontinue participation in this research at any time without prejudice to me.

I understand that in the event of physical injury resulting from this research procedure in which I am to participate, no forms of compensation are available. Medical treatment may be provided at my own expense or at the expense of my health care insurer (i.e., Medicare, Medicaid, BC/BS, etc.).

I have been informed of the various contraindications which would keep me from participating in this study. These include cardio-vascular problems and pacemakers. (I have also filled out and turned in a health history form to be reviewed by a physician to check for any medical reasons which may keep me from participating in this study—for student volunteers only)

I authorize Dr. Dean Currier, Cynthia Reed, and the Department of

Physical Therapy to keep, preserve, use, and dispose of the findings from this research with the provision that my name will not be associated with any of the results.

I have been given the right to ask, and have answered, any questions concerning the procedures to be used during this research.

Questions have been answered to my satisfaction. I have read and understand the contents of this form and have received a copy.

Witness	Date	Participant	Date

I have explained and defined in detail the research procedure to which the subject has consented to participate.

Signature	Date

Table C _____

THE *t* DISTRIBUTION (VALUES OF t_α)*

		Two-Tailed				
d.f.	$t_{.200}$	$t_{.100}$	$t_{.050}$	$t_{.020}$	$t_{.010}$	d.f.
		One-Tailed				
d.f.	$t_{.100}$	$t_{.050}$	$t_{.025}$	$t_{.010}$	$t_{.005}$	d.f.
1	3.078	6.314	12.706	31.821	63.657	1
2	1.886	2.920	4.303	6.965	9.925	2
3	1.638	2.353	3.182	4.541	5.841	3
4	1.533	2.132	2.776	3.747	4.604	4
5	1.476	2.015	2.571	3.365	4.032	5
6	1.440	1.943	2.447	3.143	3.707	6
7	1.415	1.895	2.365	2.998	3.499	7
8	1.397	1.860	2.306	2.896	3.355	8
9	1.383	1.833	2.262	2.821	3.250	9
10	1.372	1.812	2.228	2.764	3.169	10
11	1.363	1.796	2.201	2.718	3.106	11
12	1.356	1.782	2.179	2.681	3.055	12
13	1.350	1.771	2.160	2.650	3.012	13
14	1.345	1.761	2.145	2.624	2.977	14
15	1.341	1.753	2.131	2.602	2.947	15
16	1.337	1.746	2.120	2.583	2.921	16
17	1.333	1.740	2.110	2.567	2.898	17
18	1.330	1.734	2.101	2.552	2.878	18
19	1.328	1.729	2.093	2.539	2.861	19
20	1.325	1.725	2.086	2.528	2.845	20
21	1.323	1.721	2.080	2.518	2.831	21
22	1.321	1.717	2.074	2.508	2.819	22
23	1.319	1.714	2.069	2.500	2.807	23
24	1.318	1.711	2.064	2.492	2.797	24
25	1.316	1.708	2.060	2.485	2.787	25
26	1.315	1.706	2.056	2.479	2.779	26
27	1.314	1.703	2.052	2.473	2.771	27
28	1.313	1.701	2.048	2.467	2.763	28
29	1.311	1.699	2.045	2.462	2.756	29
inf.	1.282	1.645	1.960	2.326	2.576	inf.

* Table C is taken from Table III of Fisher and Yates: *Statistical Tables for Biological, Agricultural and Medical Research,* published by Longman Group Ltd., London (previously published by Oliver & Boyd, Edinburgh), by permission of the authors and publishers.

Table D

THE F DISTRIBUTION (VALUES OF $F_{.05}$)*

	\multicolumn{19}{c}{Degrees of freedom for numerator}
	1	2	3	4	5	6	7	8	9	10	12	15	20	24	30	40	60	120	∞
1	161	200	216	225	230	234	237	239	241	242	244	246	248	249	250	251	252	253	254
2	18.5	19.0	19.2	19.2	19.3	19.3	19.4	19.4	19.4	19.4	19.4	19.4	19.4	19.5	19.5	19.5	19.5	19.5	19.5
3	10.1	9.55	9.28	9.12	9.01	8.94	8.89	8.85	8.81	8.79	8.74	8.70	8.66	8.64	8.62	8.59	8.57	8.55	8.53
4	7.71	6.94	6.59	6.39	6.26	6.16	6.09	6.04	6.00	5.96	5.91	5.86	5.80	5.77	5.75	5.72	5.69	5.66	5.63
5	6.61	5.79	5.41	5.19	5.05	4.95	4.88	4.82	4.77	4.74	4.68	4.62	4.56	4.53	4.50	4.46	4.43	4.40	4.37
6	5.99	5.14	4.76	4.53	4.39	4.28	4.21	4.15	4.10	4.06	4.00	3.94	3.87	3.84	3.81	3.77	3.74	3.70	3.67
7	5.59	4.74	4.35	4.12	3.97	3.87	3.79	3.73	3.68	3.64	3.57	3.51	3.44	3.41	3.38	3.34	3.30	3.27	3.23
8	5.32	4.46	4.07	3.84	3.69	3.58	3.50	3.44	3.39	3.35	3.28	3.22	3.15	3.12	3.08	3.04	3.01	2.97	2.93
9	5.12	4.26	3.86	3.63	3.48	3.37	3.29	3.23	3.18	3.14	3.07	3.01	2.94	2.90	2.86	2.83	2.79	2.75	2.71
10	4.96	4.10	3.71	3.48	3.33	3.22	3.14	3.07	3.02	2.98	2.91	2.85	2.77	2.74	2.70	2.66	2.62	2.58	2.54
11	4.84	3.98	3.59	3.36	3.20	3.09	3.01	2.95	2.90	2.85	2.79	2.72	2.65	2.61	2.57	2.53	2.49	2.45	2.40
12	4.75	3.89	3.49	3.26	3.11	3.00	2.91	2.85	2.80	2.75	2.69	2.62	2.54	2.51	2.47	2.43	2.38	2.34	2.30
13	4.67	3.81	3.41	3.18	3.03	2.92	2.83	2.77	2.71	2.67	2.60	2.53	2.46	2.42	2.38	2.34	2.30	2.25	2.21
14	4.60	3.74	3.34	3.11	2.96	2.85	2.76	2.70	2.65	2.60	2.53	2.46	2.39	2.35	2.31	2.27	2.22	2.18	2.13
15	4.54	3.68	3.29	3.06	2.90	2.79	2.71	2.64	2.59	2.54	2.48	2.40	2.33	2.29	2.25	2.20	2.16	2.11	2.07
16	4.49	3.63	3.24	3.01	2.85	2.74	2.66	2.59	2.54	2.49	2.42	2.35	2.28	2.24	2.19	2.15	2.11	2.06	2.01
17	4.45	3.59	3.20	2.96	2.81	2.70	2.61	2.55	2.49	2.45	2.38	2.31	2.23	2.19	2.15	2.10	2.06	2.01	1.96
18	4.41	3.55	3.16	2.93	2.77	2.66	2.58	2.51	2.46	2.41	2.34	2.27	2.19	2.15	2.11	2.06	2.02	1.97	1.92
19	4.38	3.52	3.13	2.90	2.74	2.63	2.54	2.48	2.42	2.38	2.31	2.23	2.16	2.11	2.07	2.03	1.98	1.93	1.88
20	4.35	3.49	3.10	2.87	2.71	2.60	2.51	2.45	2.39	2.35	2.28	2.20	2.12	2.08	2.04	1.99	1.95	1.90	1.84
21	4.32	3.47	3.07	2.84	2.68	2.57	2.49	2.42	2.37	2.32	2.25	2.18	2.10	2.05	2.01	1.96	1.92	1.87	1.81
22	4.30	3.44	3.05	2.82	2.66	2.55	2.46	2.40	2.34	2.30	2.23	2.15	2.07	2.03	1.98	1.94	1.89	1.84	1.78
23	4.28	3.42	3.03	2.80	2.64	2.53	2.44	2.37	2.32	2.27	2.20	2.13	2.05	2.01	1.96	1.91	1.86	1.81	1.76
24	4.26	3.40	3.01	2.78	2.62	2.51	2.42	2.36	2.30	2.25	2.18	2.11	2.03	1.98	1.94	1.89	1.84	1.79	1.73
25	4.24	3.39	2.99	2.76	2.60	2.49	2.40	2.34	2.28	2.24	2.16	2.09	2.01	1.96	1.92	1.87	1.82	1.77	1.71
30	4.17	3.32	2.92	2.69	2.53	2.42	2.33	2.27	2.21	2.16	2.09	2.01	1.93	1.89	1.84	1.79	1.74	1.68	1.62
40	4.08	3.23	2.84	2.61	2.45	2.34	2.25	2.18	2.12	2.08	2.00	1.92	1.84	1.79	1.74	1.69	1.64	1.58	1.51
60	4.00	3.15	2.76	2.53	2.37	2.25	2.17	2.10	2.04	1.99	1.92	1.84	1.75	1.70	1.65	1.59	1.53	1.47	1.39
120	3.92	3.07	2.68	2.45	2.29	2.18	2.09	2.02	1.96	1.91	1.83	1.75	1.66	1.61	1.55	1.50	1.43	1.35	1.25
∞	3.84	3.00	2.60	2.37	2.21	2.10	2.01	1.94	1.88	1.83	1.75	1.67	1.57	1.52	1.46	1.39	1.32	1.22	1.00

Degrees of freedom for denominator

THE F DISTRIBUTION (VALUES OF $F_{.01}$)*

df denom \ Degrees of freedom for numerator	1	2	3	4	5	6	7	8	9	10	12	15	20	24	30	40	60	120	∞
1	4,052	5,000	5,403	5,625	5,764	5,859	5,928	5,982	6,023	6,056	6,106	6,157	6,209	6,235	6,261	6,287	6,313	6,339	6,366
2	98.5	99.0	99.2	99.2	99.3	99.3	99.4	99.4	99.4	99.4	99.4	99.4	99.4	99.5	99.5	99.5	99.5	99.5	99.5
3	34.1	30.8	29.5	28.7	28.2	27.9	27.7	27.5	27.3	27.2	27.1	26.9	26.7	26.6	26.5	26.4	26.3	26.2	26.1
4	21.2	18.0	16.7	16.0	15.5	15.2	15.0	14.8	14.7	14.5	14.4	14.2	14.0	13.9	13.8	13.7	13.7	13.6	13.5
5	16.3	13.3	12.1	11.4	11.0	10.7	10.5	10.3	10.2	10.1	9.89	9.72	9.55	9.47	9.38	9.29	9.20	9.11	9.02
6	13.7	10.9	9.78	9.15	8.75	8.47	8.26	8.10	7.98	7.87	7.72	7.56	7.40	7.31	7.23	7.14	7.06	6.97	6.83
7	12.2	9.55	8.45	7.85	7.46	7.19	6.99	6.84	6.72	6.62	6.47	6.31	6.16	6.07	5.99	5.91	5.82	5.74	5.65
8	11.3	8.65	7.59	7.01	6.63	6.37	6.18	6.03	5.91	5.81	5.67	5.52	5.36	5.28	5.20	5.12	5.03	4.95	4.86
9	10.6	8.02	6.99	6.42	6.06	5.80	5.61	5.47	5.35	5.26	5.11	4.96	4.81	4.73	4.65	4.57	4.48	4.40	4.31
10	10.0	7.56	6.55	5.99	5.64	5.39	5.20	5.06	4.94	4.85	4.71	4.56	4.41	4.33	4.25	4.17	4.08	4.00	3.91
11	9.65	7.21	6.22	5.67	5.32	5.07	4.89	4.74	4.63	4.54	4.40	4.25	4.10	4.02	3.94	3.86	3.78	3.69	3.60
12	9.33	6.93	5.95	5.41	5.06	4.82	4.64	4.50	4.39	4.30	4.16	4.01	3.86	3.78	3.70	3.62	3.54	3.45	3.36
13	9.07	6.70	5.74	5.21	4.86	4.62	4.44	4.30	4.19	4.10	3.96	3.82	3.66	3.59	3.51	3.43	3.34	3.25	3.17
14	8.86	6.51	5.56	5.04	4.70	4.46	4.28	4.14	4.03	3.94	3.80	3.66	3.51	3.43	3.35	3.27	3.18	3.09	3.00
15	8.68	6.36	5.42	4.89	4.56	4.32	4.14	4.00	3.89	3.80	3.67	3.52	3.37	3.29	3.21	3.13	3.05	2.96	2.87
16	8.53	6.23	5.29	4.77	4.44	4.20	4.03	3.89	3.78	3.69	3.55	3.41	3.26	3.18	3.10	3.02	2.93	2.84	2.75
17	8.40	6.11	5.19	4.67	4.34	4.10	3.93	3.79	3.68	3.59	3.46	3.31	3.16	3.08	3.00	2.92	2.83	2.75	2.65
18	8.29	6.01	5.09	4.58	4.25	4.01	3.84	3.71	3.60	3.51	3.37	3.23	3.08	3.00	2.92	2.84	2.75	2.66	2.57
19	8.19	5.93	5.01	4.50	4.17	3.94	3.77	3.63	3.52	3.43	3.30	3.15	3.00	2.92	2.84	2.76	2.67	2.58	2.49
20	8.10	5.85	4.94	4.43	4.10	3.87	3.70	3.56	3.46	3.37	3.23	3.09	2.94	2.86	2.78	2.69	2.61	2.52	2.42
21	8.02	5.78	4.87	4.37	4.04	3.81	3.64	3.51	3.40	3.31	3.17	3.03	2.88	2.80	2.72	2.64	2.55	2.46	2.36
22	7.95	5.72	4.82	4.31	3.99	3.76	3.59	3.45	3.35	3.26	3.12	2.98	2.83	2.75	2.67	2.58	2.50	2.40	2.31
23	7.88	5.66	4.76	4.26	3.94	3.71	3.54	3.41	3.30	3.21	3.07	2.93	2.78	2.70	2.62	2.54	2.45	2.35	2.26
24	7.82	5.61	4.72	4.22	3.90	3.67	3.50	3.36	3.26	3.17	3.03	2.89	2.74	2.66	2.58	2.49	2.40	2.31	2.21
25	7.77	5.57	4.68	4.18	3.86	3.63	3.46	3.32	3.22	3.13	2.99	2.85	2.70	2.62	2.53	2.45	2.36	2.27	2.17
30	7.56	5.39	4.51	4.02	3.70	3.47	3.30	3.17	3.07	2.98	2.84	2.70	2.55	2.47	2.39	2.30	2.21	2.11	2.01
40	7.31	5.18	4.31	3.83	3.51	3.29	3.12	2.99	2.89	2.80	2.66	2.52	2.37	2.29	2.20	2.11	2.02	1.92	1.80
60	7.08	4.98	4.13	3.65	3.34	3.12	2.95	2.82	2.72	2.63	2.50	2.35	2.20	2.12	2.03	1.94	1.84	1.73	1.60
120	6.85	4.79	3.95	3.48	3.17	2.96	2.79	2.66	2.56	2.47	2.34	2.19	2.03	1.95	1.86	1.76	1.66	1.53	1.38
∞	6.63	4.61	3.78	3.32	3.02	2.80	2.64	2.51	2.41	2.32	2.18	2.04	1.88	1.79	1.70	1.59	1.47	1.32	1.00

Degrees of freedom for denominator

Table E

THE CHI-SQUARE DISTRIBUTION (VALUES OF χ_α^2)*

d.f.	$\chi^2_{.995}$	$\chi^2_{.99}$	$\chi^2_{.975}$	$\chi^2_{.95}$	$\chi^2_{.05}$	$\chi^2_{.025}$	$\chi^2_{.01}$	$\chi^2_{.005}$	d.f.
1	.0000393	.000157	.000982	.00393	3.841	5.024	6.635	7.879	1
2	.0100	.0201	.0506	.103	5.991	7.378	9.210	10.597	2
3	.0717	.115	.216	.352	7.815	9.348	11.345	12.838	3
4	.207	.297	.484	.711	9.488	11.143	13.277	14.860	4
5	.412	.554	.831	1.145	11.070	12.832	15.086	16.750	5
6	.676	.872	1.237	1.635	12.592	14.449	16.812	18.548	6
7	.989	1.239	1.690	2.167	14.067	16.013	18.475	20.278	7
8	1.344	1.646	2.180	2.733	15.507	17.535	20.090	21.955	8
9	1.735	2.088	2.700	3.325	16.919	19.023	21.666	23.589	9
10	2.156	2.558	3.247	3.940	18.307	20.483	23.209	25.188	10
11	2.603	3.053	3.816	4.575	19.675	21.920	24.725	26.757	11
12	3.074	3.571	4.404	5.226	21.026	23.337	26.217	28.300	12
13	3.565	4.107	5.009	5.892	22.362	24.736	27.688	29.819	13
14	4.075	4.660	5.629	6.571	23.685	26.119	29.141	31.319	14
15	4.601	5.229	6.262	7.261	24.996	27.488	30.578	32.801	15
16	5.142	5.812	6.908	7.962	26.296	28.845	32.000	34.267	16
17	5.697	6.408	7.564	8.672	27.587	30.191	33.409	35.718	17
18	6.265	7.015	8.231	9.390	28.869	31.526	34.805	37.156	18
19	6.844	7.633	8.907	10.117	30.144	32.852	36.191	38.582	19
20	7.434	8.260	9.591	10.851	31.410	34.170	37.566	39.997	20
21	8.034	8.897	10.283	11.591	32.671	35.479	38.932	41.401	21
22	8.643	9.542	10.982	12.338	33.924	36.781	40.289	42.796	22
23	9.260	10.196	11.689	13.091	35.172	38.076	41.638	44.181	23
24	9.886	10.856	12.401	13.848	36.415	39.364	42.980	45.558	24
25	10.520	11.524	13.120	14.611	37.652	40.646	44.314	46.928	25
26	11.160	12.198	13.844	15.379	38.885	41.923	45.642	48.290	26
27	11.808	12.879	14.573	16.151	40.113	43.194	46.963	49.645	27
28	12.461	13.565	15.308	16.928	41.337	44.461	48.278	50.993	28
29	13.121	14.256	16.047	17.708	42.557	45.722	49.588	52.336	29
30	13.787	14.953	16.791	18.493	43.773	46.979	50.892	53.672	30

* This table is based on Table 8 of *Biometrika Tables for Statisticians, Volume I*, by permission of the *Biometrika* trustees.

Index